becoming a
nurse

a textbook for professional practice

Derek Sellman and Paul Snelling

Visit the *Becoming a Nurse* Companion Website at
www.pearsoned.co.uk/becominganurse to find valuable student
learning material including:

- Extensive links to valuable resources on the web
- Self-assessment questions to check your understanding

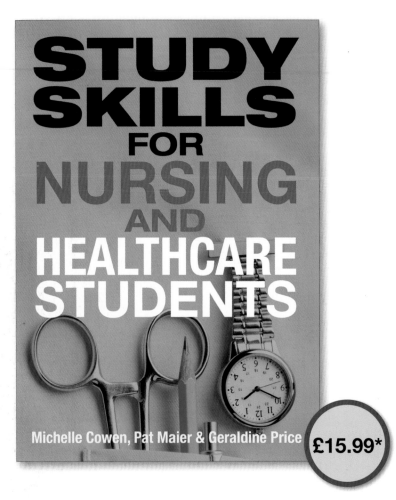
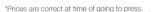

becoming a
nurse

a textbook for professional practice

Derek Sellman and Paul Snelling

PEARSON

Harlow, England • London • New York • Boston • San Francisco • Toronto • Sydney • Singapore • Hong Kong
Tokyo • Seoul • Taipei • New Delhi • Cape Town • Madrid • Mexico City • Amsterdam • Munich • Paris • Milan

Pearson Education Limited
Edinburgh Gate
Harlow
Essex CM20 2JE
England

and Associated Companies throughout the world

Visit us on the World Wide Web at:
www.pearsoned.co.uk

First published 2010

ISBN: 978-0-13-238923-5

British Library Cataloguing-in-Publication Data
A catalogue record for this book is available from the British Library

Library of Congress Cataloging-in-Publication Data
A catalog record for this book is available from the Library of Congress

10 9 8 7 6 5 4 3 2 1
13 12 11 10

Typeset in 10/12.5pt Sabon by 35
Printed and bound in China (SWTC)

The publisher's policy is to use paper manufactured from sustainable forests.

Brief Contents

List of contributors   xii

Introduction   xiv

Chapter 1   Professional issues   1

Chapter 2   Ethics   37

Chapter 3   Law   68

Chapter 4   Health policy   102

Chapter 5   Interprofessional working   138

Chapter 6   Evidence-based practice   167

Chapter 7   Assessment   198

Chapter 8   Judgement and decision-making   227

Chapter 9   Communication and interpersonal skills   252

Chapter 10   Public health   284

Chapter 11   Learning and teaching   315

Chapter 12   Management and leadership   345

Chapter 13   Personal and professional development   383

Chapter 14   Medicines management   418

Index   000

Contents

List of contributors   xii

Introduction   xiv

Derek Sellman and Paul Snelling

Chapter 1 Professional issues   1

Janet Holt

Learning outcomes   1
Related NMC Standards of Proficiency for Pre-registration Nursing Education (NMC 2004a)   2
Introduction   3

Part 1: Outlining professional issues   3
Part 2: Explaining professional issues   7
Part 3: Exploring professional issues   23

Conclusion   27
Suggested further reading   33
References   33

Chapter 2 Ethics   37

Paul Snelling

Learning outcomes   37
Related NMC Standards of Proficiency for Pre-registration Nursing Education (NMC 2004a)   38
Introduction   39

Part 1: Outlining ethics   39
Part 2: Explaining ethics   41
Part 3: Exploring ethics   56

Conclusion   62
Suggested further reading   63
References   63

Chapter 3 Law   68

Richard Thomas and Paul Snelling

Learning outcomes   68
Related NMC Standards of Proficiency for Pre-registration Nursing Education (NMC 2004)   69
Introduction   70

Part 1: Outlining the law   70
Part 2: Explaining the law   74
Part 3: Exploring the law   93

Conclusion   98
Suggested further reading   99
References   100

Chapter 4 Health policy   102

Iain Snelling

Learning outcomes   102
Related NMC Standards of Proficiency for Pre-registration Nursing Education (NMC 2004)   103
Introduction   104

Part 1: Outlining health policy   104
Part 2: Explaining health policy   109
Part 3: Exploring health policy   131

Conclusion   134
Suggested further reading   135
References   136

Chapter 5 Interprofessional working   138

Katherine Pollard and Francesca Harris

Learning outcomes   138
Related NMC Standards of Proficiency for Pre-registration Nursing Education (NMC 2004)   139
Introduction   140

Part 1: Outlining interprofessional working   140
Part 2: Explaining interprofessional working   142
Part 3: Exploring interprofessional working   153

Conclusion   163
Suggested further reading   163
References   163

Chapter 6 Evidence-based practice   167

Mark Broom and Derek Sellman

Learning outcomes   167
Related NMC Standards of Proficiency for Pre-registration Nursing Education (NMC 2004)   168
Introduction   169

Part 1: Outlining evidence-based practice
Part 2: Explaining evidence-based practice   169
Part 3: Exploring evidence-based practice   171
                                                     180

Conclusion
Suggested further reading   195
References   195
                                                     196

Chapter 7 Assessment

198

Derek Sellman, Stephen Evans and Jackie Younker

Learning outcomes
Related NMC Standards of Proficiency for Pre-registration Nursing Education (NMC 2004)   198
Introduction   199
                                                                                         200

Part 1: Outlining assessment
Part 2: Explaining assessment   200
Part 3: Exploring assessment   203
                                                     215

Conclusion
Suggested further reading   224
References   225
                                                     225

Chapter 8 Judgement and decision-making

227

P. Anne Scott, Pádraig MacNeela, Gerard Clinton and David Pontin

Learning outcomes
Related NMC Standards of Proficiency for Pre-registration Nursing Education (NMC 2004)   227
Introduction   228
                                                                                         229

Part 1: Outlining judgement and decision-making
Part 2: Explaining judgement and decision-making   229
Part 3: Exploring judgement and decision-making   232
                                                     238

Conclusion
Suggested further reading   247
References   247
                                                     247

Chapter 9 Communication and interpersonal skills

252

Victoria Lavender

Learning outcomes
Related NMC Standards of Proficiency for Pre-registration Nursing Education (NMC 2004)   252
Introduction   253
                                                                                         254

Part 1: Outlining communication and interpersonal skills
Part 2: Explaining communication and interpersonal skills   254
Part 3: Exploring communication and interpersonal skills   257
                                                              266

Conclusion
Suggested further reading   279
References   279
                                                     280

Chapter 10 Public health

284

Jane Thomas

Learning outcomes	284
Related NMC Standards of Proficiency for Pre-registration Nursing Education (NMC 2004)	285
Introduction	286
Part 1: Outlining public health	286
Part 2: Explaining public health	288
Part 3: Exploring public health	298
Conclusion	312
Suggested further reading	312
References	313

Chapter 11 Learning and teaching

315

Derek Sellman and Jane Tarr

Learning outcomes	315
Related NMC Standards of Proficiency for Pre-registration Nursing Education (NMC 2004)	316
Introduction	317
Part 1: Outlining learning and teaching	317
Part 2: Explaining learning and teaching	320
Part 3: Exploring learning and teaching	335
Conclusion	342
Suggested further reading	343
References	343

Chapter 12 Management and leadership

345

Iain Snelling, Cathryn Havard and David Pontin

Learning outcomes	345
Related NMC Standards of Proficiency for Pre-registration Nursing Education (NMC 2004)	346
Introduction	347
Part 1: Outlining management and leadership	347
Part 2: Explaining management and leadership	353
Part 3: Exploring management and leadership	378
Conclusion	380
Suggested further reading	380
References	381

Chapter 13 Personal and professional development

383

Clare Hopkinson

Learning outcomes	383
Related NMC Standards of Proficiency for Pre-registration Nursing Education (NMC 2004)	384
Introduction	385

Part 1: Outlining personal and professional development   385
Part 2: Explaining personal and professional development   389
Part 3: Exploring personal and professional development   399

Conclusion   413
Suggested further reading   413
References   414

Chapter 14 Medicines management   418

Claire Fullbrook-Scanlon

Learning outcomes   418
Related NMC Standards of Proficiency for Pre-registration Nursing Education (NMC 2004)   419
Introduction   420

Part 1: Outlining medicines management   420
Part 2: Explaining medicines management   426
Part 3: Exploring medicines management   447

Conclusion   453
Suggested further reading   453
References   454

Index   456

List of Contributors

Mark Broom is Senior Lecturer in Child Health, Faculty of Health, Sports and Sciences, University of Glamorgan. Mark's interests are in promoting high-quality care for acutely ill children, clinical reasoning and the use of I.T in nurse education.

Gerard Clinton works as a Lecturer at the School of Nursing, Dublin City University (DCU). He is a Registered Psychiatric Nurse & Registered Nurse Tutor with a BSc in Nursing Practice Development, MSc in Nursing Education and Graduate Diploma in Statistics. Before working in DCU he worked at the School of Psychiatric Nursing, St. Ita's Hospital, Portrane.

Stephen Evans MA, PGDipOT, BSc(Hons), is Senior Lecturer in Occupational Therapy, School of Health and Social Care, University of the West of England. Stephen's current interests are in inclusive design in the built environment and the social model of disability.

Claire Fullbrook-Scanlon RGN RHV BSc(Hons) MSc PGCertED, has worked predominantly in nursing older people. She is currently non medical prescribing lead and consultant nurse in acute stroke care at Royal United Hospital, Bath. Claire is also Senior Lecturer at the University of the West of England where she leads the non medical prescribing programme.

Francesca Harris is a Health Visitor, NHS South Gloucestershire. Francesca has worked as a midwife in the NHS, a midwife trainer in international development and has held a development research post at the University of the West of England. Her areas of interest include the health needs of gypsies and travellers, public health and primary care.

Cathryn Havard MSc BA (Hons) RN; FETC; is Senior Lecturer in nursing, School of Health and Social Care, University of the West of England. Cathryn teaches nursing management and leadership. Her interests and research activities relate to the experience of international students in Higher Education and the facilitation of work-based learning projects in her specialist practice area of cancer care.

Janet Holt BA, MPhil, PhD, RN, RM. is a Senior Lecturer in the School of Health Care at the University of Leeds, UK. Janet's research interests and publications are within the disciplines of Health Care Ethics and Law and Nursing Philosophy, and she is currently chair of the International Philosophy of Nursing Society.

Clare Hopkinson, RN, MSc, BA(Hons), RNT, CHSM, is Senior Lecturer, School of Health and Social Care, University of the West of England. Clare has worked as a surgical adult senior nurse and in health education. Her interests include reflective practice, arts and health, collaborative action research, and the emotional cost of caring.

Victoria Lavender, MA (Phil), BA (Hons), RMN, is Senior Lecturer in the School of Health and Social Care, University of the West of England. Victoria has worked as a Mental Health Nurse. Her areas of interest are the mental health of women and the history of mental health care provision.

Pádraig MacNeela, College Lecturer at the School of Psychology, Faculty of Arts, Social Sciences, and Celtic Studies, National University of Ireland, Galway. Pádraig is a psychologist interested in psychosocial and informal aspects of health care, especially in nursing, and their relationship to judgement and decision-making.

Katherine Pollard, Research Fellow, School of Health and Social Care, University of the West of England. Katherine worked as a midwife in the NHS before embarking on a research career. Her areas of interest include interprofessional issues, workforce development and service delivery in health and social care.

David Pontin, RN, RCSP, PhD, Reader in Nursing and Professional Practice. David has worked in a number of senior leadership roles in the NHS in England and Wales, and in the UK University sector. He is currently Director of the Graduate School Faculty of Health and Life Sciences, University of the West of England.

P. Anne Scott, is Professor of Nursing and Deputy President of Dublin City University. Anne is a nurse and philosopher. Her main research interests are in the philosophy and ethics of health care and in judgement and decision-making.

Derek Sellman, PhD, MA, BSc(Hons), RGN, RMN, is Principal Lecturer, School of Health and Social Care, University of the West of England. Derek's interests include education for professional practice, health care ethics, and philosophy of nursing. Derek is currently editor of the journal *Nursing Philosophy*.

Iain Snelling, BA, MA, DipHSM, MIHM is Principal Lecturer in the Centre for Professional and Organisation Development, Faculty of Health and Wellbeing, Sheffield Hallam University. Before joining the University in 2002, Iain was an NHS manager in a number of Acute Hospitals.

Paul Snelling, BSc(Hons), MA, RGN, is Senior Lecturer in the School of Health and Social Care, University of the West of England. Paul teaches principally on the pre-registration nursing programme, and was formerly Programme Leader for the adult branch. His research interests are nurse education, professional ethics, and personal responsibility for health.

Jane Tarr, PhD, is Principal Lecturer, School of Education, University of the West of England. Jane is Director of Training for Children and Young People in the Wider Workforce with responsibility for programmes designed for educational staff based in formal and informal educational settings and in her research seeks to enable partnerships between educational institutions and the communities they serve.

Jane Thomas, Deputy Head of School, Academic and Professional Issues, School of Health Science, Swansea University. Jane has a working background in Primary Care and Public Health and was responsible for establishing postgraduate provision in this area at Swansea. She links with the Wales Centre for Health on national issues.

Richard Thomas, RGN, RNT, DN, BA, LLM, is Senior Lecturer, School of Health and Social Care, University of the West of England. Richard teaches health care law and has a particular interest in legal principles underpinning clinical judgement-making and how clinical interventions are constructed as reasonable in law.

Jackie Younker, RN, MSN, PG Cert Ed, is Senior Lecturer in Adult Nursing, School of Health and Social Care, University of the West of England. Jackie has a background in critical care nursing. Her areas of interest are critical care nursing, advanced practice nursing, and resuscitation.

Introduction

Derek Sellman and Paul Snelling

As we near completion of the first decade of the twenty-first century, the pace of change of health care seems to be increasing. In the last twenty or so years there has been continual upheaval in nursing and nurse education. In the early 1990s nurse education moved away from the traditional 'apprenticeship' hospital-based model into universities, and at the higher minimum academic level of Diploma. There was some criticism of the move; in celebrating the practical nature of traditional nursing some saw the increasing academic level and status as a threat to the practise of nursing.

As if to emphasise the changing nature of nursing, the very day we write this introduction on New Years Day 2009, the governing body of nursing, the Nursing and Midwifery Council (NMC) introduces a new constitution in response to Government policy and legislation. Following a consultation exercise held during 2008, the NMC has affirmed that, in principle, the minimum academic level of preparation for nurse registration will be degree level, putting pre-registration nursing education in England on a par with other health care professionals including physiotherapists, radiographers and dieticians. As we write the NMC continues to work on the structure and content of new programmes, and even if implementation dates for the new curricula are not yet known, the direction of travel is clear.

There has also been change within educational institutions. As the level of academic engagement increases, so education for the practical skills of nursing also develops with, for example, greater use of computers and simulation. Those who see conflict between the practical and the theoretical will no doubt criticise the increased academic level. As discussed in Chapter 1, organisations were broadly in favour of the change, while individual respondents to the consultation tended to be less enthusiatic. But we are confident that a requirement to be more knowledgeable, more analytical and more critical about nursing practice will enhance rather than detract from practical skills. We see no conflict. Nursing has been and will continue to be flexible and adaptive in evolving to meet the needs of patients. Today's complex system of health care requires critically aware, graduate nurses, and a robust system is required in order to provide suitable educational experiences.

Unlike school education, preparation for nursing does not have a national curriculum as such. The NMC does not say *exactly* what all programmes must cover. If it did, the curriculum would have to change with every new development in practice. Instead the NMC has produced a broad set of 'proficiencies' (NMC 2004) which must be met in one of the branches of nursing. There are only 17 'overarching' standards of proficiency which define the principles of being able to practise as a nurse, though each is elaborated upon so that there is a total of 62 standards, organised in four domains: professional and ethical practice; care delivery; care management; and personal and professional development. Approved educational programmes are measured against these standards, and must demonstrate how the standards are met. The NMC has more recently introduced 'skills clusters' (NMC 2007) which give further details of what a student must be able to do in order to complete their programme of preparation and thus be eligible to register as a nurse. Both of these NMC documents are available via the NMC website, and though we always recommend that students should be thoroughly familiar with these documents, we do not know how many follow such advice. We have reproduced the standards in full at the end of this introduction. A read through them shows that there is no clinical or practical content. They are generic, covering for example, ethics, law, interprofessional working, personal development, and practice in all four branches of UK nursing (adult, children's, learning disabilities and mental health).

Many nursing textbooks are available, including several large and impressively produced single volumes which claim to cover the curriculum. In recommending some of these to our students we have found that the clinical and skills orientation of the texts does not always address the wider aspects of the context of nursing as presented by the NMC standards of proficiency. Of course, there are many single issue books about, for example, ethics and law, interprofessional working, personal development, and so on, but few that cover the wide range of generic knowledge and skills that the NMC requires. This volume has been developed in response to what we perceive as a need for a text that provides the wider range of topics indicated in the NMC standards of proficiencies. We hope that, in this collection, we have brought together valuable contributions from a number of different authors who can offer students of nursing a wide perspective approaching that required by the NMC standards. The discerning reader will notice that we have not covered every topic that appears in the proficiencies but in introducing the major topic areas we are confident that the majority of the NMC standards are addressed. Students looking for a book which discusses, for example, childhood intercranial pressure or diseases of the abdomen are invited to look elsewhere.

The structure of the book

Each chapter in the book is presented in three parts:

- In the first part, the chapter topic is outlined and introduced in a broad sense.
- In the second and longest part the subject matter is explained further.
- In the third part the subject is explored, and in some instances alternative explanations are offered.

While every chapter has its individual style, they all share some common features including:

- Each chapter opens by identifying learning outcomes and the relevant NMC standards of proficiency.
- Each chapter introduces a case to illustrate how the subject matter relates to nursing practice. In some chapters a single case is developed; in other chapters a number of different cases are utilised.
- Each chapter includes activities which aim to assist reflective and active reading. Many of these activities are designed to be undertaken in small groups in order to enhance learning.
- Each chapter offers some suggestions for further reading.

A note on terminology

We acknowledge that nursing is predominantly a female profession and we are keen to avoid promoting stereotypes. We find the constant use of: 'he or she'; 's/he'; or 'his or her' unsatisfactory in this regard: it may avoid promoting stereotypes but it gets in the way of fluid and accessible writing styles. In this volume we have chosen to adopt a convention of using either 'she' or 'he' (or 'hers' or 'his') interchangeably. No gender bias or stereotypical view should be read into the choices made, as these have been purely arbitrary throughout.

The NMC as a valuable source of information for students and practitioners of nursing

One of the most important places students can look for information is via the NMC. Though it takes a while to navigate, the NMC website provides a wealth of informative documents, which more importantly, also give 'official advice' and provide standards against which practice is measured.

In this book we have quoted extensively from relevant NMC documents, and have reproduced in full the most important of all: **The Code: Standards of conduct, performance and ethics for nurses and midwives.** We are grateful that the copyright arrangements of the NMC permits such extensive reproduction of extracts from the many valuable documents that can be found on the NMC website.

The NMC standards of proficiency for pre-registration nursing education

This volume is based on the NMC standards of proficiency. These standards are contained within a larger explanatory document which sets out the requirements for an approved pre-registration nursing programme, including, for example, how much time is to be spent in practice placements. Approved courses are of a minimum duration of three years, the first, termed the Common Foundation Programme (CFP), provides the foundation for entry to any of the four UK branches of: adult nursing; children's nursing; learning disabilities nursing; or mental health nursing. Recently introduced regulations require successful completion of the CFP prior to progression to a branch programme. Each of the overarching standards of proficiency has two sets of standards:

1. Standards of education and outcomes for entry to the branch programme, that is standards that must be completed by the end of the first year, allowing progress on the way towards meeting the standards.
2. Standards of proficiency which must be successfully completed by the end of the programme to allow entry to the NMC register of nurses.

In the tables below the overarching standards are reproduced in the left-hand column, and the related standards of proficiency for entry to the register can be found in the right-hand column. The relevant standards from this right-hand column are identified at the start of each chapter. The full document is available at www.nmc-uk.org.

Standards of proficiency for pre-registration nursing education

Domain – Professional and Ethical Practice

Manage oneself, one's practice, and that of others, in accordance with the *NMC code of professional conduct: standards for conduct, performance and ethics*, recognising one's own abilities and limitations	• practise in accordance with the *NMC code of professional conduct: standards for conduct, performance and ethics* • use professional standards of practice to self-assess performance • consult with a registered nurse when nursing care requires expertise beyond one's own current scope of competence • consult other health care professionals when individual or group needs fall outside the scope of nursing practice • identify unsafe practice and respond appropriately to ensure a safe outcome • manage the delivery of care services within the sphere of one's own accountability.
Practise in accordance with an ethical and legal framework which ensures the primacy of patient and client interest and well-being and respects confidentiality	• demonstrate knowledge of legislation and health and social policy relevant to nursing practice • ensure the confidentiality and security of written and verbal information acquired in a professional capacity • demonstrate knowledge of contemporary ethical issues and their impact on nursing and health care • manage the complexities arising from ethical and legal dilemmas • act appropriately when seeking access to caring for patients and clients in their own homes.
Practise in a fair and anti-discriminatory way, acknowledging the differences in beliefs and cultural practices of individuals or groups	• maintain, support and acknowledge the rights of individuals or groups in the health care setting • act to ensure that the rights of individuals and groups are not compromised • respect the values, customs and beliefs of individuals and groups • provide care which demonstrates sensitivity to the diversity of patients and clients.

Domain - Care Delivery

Engage in, develop and disengage from therapeutic relationships through the use of appropriate communication and interpersonal skills	• utilise a range of effective and appropriate communication and engagement skills • maintain, and where appropriate, disengage from professional caring relationships that focus on meeting the patient's or client's needs within professional therapeutic boundaries.
Create and utilise opportunities to promote the health and well-being of patients, clients and groups	• consult with patients, clients and groups to identify their need and desire for health promotion advice • provide relevant and current health information to patients, clients and groups in a form which facilitates their understanding and acknowledges choice/individual preference • provide support and education in the development and/or maintenance of independent living skills • seek specialist/expert advice as appropriate.
Undertake and document a comprehensive, systematic and accurate nursing assessment of the physical, psychological, social and spiritual needs of patients, clients and communities	• select valid and reliable assessment tools for the required purpose • systematically collect data regarding the health and functional status of individuals, clients and communities through appropriate interaction, observation and measurement • analyse and interpret data accurately to inform nursing care and take appropriate action.
Formulate and document a plan of nursing care, where possible in partnership with patients, clients, their carers and family and friends, within a framework of informed consent	• establish priorities for care based on individual or group needs • develop and document a care plan to achieve optimal health, habilitation and rehabilitation based on assessment and current nursing knowledge • identify expected outcomes, including a time frame for achievement and/or review in consultation with patients, clients, their carers and family and friends and with members of the health and social care team.
Based on the best available evidence, apply knowledge and an appropriate repertoire of skills indicative of safe and effective nursing practice	• ensure that current research findings and other evidence are incorporated in practice • identify relevant changes in practice or new information and disseminate it to colleagues • contribute to the application of a range of interventions which support and optimise the health and well-being of patients and clients • demonstrate the safe application of the skills required to meet the needs of patients and clients within the current sphere of practice • identify and respond to patients and clients' continuing learning and care needs • engage with, and evaluate, the evidence base that underpins safe nursing practice.
Provide a rationale for the nursing care delivered which takes account of social, cultural, spiritual, legal, political and economic influences	• identify, collect and evaluate information to justify the effective utilisation of resources to achieve planned outcomes of nursing care.
Evaluate and document the outcomes of nursing and other interventions	• collaborate with patients and clients and, when appropriate, additional carers to review and monitor the progress of individuals or groups towards planned outcomes • analyse and revise expected outcomes, nursing interventions and priorities in accordance with changes in the individual's condition, needs or circumstances.
Demonstrate sound clinical judgement across a range of differing professional and care delivery contexts	• use evidence based knowledge from nursing and related disciplines to select and individualise nursing interventions • demonstrate the ability to transfer skills and knowledge to a variety of circumstances and settings • recognise the need for adaptation and adapt nursing practice to meet varying and unpredictable circumstances • ensure that practice does not compromise the nurse's duty of care to individuals of the safety of the public.

Domain – Care Management

Contribute to public protection by creating and maintaining a safe environment of care through the use of quality assurance and risk management strategies	• apply relevant principles to ensure the safe administration of therapeutic substances • use appropriate risk assessment tools to identify actual and potential risks • identify environmental hazards and eliminate and/or prevent where possible • communicate safety concerns to a relevant authority • manage risk to provide care which best meets the needs and interests of patients, clients and the public.
Demonstrate knowledge of effective inter-professional working practices which respect and utilise the contributions of members of the health and social care team	• establish and maintain collaborative working relationships with members of the health and social care team and others • participate with members of the health and social care team in decision-making concerning patients and clients • review and evaluate care with members of the health and social care team and others.
Delegate duties to others, as appropriate, ensuring that they are supervised and monitored	• take into account the role and competence of staff when delegating work • maintain one's own accountability and responsibility when delegating aspects of care to others • demonstrate the ability to co-ordinate the delivery of nursing and health care.
Demonstrate key skills	• literacy – interpret and present information in a comprehensible manner • numeracy – accurately interpret numerical data and their significance for the safe delivery of care • information technology and management – interpret and utilise data and technology, taking account of legal, ethical and safety considerations, in the delivery and enhancement of care • problem solving – demonstrate sound clinical decision-making which can be justified even when made on the basis of limited information.

Domain – Personal and Professional Development

Demonstrate a commitment to the need for continuing professional development and personal supervision activities in order to enhance knowledge, skills, values and attitudes needed for safe and effective nursing practice	• identify one's own professional development needs by engaging in activities such as reflection in, and on, practice and lifelong learning • develop a personal development plan which takes into account personal, professional and organisational needs • share experience with colleagues and patients and clients in order to identify the additional knowledge and skills needed to manage unfamiliar or professionally challenging situations • take action to meet any identified knowledge and skills deficit likely to affect the delivery of care within the current sphere of practice.
Enhance the professional development and safe practice of others through peer support, leadership, supervision and teaching	• contribute to creating a climate conducive to learning • contribute to the learning experiences and development of others by facilitating the mutual sharing of knowledge and experience • demonstrate effective leadership in the establishment and maintenance of safe nursing practise.

References

NMC (Nursing and Midwifery Council). (2004) *Standards of Proficiency for Pre-registration Nursing Educaton*, London: NMC.

NMC. (2007) *Essential Skills Clusters (ESCs) for Pre-Registration Nursing Programme*, Annexe 2 to NMC circular 07/2007. London: NMC.

Supporting resources

Visit **www.pearsoned.co.uk/becominganurse** to find valuable online resources

Companion Website for students

- Extensive links to valuable resources on the web
- Self-assessment questions to check your understanding

For instructors

- PowerPoint slides that can be downloaded and used for presentations

For more information please contact your local Pearson Education sales representative or visit **www.pearsoned.co.uk/becominganurse**

Guided Tour

Related NMC Standards of Proficiency for Pre-registration Nursing Education (NMC 2004a)

● Ensure the confidentiality and security of written and verbal information acquired in a professional capacity.

● Demonstrate knowledge of contemporary ethical issues and their impact on nursing and health care.

● Manage the complexities arising from ethical and legal dilemmas.

● Maintain, support and acknowledge the rights of individuals or groups in the health care setting.

● Act to ensure that the rights of individuals and groups are not compromised.

● Respect the values, customs and beliefs of individuals and groups.

● Provide care which demonstrates sensitivity to the diversity of patients and clients.

● Identify, collect and evaluate information to justify the effective utilisation of resources to achieve planned outcomes of nursing care.

● Information technology and management – interpret and utilise data and technology, taking account of legal, ethical and safety considerations, in the delivery and enhancement of care.

NMC Standards of Proficiency for Pre-registration Nursing Education. Each chapter is tied in to the NMC code.

Introduction

Nursing has a long and distinguished history, but it is only within the last 100 years or so that it has emerged as a distinct profession. The progression of health care in modern times has caused nursing to evolve continually with other professional groups, whilst remaining distinct from them. This chapter considers issues of the place of nursing as a profession in the modern health care system.

The chapter is divided into three parts.

In Part 1, the history of nursing and its emergence as a profession is outlined, and there is discussion about how professional issues are linked to ethical and legal considerations guiding professional practice.

In Part 2, the question of whether nursing can be fully considered to be a profession is discussed. Professional self-regulation is discussed, and the ways in which this is undertaken by the Nursing and Midwifery Council is explained.

In Part 3, a more critical approach is taken, and critiques of *The Code* are explored.

Part 1: Outlining professional issues

Case 1.1

Mairi is a newly qualified staff nurse working on a busy medical ward. In addition to the patients she is already caring for, the ward manager asks her to also look after an elderly woman admitted following a cerebrovascular accident (CVA). The patient is conscious, but confused and on Mairi's assessment, needs a considerable amount of nursing care. The patient is having intravenous medication through a pump that she is unfamiliar with. Mairi asks the ward manager either to allocate this patient or some of her other patients to someone else as she feels unable to address her needs adequately. The ward manager tells Mairi that she cannot give the patient to another nurse and that she will just have to prioritise and do the best she can.

Health care is changing rapidly for many reasons, including the development of new technologies and the emergence of an ageing population with multiple health needs. Nursing is fundamental to the delivery of good health care, and while this has been the case for many hundreds of years, the concept of nursing as a distinct *profession* started about 150 years or so ago. The pace of change has accelerated, particularly in the last decade, and looks set to continue as policy develops in response to changing health care needs.

Development of the nursing profession

The history of nursing is long and complex, and in recent years, there have been a number of substantial changes in the development of the profession. In the Middle Ages, care was undertaken in the home or by religious orders, hence

Cases. Provide a range of scenarios across all branches of nursing, and demonstrate the role of psychology in nursing practice.

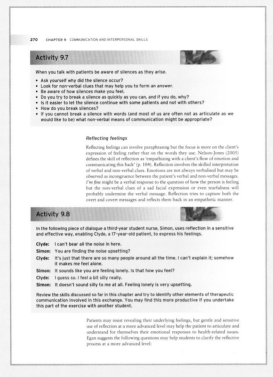

Activity 9.7

When you talk with patients be aware of silences as they arise.

- Ask yourself why did the silence occur?
- Look for non-verbal clues that may help you to form an answer.
- Be aware of how silences make you feel.
- Do you try to break a silence as quickly as you can, and if you do, why?
- Is it easier to let the silence continue with some patients and not with others?
- How do you break silences?
- If you cannot break a silence with words (and most of us are often not as articulate as we would like to be) what non-verbal means of communication might be appropriate?

Reflecting feelings

Reflecting feelings can involve paraphrasing but the focus is more on the client's expression of feeling rather that on the words they use. Nelson-Jones (2005) defines the skill of reflection as 'empathizing with a client's flow of emotion and communicating this back' (p. 104). Reflection involves the skilled interpretation of verbal and non-verbal clues. Emotions are not always verbalised but may be observed as incongruence between the patient's verbal and non-verbal messages. *I'm fine* might be a verbal response to the question of how the person is feeling but the non-verbal clues of a sad facial expression or even tearfulness will probably undermine the verbal message. Reflection tries to capture both the overt and covert messages and reflects them back in an empathetic manner.

Activity 9.8

In the following piece of dialogue a third-year student nurse, Simon, uses reflection in a sensitive and effective way, enabling Clyde, a 17-year-old patient, to express his feelings.

Clyde: I can't bear all the noise in here.
Simon: You are finding the noise upsetting?
Clyde: It's just that there are so many people around all the time. I can't explain it; somehow it makes me feel alone.
Simon: It sounds like you are feeling lonely. Is that how you feel?
Clyde: I guess so. I feel a bit silly really.
Simon: It doesn't sound silly to me at all. Feeling lonely is very upsetting.

Review the skills discussed so far in this chapter and try to identify other elements of therapeutic communication involved in this exchange. You may find this more productive if you undertake this part of the exercise with another student.

Patients may resist revealing their underlying feelings, but gentle and sensitive use of reflection at a more advanced level may help the patient to articulate and understand for themselves their emotional responses to health-related issues. Egan suggests the following questions may help students to clarify the reflective process at a more advanced level:

Activity boxes. Encourage self-reflection and self-awareness in relation to practice.

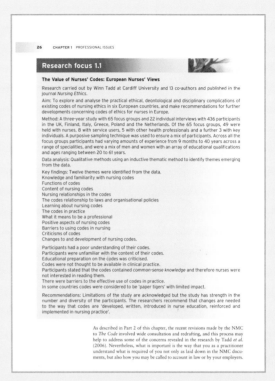

Research focus 1.1

The Value of Nurses' Codes: European Nurses' Views

Research carried out by Winn Tadd at Cardiff University and 13 co-authors and published in the journal *Nursing Ethics*.

Aim: To explore and analyse the practical ethical, deontological and disciplinary complications of existing codes of nursing ethics in six European countries, and make recommendations for further developments concerning codes of ethics for nurses in Europe.

Method: A three-year study with 65 focus groups and 22 individual interviews with 436 participants in the UK, Finland, Italy, Greece, Poland and the Netherlands. Of the 65 focus groups, 49 were held with nurses, 8 with service users, 5 with other health professionals and a further 3 with key individuals. A purposive sampling technique was used to ensure a mix of participants. Across all the focus groups participants had varying amounts of experience from 9 months to 40 years across a range of specialities, and were a mix of men and women with an array of educational qualifications and ages ranging between 20 to 61 years.

Data analysis: Qualitative methods using an inductive thematic method to identify themes emerging from the data.

Key findings: Twelve themes were identified from the data.
Knowledge and familiarity with nursing codes
Functions of codes
Content of nursing codes
Nursing relationships in the codes
The codes relationship to laws and organisational policies
Learning about nursing codes
The codes in practice
What it means to be a professional
Positive aspects of nursing codes
Barriers to using codes in nursing
Criticisms of codes
Changes to and development of nursing codes.

Participants had a poor understanding of their codes.
Participants were unfamiliar with the content of their codes.
Educational preparation on the codes was criticised.
Codes were not thought to be available in clinical practice.
Participants stated that the codes contained *common-sense knowledge* and therefore nurses were not interested in reading them.
There were barriers to the effective use of codes in practice.
In some countries codes were considered to be 'paper tigers' with limited impact.

Recommendations: Limitations of the study are acknowledged but the study has strength in the number and diversity of the participants. The researchers recommend that changes are needed to the way that codes are 'developed, written, introduced in nurse education, reinforced and implemented in nursing practice'.

As described in Part 2 of this chapter, the recent revisions made by the NMC to *The Code* involved wide consultation and redrafting, and this process may help to address some of the concerns revealed in the research by Tadd *et al.* (2006). Nevertheless, what is important is the way that you as a practitioner understand what is required of you not only as laid down in the NMC documents, but also how you may be called to account in law or by your employers.

Research focus. These boxes give examples of recent research in psychology, and show the relevance of this research to nursing practice.

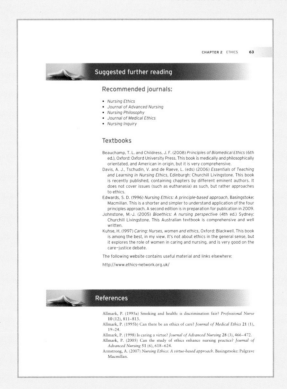

Suggested further reading

Recommended journals:

- *Nursing Ethics*
- *Journal of Advanced Nursing*
- *Nursing Philosophy*
- *Journal of Medical Ethics*
- *Nursing Inquiry*

Textbooks

Beauchamp, T. L. and Childress, J. F. (2008) *Principles of Biomedical Ethics* (6th ed.), Oxford: Oxford University Press. This book is medically and philosophically orientated, and American in origin, but it is very comprehensive.

Davis, A. J., Tschudin, V. and de Raeve, L. (eds) (2006) *Essentials of Teaching and Learning in Nursing Ethics*, Edinburgh: Churchill Livingstone. This book is recently published, containing chapters by different eminent authors. It does not cover issues (such as euthanasia) as such, but rather approaches to ethics.

Edwards, S. D. (1996) *Nursing Ethics: A principle-based approach*, Basingstoke: Macmillan. This is a shorter and simpler to understand application of the four principles approach. A second edition is in preparation for publication in 2009.

Johnstone, M.-J. (2005) *Bioethics: A nursing perspective* (4th ed.) Sydney: Churchill Livingstone. This Australian textbook is comprehensive and well written.

Kuhse, H. (1997) *Caring: Nurses, women and ethics*, Oxford: Blackwell. This book is among the best, in my view. It's not about ethics in the general sense, but it explores the role of women in caring and nursing, and is very good on the care-justice debate.

The following website contains useful material and links elsewhere:

http://www.ethics-network.org.uk/

References

Allmark, P. (1995a) Smoking and health: is discrimination fair? *Professional Nurse* 10 (12), 811–813.
Allmark, P. (1995b) Can there be an ethics of care? *Journal of Medical Ethics* 21 (1), 19–24.
Allmark, P. (1998) Is caring a virtue? *Journal of Advanced Nursing* 28 (3), 466–472.
Allmark, P. (2005) Can the study of ethics enhance nursing practice? *Journal of Advanced Nursing* 51 (6), 618–624.
Armstrong, A. (2007) *Nursing Ethics: A virtue-based approach*. Basingstoke: Palgrave Macmillan.

Suggested further reading and web links.
These will point the way forward for continued and more in-depth study.

For Louise and Imogen for their forbearance, and for Thomas and Joe, with love (DS)

For Agnes and John (aka mum and dad), with love and thanks (PS)

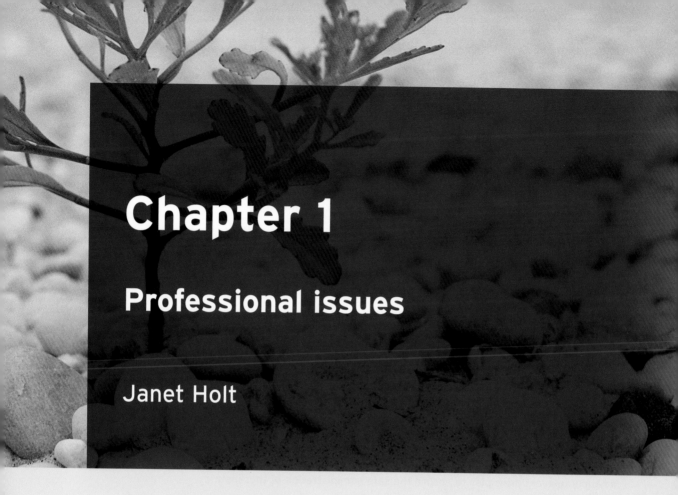

Chapter 1

Professional issues

Janet Holt

Learning outcomes

After reading and reflecting on this chapter, you should be able to:

- Explain the importance of accountability for professional practice;
- Identify the role and functions of professional self-regulation;
- Outline the role of the Nursing and Midwifery Council;
- Identify how to access professional advice from the Nursing and Midwifery Council;
- Discuss how the Nursing and Midwifery Council calls nurses to account.

Related NMC Standards of Proficiency for Pre-registration Nursing Education (NMC 2004a)

- Practise in accordance with the NMC code of professional conduct: standards for conduct, performance and ethics.

- Use professional standards of practice to self-assess performance.

- Consult with a registered nurse when nursing care requires expertise beyond one's own current scope of competence.

- Consult other health care professionals when individual or group needs fall outside the scope of nursing practice.

- Identify unsafe practice and respond appropriately to ensure a safe outcome.

- Manage the delivery of care services within the sphere of one's own accountability.

- Demonstrate the safe application of the skills required to meet the needs of patients and clients within the current sphere of practice.

- Recognise the need for adaptation and adapt nursing practice to meet varying and unpredictable circumstances.

- Ensure that practice does not compromise the nurse's duty of care to individuals or the safety of the public.

- Apply relevant principles to ensure the safe administration of therapeutic substances.

- Communicate safety concerns to the relevant authority.

- Take into account the role and competence of staff when delegating work.

- Maintain one's own accountability and responsibility when delegating aspects of care to others.

- Take action to meet any identified knowledge and skills deficit likely to affect the delivery of care within the current sphere of practice.

Introduction

Nursing has a long and distinguished history, but it is only within the last 100 years or so that it has emerged as a distinct profession. The progression of health care in modern times has caused nursing to evolve continually with other professional groups, whilst remaining distinct from them. This chapter considers issues of the place of nursing as a profession in the modern health care system.

The chapter is divided into three parts.

In Part 1, the history of nursing and its emergence as a profession is outlined, and there is discussion about how professional issues are linked to ethical and legal considerations guiding professional practice.

In Part 2, the question of whether nursing can be fully considered to be a profession is explored. Professional self-regulation is discussed, and the ways in which this is undertaken by the Nursing and Midwifery Council is explained.

In Part 3, a more critical approach is taken, and critiques of *The Code* are explored.

Part 1: Outlining professional issues

Case 1.1

Mairi is a newly qualified staff nurse working on a busy medical ward. In addition to the patients she is already caring for, the ward manager asks her to also look after an elderly woman admitted following a cerebrovascular accident (CVA). The patient is conscious, but confused and on Mairi's assessment, needs a considerable amount of nursing care. The patient is having intravenous medication through a pump that she is unfamiliar with. Mairi asks the ward manager either to allocate this patient or some of her other patients to someone else as she feels unable to address her needs adequately. The ward manager tells Mairi that she cannot give the patient to another nurse and that she will just have to prioritise and do the best she can.

Health care is changing rapidly for many reasons, including the development of new technologies and the emergence of an ageing population with multiple health needs. Nursing is fundamental to the delivery of good health care, and while this has been the case for many hundreds of years, the concept of nursing as a distinct *profession* started about 150 years or so ago. The pace of change has accelerated, particularly in the last decade, and looks set to continue as policy develops in response to changing health care needs.

Development of the nursing profession

The history of nursing is long and complex, and in recent years, there have been a number of substantial changes in the development of the profession. In the Middle Ages, care was undertaken in the home or by religious orders, hence the title 'Sister' which has persisted since this time. Florence Nightingale (1820–1910) is usually credited with initiating the reform of nursing and nursing education (Abbott and Wallace 1998). While she only had a small amount of training herself, she came from a well-connected and wealthy family and in 1854 was asked by the Minister of War, Sidney Herbert, to oversee the introduction of female nurses into the military hospitals of Turkey. The military hospitals were full of casualties from the Crimean war and it is for this work that Nightingale is perhaps best remembered. She was single-minded in pursuing policies which today may be recognised as fundamental nursing care, prioritising cleanliness and nutrition. In two years the death rate fell from 40 per cent to 2 per cent (Porter 1997), and when she returned home in 1856 she was already a national hero. A public appeal produced the funds to establish a school of nursing at St Thomas', London. While Nightingale appreciated the need for training, she did not regard nurses as autonomous practitioners, but as working under the direction of doctors. For Nightingale, male doctors controlled the activities of female nurses.

According to McGann (2004), 1887 was the turning point in the emergence of the profession of nursing, with the formation of the British Nurses' Association (BNA), which campaigned for the formation of a register of nurses. In 1905, the Select Committee on the Registration of Nurses recommended three year education and registration, but this failed to gain Government support. Along with other important social changes, the First World War (1914–1918) acted as the main catalyst to progress. The Nurses' Registration Act became law in 1919, setting up the first General Nursing Council with the following duties (Baly 1995):

- To complete a syllabus of instruction.
- To compile a syllabus for subjects for examination.
- To compile a register of qualified nurses.

The International Council of Nurses (ICN) began work on a code of ethics for nurses in 1923, but it was not finally accepted until 1953 (Fry and Johnstone 2002). The clause in this code which required obedience to the doctor was only removed in 1973, at the behest of some student nurses from Canada (Chiarella 2002). The UK published its first Code of Conduct in 1983 and in 2002, the Nursing and Midwifery Council (NMC), the body which regulates nursing and midwifery, was established.

The profession of nursing continues to change and develop. For example, in England, there has been consultation about nursing becoming an all-graduate profession, bringing English nursing in line with other health professionals and countries including Scotland, Wales and Eire. Many nurses routinely undertake tasks that until recently were considered to belong in the domain of medical practice such as venepuncture, cannulation, the performance of minor operations, and the prescription of almost all medicines. Consequently, the practice of nursing is increasingly complex and requires highly developed skills for which a knowledge base is required. While this knowledge base will include relevant anatomical, physiological and psychological information, any nurse working in current health care practice also needs an understanding of responsibility and accountability.

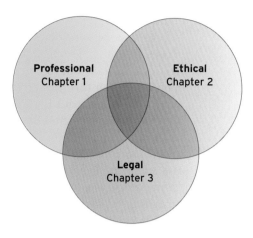

Figure 1.1 The relationship between ethics, law, and professional accountability.

Being accountable means being asked to give reasons for your actions.

It has been suggested that accountability is 'one of those delightfully para-doxical words because no-one knows what it means' (Jacobs 2004 p. 21). However, even if the precise nature of accountability is problematic, its applica-tion needs to be straightforward. It is a real issue for nurses and patients and clients and to a large extent governs practice. The concept of **being accountable** is discussed by Fletcher and colleagues (1995), but as will be explained in this chapter, for nurses in practice there are different types of accountability. The cornerstone of accountability is *professional* accountability to the regulatory body, and the NMC provides practical advice and guidance as well as the means by which nurses can be held to account for their actions or omissions.

There is much more to being professionally accountable than following pro-fessional advice, however authoritative it appears to be. There are other sources which guide action and can be referred to where accountability is required, and these can be categorised in a number of different ways. In this book the differ-ent facets of accountability are discussed not only in this chapter, but also in the two following chapters exploring ethics and law in professional practice. These three influences on practice often correspond, as represented in the Venn diagram (Figure 1.1).

A clause in *The Code* informs registrants that 'you must adhere to the laws of the country in which you are practising' (NMC 2008a). However, this may not be quite as straightforward as it seems, as different criteria may be used to judge different actions. For example, professional criteria are contained within *The Code* and other publications from the NMC, legal requirements can be found within the law, but ethical standards can originate from a number of sources. Take for example the medical procedure of termination of pregnancy. In England, Wales and Scotland abortion is unlawful except under the circumstances laid down in the Abortion Act 1967 (amended by the Human Fertilisation and Embryology Act 1990). Despite being a lawful procedure in certain circum-stances, some individuals and 'pro-life' organisations believe abortion to be morally wrong irrespective of the circumstances or the law. The law gives health care professionals, including nurses, the right to refuse to participate on grounds of conscientious objection, although it should be noted that this is not an absolute right, (that is, one that cannot be overridden in any circumstance) and there are limits placed on this (Lesser 2002). Hence, an abortion may be lawful, but a nurse may consider it to be an immoral act and may, with the support of the NMC, refuse to participate in most circumstances (NMC 2008b). This example shows the complex nature of professional accountability even when the initial edict, adherence to the law, appears on the face of it to be straightforward. The case study at the beginning of the chapter presents a similar dilemma for the nurse. On one hand she has a professional duty of care (based in law) for the delivery of care to all of the patients she is responsible for. However, Mairi also has concerns about her ability to deliver care of an adequate standard. While the repercussions of compromising care can result in the nurse being called to account in a professional or legal capacity, the heart of Mairi's concerns in this case is probably neither professional or legal in nature but based upon the ethical concern of how best to care for other people. Nevertheless, nurses will be held accountable professionally for their actions, and in other situations poor practice may be considered unprofessional, but not necessarily sufficiently serious to have a chance of successful legal redress. Even if the influences are mutually supportive, their standards are not the same. Legal standards are the lowest, professional standards are higher, and ethical standards higher still (Lesser 2002) (see Figure 1.2).

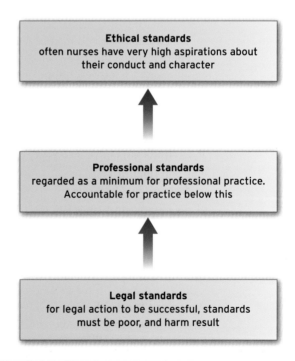

Figure 1.2 Different standards informing nursing practice.

Activity 1.1

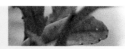

Write a list of contemporary nurses that appear in TV dramas like *Holby City* and *Casualty*. Are they good role models for you as a student nurse? Can you think of any instances where their professional behaviour might be questioned?

Part 2: Explaining professional issues

The profession of nursing

The term 'professional' is not restricted to health care professions or others such as doctors or lawyers traditionally thought of as belonging to the professions. For example plumbers may offer a 'professional plumbing service' and sportsmen and women such as footballers, golfers and athletes are also described as professionals. These forms of professionalism differ from its understanding in health care. The term 'professional' is used in sport simply to mean that individuals are paid for their services, while if a plumber offers a professional service, you could reasonably expect the work to be completed efficiently and competently. While some professions such as medicine and the law have been long established in society, there is much speculation over whether nursing can be accurately described as a profession. Professional identity has traditionally focused on the traits or characteristics that professionals were expected to demonstrate. The traits or characteristics defining a profession include:

- Altruism
- Trustworthiness
- Specialist skills
- A body of knowledge
- Competence
- Professional autonomy.

In addition, professions organise themselves into associations (such as Royal Colleges) and have a culture and etiquette that bind professionals together guided by codes of conduct. Professions are also seen to have power through their influence on policy making (Finlay 2000). Other accounts of professionalism have been described as functionalist, that is focusing on the role played by the professionals rather than their characteristics. In functionalist accounts, professions such as medicine directly help to maintain the social order by what Morrall (2001) describes as 'controlling entry to the sick role' (p. 83).

Activity 1.2

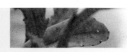

Discuss the criteria for professional status as set out above. Does nursing fulfil these criteria? Can nursing be fully described as a profession?

Both trait and functionalist accounts of professionalism are criticised by Morrall (2001) because 'they appear to reflect what those who consider themselves to be professionals believe are the characteristics of a profession. Therefore there is a strong element of self-justification in describing the professions in this way' (p. 83). While acknowledging the improved social status of nursing, Morrall (2001) is unconvinced of the professional status of nursing because he considers power to be central to the understanding of professions. In comparison to the power exercised by medicine, nursing appears to be powerless. There are also numerous occasions where, despite claims of professional autonomy, nursing activity is directed by doctors. Thus, on this account, nursing is regarded as a semi-profession complicated by unequal power relations.

An alternative approach to explaining professional identity in health care is examined by Colyer (2004), who discusses the five stages of professionalisation identified by Wilensky (1964). This process begins with the emergence of an occupational group, the establishment of a training and selection programme, the formation of a professional association, the development of a code of ethics, and political activity to establish recognition and protection of professional work. Using this definition, nursing can accurately be considered a profession as there is a clearly defined professional group, a training and selection programme, and a code of conduct overseen by the NMC. The recognition and protection of professional work is governed by the Nurses and Midwives Act (1979) and its subsequent amendment in 1992. There is also a professional association, The Royal College of Nursing, which represents approximately half of the registered nurses in the UK (Box 1.1). Other nurses are represented by trades unions such as Unison.

Box 1.1   The Royal College of Nursing

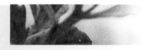

 The Royal College of Nursing (RCN) was established in 1916 and currently has around 395,000 members including health care assistants and students. The RCN represents about half of registered nurses in the UK. The RCN's homepage claims that it 'represents nurses and nursing, promotes excellence in practice and shapes health policies'. So it is more than just a trade union, which has narrower interests, though the RCN also fulfils this function, offering indemnity insurance, individual representation, and other membership benefits, similar to other trade unions representing nurses. In addition, it offers guidance on practice issues, distance learning courses in collaboration with the Open University and has a research institute based at the University of Warwick. There is a student section at the RCN, the Association of Nursing Students. The most senior officer is the Chief Executive and General Secretary, but the College is governed by a representative council.

The question of whether nursing can be truly considered to be a profession on an equal basis with one such as medicine, for example, remains largely unresolved. Furthermore, the assumption that the professionalisation of nursing is necessarily beneficial to both society and to nursing has also been questioned. In the pursuit of professionalisation, nurses could be in danger of becoming elitist and subsequently compromise their inclusive, caring philosophies (Gerrish *et al.* 2003). Despite this lack of consensus, there are some elements of professional identity that are clearly evident in the organisation of nursing. One of the most important of these is the concept of self-regulation.

Professional body	Professions regulated
General Chiropractic Council (GCC)	Chiropractors
General Dental Council (GDC)	Dentists, dental hygienists and dental therapists
General Medical Council (GMC)	Doctors
General Optical Council (GOC)	Dispensing opticians and optometrists
General Osteopathic Council (GOsC)	Osteopaths
Health Professions Council (HPC)	Arts therapists Biomedical scientists Chiropodists/podiatrists Clinical scientists Dietitians Occupational therapists Operating department practitioners Orthoptists Paramedics Physiotherapists Prosthetists/orthotists Radiographers Speech and language therapists
Nursing and Midwifery Council (NMC)	Nurses, midwives and specialist community public health nurses
Pharmaceutical Society of Northern Ireland (PSNI)	Pharmacists
Royal Pharmaceutical Society of Great Britain (RPSGB)	Pharmacists

Figure 1.3 Professional regulatory bodies in the United Kingdom.

Self-regulation

Self-regulating professions have a majority of members of the profession on the regulating body.

Self-regulation, through the establishment of regulatory bodies, is usually a feature of professions that have potential to cause harm to individuals or groups of people (Pearson 2005). There are a number of regulatory bodies in the UK which provide guidance and set standards for the profession they regulate (Figure 1.3). Nurses and midwives are regulated by the NMC. The operation of each regulatory body varies, but their main function is to protect the public. However, the government has recently instigated change in the regulation of health professionals following the white paper, Trust Assurance and Safety (DH 2007). From 1 January 2009, there has been a minimum parity of membership between lay and professional members of the NMC, undermining the claim of nurses, and other health professions, to self-regulation. The NMC opposed this change in its response to the consultation preceding the publication of the white paper (NMC 2006).

The Council for Health Care Regulatory Excellence is the statutory body co-ordinating the regulatory bodies of all health professions.

Recent developments in health care regulation also include the establishment, in 2003, of a co-ordinating body, **The Council for Health Care Regulatory Excellence** (CHRE). The functions of the CHRE include setting standards for professional regulation, and promoting good practice (CHRE 2008). All decisions taken by the Conduct and Competence Committee of the NMC are referred to the CHRE, which can appeal if it thinks that a decision is too lenient.

The Nursing and Midwifery Council

Nurses from all four branches of nursing, specialist community public health nurses and midwives are regulated by the NMC. The NMC states that

> *The core function of the NMC is to establish standards of education, training, conduct and performance for nursing and midwifery and to ensure those standards are maintained, thereby safeguarding the health and well-being of the public.*
>
> NMC (undated a)

The organisation is known as the Nursing and Midwifery Council, and the word 'Council' also refers to the board which governs the activity of the NMC. Prior to the recent changes in its governance arrangements, the Council was made up of 12 elected members representing each of the professions (nurses, specialist community public health nurses and midwives) across each of the four UK countries, and 11 lay members appointed by the Appointments Commission on behalf of the Privy Council. Lay members come from a wide variety of backgrounds and include individuals from business, health care, education, the law and consumer groups. There are now to be no more elections to Council. From January 2009, the council is smaller, consisting of seven registrant members and seven lay members, all of whom are appointed by the Appointments Commission. Meetings are held in public and the minutes and associated documents are published on the NMC website (http://www.nmc-uk.org).

There are a range of other committees of the Council, four of which are Statutory Committees required by law and established under the Nursing and Midwifery Order 2001. These committees are responsible for fitness to practice and are:

1. The Conduct and Competence Committee
2. The Health Committee
3. The Investigating Committee
4. The Midwifery Committee.

In addition, under the Order, the Council may establish other committees where it feels there is a need to do so. Currently there are eight further committees:

1. The Audit and Risk Committee
2. The Governance Committee
3. The Nursing Committee
4. The Performance and Business Planning Committee
5. The Quality Assurance Committee

6. The Registration Committee
7. The Remuneration and Appointments Committee
8. The Specialist Community Public Health Nursing Committee.

The NMC Chief Executive and Registrar is an appointed position, accountable to the Council, with responsibility for leading and managing the Council's professional, management and business affairs. The NMC, through the workings of its committees, the Council members and appointed members of staff, upholds the standards of nursing and midwifery practice and can call to account those deemed to have compromised standards of care. For self-regulation to be effective, the regulatory bodies must be impartial and the needs of patients and clients must clearly be observed to be paramount to those of practitioners. Affara (2005) considers self-regulation a privilege to be valued, and one that should not promote self-interest, be carried out behind closed doors or maintain indefensible structures. The Conduct and Competence Committee of the NMC for example generally holds hearings in public, believing that the openness of the proceedings reflects the NMC's public accountability (NMC 2004b).

To achieve its aims, the NMC has five key tasks (NMC undated a):

1. Maintain a register of nurses and midwives eligible to practise in the UK.
2. Set standards and information for nursing and midwifery conduct, performance and ethics.
3. Quality assure nursing and midwifery education.
4. Consider allegations of misconduct, lack of competence or unfitness to practise due to ill health.
5. Set standards and provide guidance for local supervising authorities for midwives.

The final task in the list applies exclusively to midwives, so will not be considered here. The other tasks will be explained in more detail.

Maintain a register of nurses and midwives eligible to practise in the UK

The maintenance of the professional register is an important task and recognised as central to the professional aspirations of nurses 100 years ago. The most recent data published by the NMC (year ending 31 March 2007) shows 686,886 nurses on the register, of which 27,704 registered for the first time and would mainly consist of students registering at the end of their programme of study (NMC 2007a). Only an individual who is registered as a nurse with the NMC is entitled to describe themselves as a registered nurse, and it is a criminal offence falsely to claim registration.

The word 'nurse' was used more frequently previously when health care workers who assisted nurses were often given the title 'auxiliary nurse'. Today these workers are more often entitled 'health care assistants', and more qualified workers are often entitled 'assistant practitioners'. Although these individuals may undertake tasks and procedures recognised as nursing care such as washing and dressing patients and clients, the use of the word 'nurse' does not appear in job titles, job descriptions or name badges. For patients and clients, who may be bewildered by the range of different professionals contributing to their care, this helps to clarify that the term 'nurse' refers to registered nurses working within agreed standards of professional practice.

Set standards and information for nursing and midwifery conduct performance and ethics

There are a number of standards published by the NMC on, amongst other things, medicines management, records and record keeping, and these serve as guides for practice. The most important of these is *The Code*.

The Code. Standards of conduct, performance and ethics for nurses and midwives

An important feature of professions is the existence of a code of ethics. The NMC regards *The Code* as a key document which summarises the duties and obligations of registered nurses and midwives. The first Code of Conduct for UK nurses was published in 1983 by the forerunner of the NMC, The United Kingdom Central Council for Nurses, Midwives and Health Visitors (UKCC). It was revised several times and following the establishment of the NMC, a new version was produced in 2002. Further amendments were made in 2004. Following wide consultation the latest version of *The Code* was published by the NMC in 2008, and is now entitled *The Code. Standards of conduct, performance and ethics for nurses and midwives*.

The Code is divided into four sections:

- Make the care of people your first concern, treating them as individuals and respecting their dignity.
- Work with others to protect and promote the health and well-being of those in your care, their families and carers, and the wider community.
- Provide a high standard of practice and care at all times.
- Be open and honest, act with integrity and uphold the reputation of your profession.

(NMC 2008a)

Within each section there are a number of standard statements which nurses have a duty to uphold. In the first section, the issues are directed towards patient care such as respecting confidentiality, gaining informed consent, collaborating with those in your care and treating people as individuals. The standards of the second section are focused on team working and include sharing information with your colleagues, working effectively as part of a team, delegating effectively and managing risk. Section three details the obligations of the practitioner to keep skills and knowledge up to date and to keep clear and accurate records. The final section is concerned with not bringing the profession into disrepute and requires practitioners to act with integrity, deal with problems, be impartial and uphold the reputation of the profession. *The Code* is reproduced in full at the end of this chapter.

Codes of conduct generally are either aspirational or prescriptive (Johnstone 2005). Aspirational codes tend to be directed at virtue, stating aims rather than prescribing behaviour and subsequently concentrating on the characteristics of individuals. Prescriptive codes are more orientated to duties. The NMC Code can be said to be a prescriptive code; its language is directive, telling registrants what they *must* do, for example, 'you *must* respect a person's right to confidentiality'. In this sense the code sets out *minimum* standards, below which registrants run the risk of censure and being called to account.

Case 1.1 (continued)

Mairi thinks that it is unfair on her and more importantly her other patients to be asked to care for the new admission. In her discussions with the ward manager she quotes from *The Code*, in particular the following clauses:

- You must act without delay if you believe that you, a colleague or anyone else may be putting someone at risk.
- You must inform someone in authority if you experience problems that prevent you from working within this Code or other nationally agreed standards.
- You must report your concerns in writing if problems in the environment of care are putting people at risk.

The ward manager, also a nurse, recognises these concerns, but the hospital is full and she has been required to accept the patient. Together they telephone the duty manager to explain that the transfer is not safe and that the patient will be at risk. They agree that this will be followed up with a letter as soon as it is possible. Mairi does make it clear, however, that she cannot operate the IV pump, because she doesn't know how it works. *The Code* states that:

- You must recognise and work within the limits of your competence.

Wainwright and Pattison (2004) note that Codes of Conduct are produced 'having the full weight of anonymous corporate authority without any hint that their production might have involved dispute and discussion' (p. 110). However, the creation and subsequent revision of the latest version of *The Code* has been conducted with more openness and discussion than previous versions. The degree of consultation may reflect a spirit of openness in the regulatory affairs of the NMC, facilitated by use of the Internet to disseminate and publish information.

The review of *The Code* began in January 2006 with a call for ideas. A small internal group of the NMC was convened to review the ideas and to assemble the elements in a new way. An initial draft was produced:

- Version 1 was produced and used as the basis for consultation. Focus groups and seminars were held, and a total of 1,459 valid responses to a questionnaire were received, including from around 170 students.
- Amendments were made to the draft (version 2) and a report was written by Jane Ball of Employment Research Ltd detailing the responses (Ball 2007).
- Further amendments were made to the draft (now version 3) and these can be tracked on a document available from the NMC website (NMC 2007b). An example of a change made following consultation is that 'You must refuse any gifts, favours, or hospitality that you are offered in the course of your work', was changed to 'You must refuse any gifts, favours or hospitality that might be interpreted as an attempt to gain preferential treatment'.
- Further consultation was carried out including:
  1. A random sample of 5,500 UK-based registrants was sent a questionnaire
  2. A questionnaire was sent to a range of stakeholder organisations:
     i. Organisations representing nurses and midwives
     ii. Organisations representing service users
     iii. Major employers
     iv. Other regulators

    3. An online consultation for everyone, highlighted in the media.
    4. Focus groups.
    5. A specific event for members of the public.
    6. Employers summits.

- A further report compiling the findings of the consultation was produced by Employment Research Limited.
- The final version was presented to the NMC at its December 2007 meeting.
- The new *Code* was published online and a paper copy sent to all registrants.

Quality assure nursing and midwifery education

The NMC is required to validate all courses leading to registration as a registered nurse. When students complete these validated courses, they are able to apply to be admitted to the register. Institutions offering the educational award are regularly audited by the NMC or other organisations acting on behalf of the NMC, and any changes to courses must be approved. Validated courses must be able to demonstrate how the proficiencies for pre-registration nursing are met. The NMC, through its *Standards to Support Learning and Assessment in Practice* (NMC 2008c) also stipulates who is able to assess students in practice, and universities are required to demonstrate their processes in meeting these standards. The regulation of courses evolves over time, for example, in 2006 the NMC implemented a rule that students must pass all of the first year Common Foundation Programme before starting the branch programme in adult, child, learning disability or mental health nursing. There are also periodic major reviews of the curriculum, involving extensive public consultation. The most recent review was launched in November 2007, and revised proficiencies will follow. The public consultation showed that a majority of key stakeholder organisations and other organisations were in favour of nurse education being at a minimum of degree level, though a majority of the approximately 3,000 individuals who responded to the survey thought that the minimum level should remain as Diploma in Higher Education (Mitchell 2008). The NMC has indicated in principles agreed at its September 2008 council meeting that the minimum academic level will be at degree level (NMC 2008c). So, while there is no national curriculum as such, with universities deciding the content and assessment for their courses, initial and periodic validation, and the imposition of extra rules and regulation mean that the NMC takes an active role in the regulation of nursing and midwifery education.

Consider allegations of misconduct, lack of competence or unfitness to practise due to ill health

Caulfield (2005) describes professional accountability as the first pillar of accountability, 'at the heart of nursing practice . . . [and] . . . based on promoting the welfare and wellbeing of patients through nursing care' (p. 4). The NMC has defined 'accountable' as being 'responsible for something or to someone' (NMC 2004c). However, this is a somewhat simplistic account, and before the process by which the NMC holds nurses to account is considered, further discussion about the concepts of responsibility and accountability is required.

Responsibility

While as citizens we all have responsibilities in society such as paying taxes, upholding the law and keeping promises, health professionals have special responsibilities as part of their professional role. For example according to *The Code* (NMC 2008a), nurses are expected to respect an individual's right to confidentiality, not to discriminate against those in their care, and recognise and work within the limits of their competence. This type of responsibility has been described by Hart (1968) as role responsibility. Hart suggests that if a person occupies an office or distinctive place within society, such as a nurse, then they are responsible for fulfilling whatever duties are recognised as part of that role. The duties attached to the role of the nurse may vary according to the area of clinical practice that they may work in. For example, the duties expected of a nurse working in an intensive care unit might be quite different to those expected of a nurse practising in the community. Nevertheless, each nurse will have a role with corresponding responsibilities attached to it determined either by the NMC or the nurse's employer.

While duties determined by the nurses' employers are likely to be contractual responsibilities, role responsibility may have legal or moral implications. In many respects, contractual duties are straightforward relating to, for example, hours of work and holiday entitlement. In addition, depending on the level of seniority, the nurse will have other more specific contractual obligations. A ward manager, for example, will have leadership and management responsibilities not expected of a more junior member of the ward team. However, the idea of nursing as a moral activity is a recurring theme in the nursing literature (Gallagher 2007, Gastmans 1999, Nortvedt 1998, Watson 1999), and this implies a moral dimension to role responsibility. Therefore the morally responsible nurse does not just carry out what they are contractually or legally required to do, but also as Pattison (2001) suggests has 'an eye to the larger and more universal ethical principles applying to human existence and behaviour' (Pattison 2001 p.7). This is a much more stringent form of responsibility which can cause difficulties and conflict for the practitioner. An example of this can be seen in the case study at the beginning of the chapter where the nurse is concerned about the level of care that she can offer the new patient.

Other situations can arise that are equally difficult to resolve, but may be more directly related to the nurse's contractual responsibilities.

Case 1.2

Suppose that John, a student nurse, has asked Robert his mentor to spend some time with him to complete records of evidence for his portfolio of clinical practice. Robert knows that it is important that John completes this today. When he made the arrangements with Robert several days ago, John informed him that they need to be submitted to the university for verification. However, the clinical area has been exceptionally busy, and John has not been able to meet with his mentor prior to their shift ending. John tells Robert he is able to stay behind to complete the documents, but Robert wants to go shopping. He has decided to buy a new laptop and has just enough time to get there before the shop closes.

Robert may feel that as John's mentor he has a responsibility to agree to stay after work to help him and while this is clearly not a contractual responsibility (as Robert has completed the required working hours), it may be argued that Robert has a moral responsibility to help John succeed. The NMC Code states that a nurse 'must facilitate students and others to develop their competence' (NMC 2008a), so if Robert does not help John on this occasion he could be considered to be in breach of his professional requirements. Robert could simply walk away from the situation, or he may feel that he does have some moral responsibility to help John succeed and decide to postpone his shopping trip. We can see in this example that having a moral responsibility can be more onerous for the individual than legal or contractual responsibilities. Here Robert is just postponing a shopping trip, but what if he needed to collect his children from school or had made a promise to a patient rather than a student? In these situations the nurse may find it difficult if not impossible to fulfil moral responsibilities. Nevertheless, nurses need to define as closely as possible what legal, contractual and moral responsibilities are required of them because it is for these that they will be held to account.

Accountability

Being called to account means being asked to give reasons for your actions (Fletcher *et al.* 1995), and nurses may be held to account in a number of ways and by different individuals or bodies such as patients and clients, employers or the NMC. Accountability therefore assumes being answerable to another person or group of people, and as discussed above, nurses are responsible for carrying out the duties expected as part of their professional role and thus are accountable for their actions in carrying out such duties. The NMC regards nurses as personally accountable for actions and omissions in professional practice and expects practitioners to be able to justify decisions they have made. Generally speaking, nurses are accountable to:

- Patients and clients – through complaints and legal processes.
- Their employers – through contractual responsibilities.
- The NMC – through *The Code*.

Accountability in law

Nurses are expected to act within the law, and *The Code* (NMC 2008a) states that nurses must 'always act lawfully whether those laws relate to your professional practice or personal life'. In 2007–2008 almost 15 per cent of fitness to practice hearings related to allegations of misconduct occurring outside work (NMC 2008e). Therefore a nurse who is convicted of an offence in their personal life (such as driving over the permitted alcohol limit) will in addition to the punishment given to them by the courts be reported to the NMC. There has been a case where a nurse was removed from the register for numerous traffic offences (Chiarella 2002). Like all other citizens, nurses are accountable under criminal law, and if a nurse is found to have committed a crime punishable by the state they would be called to account through the courts. Examples of criminal acts are murder, manslaughter, theft and drug-related offences. It is rare for any health care professional to be accused or found guilty of criminal behaviour for negligent practice and health care professionals are more commonly held to account through the law of tort. The law of tort relates to civil actions or disputes between individuals where actions for compensation are brought in the civil courts. A complaint of wrongdoing could be made against a nurse and if proven compensation could be awarded.

Case 1.1 (continued)

If Mairi operated the intravenous pump wrongly and the patient suffered some complications as a result, she could be called to account by the patient or their relatives through the courts for her actions (see Chapter 3). Simply stating that she had been instructed to operate the pump by the ward manager would not be a plausible defence for a professional in a court of law.

Accountability to employers

Nurses may be employed in the NHS, the private sector, through agencies or be self-employed. Any nurse in employment will have a contract of employment setting out the duties of both the employer (such as paying wages, health and safety responsibilities) and the employee. In addition there will be a number of policies and protocols to which the employee is expected to conform. Some policies and protocols may directly relate to the patient, such as a tissue viability policy, maintaining confidentiality, or health and safety issues. A nurse who does not adhere to what is required of them by their employer, either through their contractual responsibilities or those required by policies and protocols, may be subject to investigation and discipline through their employer's disciplinary procedures. In the case study at the beginning of the chapter, the nurse could also find herself being called to account by her employer. Suppose the patient's relatives made a formal complaint to the hospital about the care the woman had received. The hospital would investigate this in accordance with their complaints policy and a nurse could be asked to detail and explain their actions. If found to have breached any hospital policies and/or protocols, the nurse could face disciplinary action. Mairi has acted according to *The Code*, but others may not have been so clear about their actions.

Accountability to the NMC

The most significant aspect of accountability for nurses is that of professional accountability to the professional body. The core responsibility of the NMC is to protect patients and clients by ensuring that nurses receive a suitable educational programme that enables them to be both fit for purpose and fit for registration and furthermore that they are deemed to be fit for practice. The NMC sets the standards of professional behaviour required from nurses and these standards are set out in the Council's key document, *The Code*. Anyone can complain to the NMC about a registered nurse and complaints made against practitioners by service users and carers, colleagues, employers or the police are investigated through a series of practice committees. The NMC only investigates complaints where a nurse's fitness for practice is called into question. It does not investigate local contractual breaches unless it impacts directly on the quality of patient care (NMC 2004b).

Complaints about fitness for practice

The procedure for calling practitioners to account is detailed in the NMC document *Complaints about Unfitness to Practise* (NMC 2004b). If the NMC receives a complaint about a nurse that suggests that they are unfit for practise, it will be heard first by a panel of the Investigating Committee which consists of one NMC Council member and members of the NMC registrant and lay panels. The meetings at this stage are held in private and the nurse is considered innocent until proven guilty. Having considered the evidence, the Investigating Committee panel can close the case with no further action, or refer the case to a panel of the Conduct and Competence Committee or a panel of the Health Committee, in circumstances where ill health is thought to be implicated in the allegation. In serious cases an interim order can suspend a nurse's registration or impose conditions for up to 18 months while investigations are undertaken.

At the next stage, the case is heard by a panel of the Conduct and Competence Committee usually consisting of three people, an NMC Council member and members of the registrant and lay panels. At least one member of the panel must have expertise in the same area and be registered on the same part of the register as the person against whom the allegation has been made. For example if the allegation is against a mental health nurse working in forensic psychiatry, then one of the panel members must also be a registered mental health nurse with expertise in that area of mental health. In contrast to the Investigating Committee, meetings of the Conduct and Competence Committee are usually public and a member of the NMC legal team will be in attendance to advise on points of law. The nurse may be represented by a trade union official, or choose to have legal representation from a solicitor or a barrister. The Committee will hear the evidence, information about the nurse's previous history and any relevant circumstances surrounding the allegations and must decide if the facts of the case are proven. If they find that they are not, then the panel will take no further action. If the case is proven, then the panel can decide to:

- Take no further action.
- Issue a caution (a caution order).
- Impose conditions of practise for a specified period of time up to three years (a conditions of practice order).
- Suspend the nurse's registration for up to one year (a suspension order).
- Remove the person from the register (a striking-off order).

The NMC publishes guidance about how these sanctions should be implemented (NMC undated b). This document states that a striking-off order:

> *is likely to be appropriate when the behaviour is fundamentally incompatible with being a registrant. The following list is not exhaustive.*
>
> - *Serious departure from the relevant standards as set out in* The Code *[of conduct] or other of Council's standards and/or where there is continuing risk to patients/clients or others;*
> - *Confidence in the Council would be undermined if the person is not struck off;*
> - *Serious lack of competence where there is no evidence of improvement following two years of continuous suspension or conditions of practice; and*
> - *Serious ill health where there is no evidence of improvement following two years of continuous suspension or conditions of practice;*
>
> (NMC undated b p. 4)

If the Committee removes a nurse from the register, a minimum of five years must elapse before the individual may apply for reinstatement. A panel of either the Conduct and Competence Committee or the Health Committee decides if the person may be reinstated. In 2007–2008, 10 applications for reinstatement were considered. All were rejected.

The NMC publishes an annual report giving information about the cases that have been referred and heard under the fitness for practice procedures. The most recent report published covers the period 2007–2008 during which the Council received 1,487 complaints. A total of 53 per cent of these complaints were made by employers, 9 per cent from members of the public, and a further 29 per cent were notified by the police. While many of these involved minor issues, they also included convictions for rape, violent crime, downloading pornography and dishonesty (NMC 2008f). At the time of writing, two sets of rules operate for these hearings, and taken together, the various committees heard 612 cases of alleged misconduct. Of these 153 were adjourned. Of the 459 cases that were completed, 272 (59 per cent) resulted in a striking-off order. In addition two nurses were removed from the register, and 13 suspended because of ill health. Details are available from the NMC website, where explanations and justifications for decisions made can be found.

The annual reports make uncomfortable reading, especially the selection of detailed case studies that the NMC has dealt with, but the publication of the reports demonstrates the NMC's commitment to transparency in its duty to protect the public. While it is clearly important that the public is protected from incompetent, unsafe or dangerous practitioners, the whole process of self-regulation is also important to the growth and development of the nursing profession. By ensuring practitioners are publicly accountable for their actions, and show commitment to maintaining high standards of nursing care, there are opportunities to shape nursing practice (Affara 2005).

Standard of proof

In law there are two standards of proof that can be applied to the facts of a case. In civil cases involving disputes between persons, the standard of proof is 'on the balance of probability'. In criminal cases a more stringent standard of proof is used, 'beyond reasonable doubt' (see Chapter 3). Until recently, the NMC Conduct and Competence Committee used the more stringent criminal standard of proof, beyond reasonable doubt. A consultation in 2003 on the possibility of reducing the burden of proof to the civil standard did not result in a change. However, the proposal formed part of the White Paper, Trust, Assurance and Safety (DH 2007), and from October 2008, fitness to practise hearings use the civil standard of proof. This test applies for disputed facts, and not whether the facts constitute impairment to practise, which is a matter for judgement rather than proof (NMC 2008g).

Activity 1.3

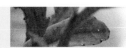

Consider the following cases:

1. A nurse is convicted of possession of cannabis
2. A nurse is convicted of possession of cannabis with intent to supply
3. A nurse is convicted of stealing money from her patients

Activity 1.3 (continued)

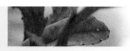

4. A nurse has given a dose of antibiotic to the wrong patient, fails to report it, and alters the drug chart in an attempt to cover up the error
5. A nurse takes 2 diazepam tablets from the drug trolley for his own use
6. A nurse is convicted of drink driving
7. A nurse is cautioned for possession of cocaine, a class A drug
8. A nurse makes inappropriate sexual comments to a fellow worker, and fails to work collaboratively with colleagues
9. A nurse is caring for a patient in a care home. The patient, who has a documented history of a serious gastric condition, vomits a large amount of brown vomit. The nurse takes no action, that is, doesn't perform any observations, and fails to notify the Matron or GP

What do you think the appropriate level of sanction is against these nurses?

Can you think of any other examples where the activities of a nurse not currently employed in practice would compromise the trust and confidence of the public? (see end of this section).

Complaints about competence

Complaints about competence are brought to the NMC's attention by employers and the process of this is detailed in the NMC document 'Reporting lack of competence' (NMC 2004d). The NMC should only be involved if all local measures have been exhausted and despite having been given opportunities and support to improve their competence, the nurse continues to give cause for concern. The process for these hearings is similar to those for complaints about unfitness to practise and the case is first put to a panel of the Investigating Committee. If it decides there is a case to answer, the case is referred to the Conduct and Competence Committee. If this Committee finds the case proven, similar to allegations of unfitness for practise, it can impose a condition of practice order, a suspension order, a striking-off order, or a caution. However, the most serious penalty, a striking-off order, can only be made *after* the nurse has been subject to either conditions of practice order or a suspension order.

Accountability and students

A common misconception is that students are not accountable for their actions. It is the case that students cannot be held to account for their actions by the NMC, as they are not registered practitioners. Students are supervised in clinical practice and if necessary, the NMC would call to account the registered practitioners with whom the student was working, not the student. This is in keeping with Hart's definition of role responsibility, discussed earlier (Hart 1968). Part of the role of registered nurses is an obligation to 'facilitate students and others to develop their competence' (NMC 2008a). If the registered nurse fails to supervise the student adequately or delegates a task beyond that expected of them at that point in their education, then the registered nurse would be accountable. Similarly where registered nurses have authority to delegate tasks to non-regulated health care staff such as care assistants, the NMC considers the nurse to retain responsibility and accountability for any delegated tasks (NMC 2008h).

Nevertheless, students are expected to work only within their 'level of understanding and competence, and always under the appropriate supervision of a registered nurse' (NMC 2002a p. 2). If a student failed to do this then they could be held to account either by their university or even in law.

Case 1.3

Jenna is a third-year student. Having examined a patient's intravenous cannula she (correctly) judges that it needs to be flushed through. Having seen her mentor do this on several occasions, Jenna feels that she would be able to carry out the action without any difficulty and therefore collects the required equipment and flushes the cannula.

Clearly this task is beyond the remit of the student even if supervised, but as the student decided to carry out the action without consulting her supervisor, she could be called to account for her actions by the university using the appropriate student conduct or disciplinary processes. Furthermore, if the patient's well-being was compromised, they could make a complaint or seek recompense in law. In this scenario it is unlikely that the student's supervisor would be culpable because the student was not acting either under their supervision or on their instructions, and therefore the student themself could be held to account in law. It is important that students always work under supervision while in practice.

Good health and good character

Similarly to the NMC fitness to practise process, universities are required to have a 'fitness to practise' panel to consider any health or character issues and to ensure that public protection is maintained (NMC 2008i). Students are required to disclose any convictions or cautions prior to admission to a course, and a Criminal Records Bureau (CRB) check will be undertaken. During the programme, students are required to disclose any cautions or convictions, and their fitness to remain on the programme will be considered by the fitness for practice panel. However, good character is more than an absence of convictions; any other behaviour that indicates dishonesty can be considered. Students are regularly required to declare that they are of good health and character, as are registered nurses, each time they renew their registration. *The Code* requires registrants 'to inform the NMC if you have been cautioned, charged, or found guilty of a criminal offence' (NMC 2008a). The NMC explains good health and good character as:

Good health
Good health is necessary to undertake practice as a nurse or midwife. Good health means that you must be capable of safe and effective practice without supervision. It does not mean the absence of any disability or health condition. Many disabled people and those with long-term health conditions are able to practise with or without adjustments to support their practice.

Long-term conditions such as epilepsy, diabetes or depression can be well managed and would then not be incompatible with registration.

Temporary health conditions do not necessarily mean a person is not fit to practise. For example having a broken leg may mean a person is not fit to work for a period of time. It does not mean they are not fit to practise as they can reasonably expect to recover fully and return to work.

Good character

Good character is important as nurses and midwives must be honest and trustworthy. Your good character is based on your conduct, behaviour and attitude. It covers examples such as someone who knowingly practises as a nurse or midwife before they are on the register, or someone who signs a student off from an educational programme while being aware of poor behaviour.

It also includes any convictions and cautions that are not considered compatible with professional registration and that might bring the profession into disrepute. Your character must be sufficiently good for you to be capable of safe and effective practice without supervision.

(NMC 2008j)

Activity 1.4

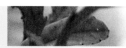

The following scenarios relate to students' behaviour while on the pre-registration programme, and both resulted in referral to the university fitness to practise panel. Do you think that the students should be allowed to remain on the course? The cases are derived from worked examples from the NMC (2008k, 2008l). The NMC guidance about the cases is given at the end of the chapter.

Case 1.4

Dorothy, a student in the beginning of her third year, plagiarised her most recent assignment by copying work from an Internet site. The plagiarism was detected and referred to the fitness to practise panel.

Case 1.5

Stephanus has completed all of the theory parts of the programme and is making up practice hours. The final two weeks of the course were planned as annual leave. While on annual leave Stephanus was involved in a fight at a nightclub. He was given a caution and informed the university, who referred the matter to the fitness to practise panel.

Other services provided by the NMC

As well as fulfilling the key tasks, the NMC provides other services. These are:

- An online registration confirmation service for employers.
- A free and confidential advice service for nurses and midwives. In 2007–2008, this service answered 594,749 calls, or an average of 3,000 per day. Contact details (Monday to Friday 0800–1800) are:
  Tel: 020 7333 9333
  Email: advice@nmc-uk.org

There are also a number of easily accessible advice sheets, available as an A-Z of advice from the homepage. These contain practical advice, cross-referenced to *The Code*, and other NMC publications. These advice sheets vary in length, but are generally around 2–4 sides of A4. They are regularly updated, easily accessible, and should be considered a good learning resource:

- Free publications keep practitioners, students and the general public informed about the Council's work.
- A range of events including exhibitions, seminars and conferences.
- *NMC News*, a quarterly news magazine, is mailed to all registrants in the UK and overseas. This is also publicly available online.

The cases in Activity 1.3 are all based on real cases presented to the NMC, and are available on their website. Details and mitigation are of great importance, but similar cases have resulted in striking of orders for cases 2, 3, 4, 5, 8 and 9.

Part 3: Exploring professional issues

What is of more importance than the existence of a code of ethics or conduct is its effectiveness in practice. This has been a subject of comment and research for over ten years and still considered to be a sufficiently important topic to be the focus of one of the papers selected for the thirtieth anniversary issue of the *Journal of Advanced Nursing* in 2006. Esterhuizen's paper 'Is the professional code the cornerstone of clinical nursing practice?' was published in the 1996 volume of the *Journal of Advanced Nursing* (Esterhuizen 1996). In this paper Esterhuizen concludes that codes of nursing do provide the base for nursing actions and are necessary for professional accountability. Ten years later in the anniversary issue, the paper was reproduced with three commentaries from contemporary authors. While acknowledging the methodological limitations of Esterhuizen's review, the question is still considered to need further research (Gastmans and Verpeet 2006, Leino-Kilpi 2006). Leino-Kilpi (2006) points out that there is little evidence to suggest that nurses who put ethical codes into practice provide better nursing care than those who do not, especially since in countries that do not have ethical codes nurses still appear to care competently for patients.

Codes of ethics?

Whether *The Code* is, or even should be, a code of ethics or a set of standards is a matter of debate. Pattison (2001) pertinently asks 'Are nursing codes of practice ethical?' and concludes that although written in ethical language, professional codes do not develop or support independent critical judgement, which Pattison deems necessary for good professionalism. Except in its title, the latest version of *The Code* does not specifically mention ethics or ethical practice, but in keeping with former versions, it continues to be written in ethical language insofar as ethics is concerned with distinguishing between good and bad actions. However, *The Code* can more accurately be considered to be a code of conduct rather than a code of ethics (Snelling and Lipscomb 2004).

The Code does not give the nurse an indication of what they must do to act morally: it simply states the standard of behaviour to which the nurse is required to conform. For example, a nurse is expected to gain informed consent before they begin any treatment or care. This is a legal as well as a professional requirement, and should a nurse fail to do this, they could be called to account for their actions. However, it is possible for the nurse to approach the patient and obtain informed consent without any sense of the moral imperative of the act. The nurse would be acting in accordance with *The Code*, but may not (or indeed not need to) justify their actions morally. If the nurse was asked why they were obtaining informed consent, they could simply say because *The Code* requires them to do so, without explaining or justifying why this is morally the right action. Gastmans and Verpeet (2006) discuss how a decade earlier, Esterhuizen's (1996) paper pointed out that the most important feature of codes is their normative function rather than their disciplinary, legal or professional functions. However, to achieve this codes would need to be designed to be both useful and effective in bringing about ethical practice (Meulenbergs *et al.* 2004).

Following this theme, Pattison (2001) raises the concern that professional codes do not develop the independent critical thought needed for good moral and professional judgement, nor do they detail why the values and principles addressed in the codes have been selected. A code of ethics has been regarded as an essential characteristic of a profession and *The Code* is the central document used by the NMC in making judgements about fitness to practise. Thus, codes may be considered simply as useful tools for social recognition, as an indicator of professional status or as instruments to control the activities of practitioners (Meulenbergs *et al.* 2004). Whether they provide guidance on ethical practice or develop a sense of ethical conduct in practitioners is open to debate. The NMC expects practitioners to act in the best interests of patients and clients, but how this may be best achieved in the many encounters with service users across a broad spectrum of practice is left to the practitioner to discern.

Good character and conduct

The NMC clearly expects practitioners not only to practise competently but also to be of good character. Students are required to make a self-declaration that they are of good health and good character, but before being admitted to the register, the NMC also requires that this is supported by a statement from a registered nurse involved in pre-registration education. Therefore, as well as completing the theoretical and clinical requirements of the programme, the student must also convince the person signing this declaration of good character (usually a designated member of the university staff) that they are a suitable candidate for inclusion on the register of nurses.

An assessment of good character requires consideration of conduct, behaviour or attitudes that are not compatible with professional registration in addition to any convictions or cautions. However, as Sellman (2007) discusses, NMC guidance for those making such character assessments is not explicit but requires the applicant to intend to comply with *The Code*, not have relevant criminal convictions, or not to have been found guilty of misconduct. Furthermore, to assess a person's character is to make a moral judgment about the person based upon the available evidence. Without this signed declaration, the application for registration as a nurse with the NMC will not be accepted. Consequently any wrongdoing on your part which may be construed as not demonstrating good character and conduct could prevent you from being admitted to the professional register even though you may have successfully completed the programme of study. Once you are registered as a nurse, how you behave in your personal life as well as when in practice will be subject to scrutiny, as demonstrated in a case brought before the Professional Conduct Committee where a nurse had been convicted of possession of cannabis with intent to supply. In this case, the committee found the nurse guilty of professional misconduct because he had failed to justify public trust and confidence and failed to uphold and enhance the good standing and reputation of the profession. His name was subsequently removed from the register (NMC 2002b).

Codes of ethics in practice

A further and perhaps more worrying concern is how nurses use codes of conduct or codes of ethics in clinical practice. Little research has been carried out to examine the usefulness of codes in nursing practice, but a comprehensive evaluation of the views of European nurses in six countries were explored in a recent study of 49 focus groups involving 311 participants (Tadd *et al.* 2006). The research suggested that nurses lacked knowledge of their codes and failed to use them to consider the moral dimensions of their practice. Most participants were unfamiliar with the context of the codes and believed they had little practical value. In the terms of *The Code*, the hallmark of a professional is the personal accountability of the nurse, but as emphasised by Tschudin (2006), 'A code can demand accountability: but, for someone who wants to be truly accountable, a code is not the first port of call' (p. 113). Despite the acknowledged shortcomings of codes of practice, *The Code* does identify the standards of practice that it expects nurses to practise in accordance with, and is therefore highly significant in making judgements when nurses are called to account for their actions.

Research focus 1.1

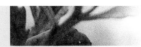

The Value of Nurses' Codes: European Nurses' Views

Research carried out by Winn Tadd at Cardiff University and 13 co-authors and published in the journal *Nursing Ethics*.

Aim: To explore and analyse the practical ethical, deontological and disciplinary complications of existing codes of nursing ethics in six European countries, and make recommendations for further developments concerning codes of ethics for nurses in Europe.

Method: A three-year study with 65 focus groups and 22 individual interviews with 436 participants in the UK, Finland, Italy, Greece, Poland and the Netherlands. Of the 65 focus groups, 49 were held with nurses, 8 with service users, 5 with other health professionals and a further 3 with key individuals. A purposive sampling technique was used to ensure a mix of participants. Across all the focus groups participants had varying amounts of experience from 9 months to 40 years across a range of specialities, and were a mix of men and women with an array of educational qualifications and ages ranging between 20 to 61 years.

Data analysis: Qualitative methods using an inductive thematic method to identify themes emerging from the data.

Key findings: Twelve themes were identified from the data.
Knowledge and familiarity with nursing codes
Functions of codes
Content of nursing codes
Nursing relationships in the codes
The codes relationship to laws and organisational policies
Learning about nursing codes
The codes in practice
What it means to be a professional
Positive aspects of nursing codes
Barriers to using codes in nursing
Criticisms of codes
Changes to and development of nursing codes.

Participants had a poor understanding of their codes.
Participants were unfamiliar with the content of their codes.
Educational preparation on the codes was criticised.
Codes were not thought to be available in clinical practice.
Participants stated that the codes contained *common-sense knowledge* and therefore nurses were not interested in reading them.
There were barriers to the effective use of codes in practice.
In some countries codes were considered to be 'paper tigers' with limited impact.

Recommendations: Limitations of the study are acknowledged but the study has strength in the number and diversity of the participants. The researchers recommend that changes are needed to the way that codes are 'developed, written, introduced in nurse education, reinforced and implemented in nursing practice'.

As described in Part 2 of this chapter, the recent revisions made by the NMC to *The Code* involved wide consultation and redrafting, and this process may help to address some of the concerns revealed in the research by Tadd *et al.* (2006). Nevertheless, what is important is the way that you as a practitioner understand what is required of you not only as laid down in the NMC documents, but also how you may be called to account in law or by your employers.

Conclusion

In this chapter, the concepts of responsibility and accountability have been explored. As a registered nurse you will be expected to adhere to the standards of practice required by the NMC and detailed in their publications, most notably in *The Code*. The primary function of the NMC is to protect the public, and it fulfils this responsibility by ensuring that nurses who are on the professional register are fit for practice and by imposing sanctions on nurses who do not meet the required standards. However, as discussed, there are different facets to accountability, and a nurse may be called to account by patients and clients through legal processes, or by their employers according to their terms and conditions of employment. The research by Tadd *et al*. (2006) showed that some codes are considered to be 'paper tigers', that is, impressive but ineffective documents. Some nurses may demonstrate poor practice, but never be challenged to give reasons for their actions. While the mechanisms of accountability are important, what lies at the heart of this issue is the integrity, honesty and trustworthiness of the practitioner, and hence a sense of the moral responsibility you have to the patients and clients in your care, your colleagues and to the profession as a whole.

Another important issue addressed in this chapter is the need to separate the issues of responsibility and accountability so you know what is expected of you in your professional role. As well as any specific aspects of practice, you will also be responsible for making judgments about what is and what is not within your scope of practice. As shown in the case study at the beginning of the chapter, if you accept responsibility for the care required by patients and clients, then this is what you are accountable for to the patient or client themselves (or their relatives), your employers and the NMC. Accountability may also extend to your personal life as well as regulating your professional life.

Nurses in the UK do not work in isolation, and if you are unsure of what to do in a given situation, it is important that you seek advice from more senior colleagues, though simply following the advice does not absolve you of personal accountability. You should also ensure that you keep clear records in case you need to refer to them at a later date. Professional responsibility and accountability is onerous for practitioners, but ensuring that only those practitioners who remain fit to practise have responsibility for patient care is the consequence of belonging to a profession with the privilege of self-regulation.

The Code: Standards of conduct, performance and ethics for nurses and midwives

Quoted in full from nmc-uk.org with permission.

The people in your care must be able to trust you with their health and well-being.

To justify that trust, you must:

- make the care of people your first concern, treating them as individuals and respecting their dignity
- work with others to protect and promote the health and wellbeing of those in your care, their families and carers, and the wider community
- provide a high standard of practice and care at all times
- be open and honest, act with integrity and uphold the reputation of your profession

As a professional, you are personally accountable for actions and omissions in your practice and must always be able to justify your decisions.

You must always act lawfully, whether those laws relate to your professional practice or personal life.

Failure to comply with this Code may bring your fitness to practise into question and endanger your registration.

This Code should be considered together with the Nursing and Midwifery Council's rules, standards, guidance and advice available from http://www.nmc-uk.org.

Make the care of people your first concern, treating them as individuals and respecting their dignity

Treat people as individuals

- You must treat people as individuals and respect their dignity
- You must not discriminate in any way against those in your care
- You must treat people kindly and considerately
- You must act as an advocate for those in your care, helping them to access relevant health and social care, information and support

Respect people's confidentiality

- You must respect people's right to confidentiality
- You must ensure people are informed about how and why information is shared by those who will be providing their care
- You must disclose information if you believe someone may be at risk of harm, in line with the law of the country in which you are practising

Collaborate with those in your care

- You must listen to the people in your care and respond to their concerns and preferences
- You must support people in caring for themselves to improve and maintain their health
- You must recognise and respect the contribution that people make to their own care and wellbeing
- You must make arrangements to meet people's language and communication needs
- You must share with people, in a way they can understand, the information they want or need to know about their health

Ensure you gain consent

- You must ensure that you gain consent before you begin any treatment or care
- You must respect and support people's rights to accept or decline treatment and care
- You must uphold people's rights to be fully involved in decisions about their care
- You must be aware of the legislation regarding mental capacity, ensuring that people who lack capacity remain at the centre of decision-making and are fully safeguarded

- You must be able to demonstrate that you have acted in someone's best interests if you have provided care in an emergency

Maintain clear professional boundaries

- You must refuse any gifts, favours or hospitality that might be interpreted as an attempt to gain preferential treatment
- You must not ask for or accept loans from anyone in your care or anyone close to them
- You must establish and actively maintain clear sexual boundaries at all times with people in your care, their families and carers

Work with others to protect and promote the health and well-being of those in your care, their families and carers, and the wider community

Share information with your colleagues

- You must keep your colleagues informed when you are sharing the care of others
- You must work with colleagues to monitor the quality of your work and maintain the safety of those in your care
- You must facilitate students and others to develop their competence

Work effectively as part of a team

- You must work co-operatively within teams and respect the skills, expertise and contributions of your colleagues
- You must be willing to share your skills and experience for the benefit of your colleagues
- You must consult and take advice from colleagues when appropriate
- You must treat your colleagues fairly and without discrimination
- You must make a referral to another practitioner when it is in the best interests of someone in your care

Delegate effectively

- You must establish that anyone you delegate to is able to carry out your instructions
- You must confirm that the outcome of any delegated task meets required standards
- You must make sure that everyone you are responsible for is supervised and supported

Manage risk

- You must act without delay if you believe that you, a colleague or anyone else may be putting someone at risk
- You must inform someone in authority if you experience problems that prevent you working within this Code or other nationally agreed standards
- You must report your concerns in writing if problems in the environment of care are putting people at risk

Provide a high standard of practice and care at all times

Use the best available evidence

- You must deliver care based on the best available evidence or best practice
- You must ensure any advice you give is evidence based if you are suggesting health care products or services
- You must ensure that the use of complementary or alternative therapies is safe and in the best interests of those in your care

Keep your skills and knowledge up to date

- You must have the knowledge and skills for safe and effective practice when working without direct supervision
- You must recognise and work within the limits of your competence
- You must keep your knowledge and skills up to date throughout your working life
- You must take part in appropriate learning and practice activities that maintain and develop your competence and performance

Keep clear and accurate records

- You must keep clear and accurate records of the discussions you have, the assessments you make, the treatment and medicines you give and how effective these have been
- You must complete records as soon as possible after an event has occurred
- You must not tamper with original records in any way
- You must ensure any entries you make in someone's paper records are clearly and legibly signed, dated and timed
- You must ensure any entries you make in someone's electronic records are clearly attributable to you
- You must ensure all records are kept securely

Be open and honest, act with integrity and uphold the reputation of your profession

Act with integrity

- You must demonstrate a personal and professional commitment to equality and diversity
- You must adhere to the laws of the country in which you are practising
- You must inform the NMC if you have been cautioned, charged or found guilty of a criminal offence
- You must inform any employers you work for if your fitness to practise is called into question

Deal with problems

- You must give a constructive and honest response to anyone who complains about the care they have received
- You must not allow someone's complaint to prejudice the care you provide for them

- You must act immediately to put matters right if someone in your care has suffered harm for any reason
- You must explain fully and promptly to the person affected what has happened and the likely effects
- You must co-operate with internal and external investigations

Be impartial

- You must not abuse your privileged position for your own ends
- You must ensure that your professional judgment is not influenced by any commercial considerations

Uphold the reputation of your profession

- You must not use your professional status to promote causes that are not related to health
- You must co-operate with the media only when you can confidently protect the confidential information and dignity of those in your care
- You must uphold the reputation of your profession at all times

Information about indemnity insurance

The NMC recommends that a registered nurse, midwife or specialist community public health nurse, in advising, treating and caring for patients/clients, has professional indemnity insurance. This is in the interests of clients, patients and registrants in the event of claims of professional negligence.

Whilst employers have vicarious liability for the negligent acts and/or omissions of their employees, such cover does not normally extend to activities undertaken outside the registrant's employment. Independent practice would not be covered by vicarious liability. It is the individual registrant's responsibility to establish their insurance status and take appropriate action.

In situations where an employer does not have vicarious liability, the NMC recommends that registrants obtain adequate professional indemnity insurance. If unable to secure professional indemnity insurance, a registrant will need to demonstrate that all their clients/patients are fully informed of this fact and the implications this might have in the event of a claim for professional negligence.

NMC scenarios of good health and character

Reproduced in full from www.nmc-uk.org. The numbers of the scenarios refer to NMC worked examples.

Scenario 5: Students on pre-registration courses - character

Dorothy, a student in the beginning of her third year, plagiarised her most recent assignment. This was reported to the External Examiner and would be considered formally by the Examination Board. The programme leader is unsure about whether she can sign the confirming declaration of good health and good character and whether Dorothy should remain on the programme until the Board meets to make a formal decision. She refers the case to the university's fitness to practise panel.

The issue

Is Dorothy capable of safe and effective practice without supervision? The university needs to consider whether Dorothy knowingly copied another individual's work and then submitted it as her own work. To knowingly plagiarise academic material is the equivalent of fraud.

Outcome

It was established that Dorothy had previously been taught the need to make reference to other people's work when writing assignments. The university's fitness to practise panel interviewed her and her teachers and found that Dorothy had already submitted several pieces of work using the correct approach, demonstrating that she did understand referencing processes. The fitness to practise panel decided that Dorothy had knowingly plagiarised and she was discontinued from the programme.

Scenario 7: UK students applying for entry to the register - character

Stephanus was recommended by the university Examination Board to be awarded a BSc (Hons) Nursing subject to completion of programme hours. The final two weeks of the course were planned as annual leave. While on annual leave Stephanus was involved in a fight at a nightclub. He was given a caution and informed the university. The programme leader was not prepared to sign his declaration of good character and took the case to the university's fitness to practise panel. The unsigned declaration of good character was forwarded to the NMC unsigned with details about the investigation. The university told Stephanus about what was happening. The panel were unable to reach a decision and decided to seek advice from the NMC.

The issue

Is Stephanus capable of safe and effective practice without supervision? A caution may indicate that he is not trustworthy and does not have the potential to apply the Code. Although the incident occurred outside of work this behaviour might be repeated if Stephanus were involved in a difficult situation at work. The NMC has to be satisfied that there is not a conflict between Stephanus' personal and professional value systems and that he will act in accordance with the Code.

Outcome

Stephanus had no previous cautions or convictions and had a positive reference from his mentor in practice. The programme leader confirmed that before this incident the university had been happy with his behaviour.

The programme leader then signed a declaration of good character and forwarded it to the NMC. Stephanus was told that he must declare the caution when applying for registration, which he did and was registered as a nurse.

Suggested further reading

The major source for further information about professional issues is the Nursing and Midwifery Council's website, http://www.nmc-uk.org All of the documents referred to in this chapter are publicly available. Navigation around the site takes a little while to master, but patience is rewarded. The material there is invaluable to understanding your responsibilities as a nurse. In addition the Department of Health website contains much useful information, especially the Chief Nurse's page.

http://www.dh.gov.uk/en/Aboutus/Chiefprofessionalofficers/Chiefnursingofficer/index.htm there are links from here to relevant documents, and you can arrange for regular newsletters to be sent.

The following books explore professional issues and accountability in more depth

Caulfield, H. (2005) *Accountability*, Oxford: Blackwell. A basic introductory textbook.

Chiarella, M. (2002) *The Legal and Professional Status of Nursing*, Edinburgh: Churchill Livingstone. This is a fascinating account of how the profession of nursing is defined in a number of different ways through judgements made in legal cases throughout the English-speaking liberal democracies.

Tilley, S. and Watson, R. (eds). *Accountability in Nursing* (2nd ed.), Oxford: Blackwell. Chapter 3 (pp. 21-37) contains an impressive discussion of accountability within a range of settings.

References

Abbott, P. and Wallace, C. (1998) Health visiting, social work, nursing and midwifery: a history. In *The Sociology of the Caring Professions* (2nd ed.), Abbot, P. and Meerabeau, L. (eds). London: UCL Press, 20–53.

Affara, F. A. (2005) Valuing professional self-regulation. *Journal of Advanced Nursing* 52 (6), 579.

Ball, J. (2007) *Responses to the NMC Consultation on the New Draft Code of Conduct*. London: Employment Research Ltd.

Baly, M. E. (1995) *Nursing and Social Change* (3rd ed.). London: Routledge.

Caulfield, H. (2005) *Accountability*. Oxford: Blackwell.

Chiarella, M. (2002) *The Legal and Professional Status of Nursing*. Edinburgh: Churchill Livingstone.

CHRE (Council for Healthcare Regulatory Excellence). (2008) *Protecting the Public: Learning from Fitness to Practice*. London: CHRE. (http://www.chre.org.uk).

Colyer, H. M. (2004) The construction and development of health professionals: where will it end? *Journal of Advanced Nursing* **48** (4), 406–412.

DH (Department of Health). (2007) *Trust, Assurance and Safety – The Regulation of Health Professionals in the 21st Century*. London: The Stationery Office.

Esterhuizen, P. (1996) Is the professional code still the cornerstone of clinical nursing practice? *Journal of Advanced Nursing* **23** (1), 25–31.

Finlay, L. (2000) The challenge of professionalism. In *Critical Practice in Health and Social Care*, Brechin, A. Brown, H. and Eby, M. A. (eds). London: Open University Press, 73–95.

Fletcher, N., Holt, J., Brazier, M. and Harris, J. (1995) *Ethics, Law and Nursing*. Manchester: Manchester University Press.

Fry, S. T. and Johnstone, M-J. (2002) *Ethics in Nursing Practice: A guide to ethical decision-making* (2nd ed.). Oxford: Blackwell.

Gallagher, A. (2007) The respectful nurse. *Nursing Ethics* **14** (3), 360–371.

Gastmans, C. (1999) Care as a moral attitude in nursing. *Nursing Ethics* **6** (3), 214–223.

Gastmans, C. and Verpeet, E. (2006) 30th anniversary commentary of Esterhuizen, P. (1996) Is the professional code still the cornerstone of clinical nursing practice? *Journal of Advanced Nursing* **53** (1), 111–112.

Gerrish, K., McManus, M. and Ashworth, P. (2003) Creating what sort of professional? Master's level nurse education as a professionalising strategy. *Nursing Inquiry* **10** (2), 103–112.

Hart, H. L. A. (1968) *Punishment and Responsibility*. Oxford: Oxford University Press.

Jacobs, K. (2004) Accountability and clinical governance in nursing; a critical overview of the topic. In *Accountability in Nursing* (2nd ed.), Tilley, S. and Watson, R. (eds). Oxford: Blackwell, 21–37.

Johnstone, M-J. (2005) *Bioethics. A Nursing Perspective* (4th ed.). Sydney: Churchill Livingstone.

Leino-Kilpi, H. (2006) 30th anniversary commentary of Esterhuizen, P. (1996) Is the professional code still the cornerstone of clinical nursing practice? *Journal of Advanced Nursing* **53** (1), 112–113.

Lesser, H. and Cribb, A. (2002) An ethical perspective – negligence and moral obligations. In *Nursing Law and Ethics* (2nd ed.), Tingle, J. and Cobb, A. (eds). Oxford: Blackwell, 90–98.

McGann, S. (2004) The development of nursing as an accountable profession. In *Accountability in Nursing* (2nd ed.), Tilley, S. and Watson, R. (eds). Oxford: Blackwell, 9–20.

Meulenbergs, T., Verpeet, E., Schotsmans, P. and Gastmans, C. (2004) Professional codes in a changing nursing context: literature review. *Journal of Advanced Nursing* **46** (3), 331–336.

Mitchell, D. (2008) *A Review of Pre-registration Education – Report of Consultation Findings*. London: NMC (http://www.nmc-uk.org).

Morrall, P. (2001) *Sociology and Nursing*. London: Routledge.

Nortvedt, P. (1998) Sensitive judgement: an inquiry into the foundations of nursing ethics. *Nursing Ethics* **5** (5), 385–386.

Nursing and Midwifery Council (NMC) (undated a) About Us http://www.nmc-uk.org NMC. (undated b) Indicative Sanctions Guidance for Panels of the Conduct and Competence and Health Committees. London: NMC (http://www.nmc-uk.org).

NMC (2002a) *An NMC Guide for Students of Nursing and Midwifery*. London: NMC (http://www.nmc-uk.org).

NMC (2002b) *Professional Conduct Annual Report 2001–2002*. London: NMC (http://www.nmc-uk.org).

NMC (2004a) *Standards of Proficiency for Pre-Registration Nursing Education*. London: NMC (http://www.nmc-uk.org).

NMC (2004b) *Complaints About Unfitness to Practise: A guide for members of the public*. London: NMC (http://www.nmc-uk.org).

NMC (2004c) *The NMC Code of Professional Conduct: Standards for conduct, performance and ethics*. London: NMC (http://www.nmc-uk.org).

NMC (2004d) *Reporting Lack of Competence: A guide for employers and managers*. London: NMC (http://www.nmc-uk.org).

NMC (2006) *Response to Department of Health Consultation*, published 14 July 2006. London: NMC (http://www.nmc-uk.org).

NMC (2007a) *Statistical Analysis of the Register 1st April 2006 to 31st March 2007* London: NMC (http://www.nmc-uk.org).

NMC (2007b) *Annex 1 of the Review of the Code of Professional Conduct*. London: NMC (http://www.nmc-uk.org).

NMC (2008a) *The Code. Standards of conduct, performance and ethics for nurses and midwives*. London: NMC (http://www.nmc-uk.org).

NMC (2008b) *Conscientious Objection*. London: NMC (http://www.nmc-uk.org).

NMC (2008c) *Standards to Support Learning and Assessment in Practice*. London: NMC (http://www.nmc-uk.org).

NMC (2008d) *Confirmed Principles to Support a New Framework for Pre-registration Nursing Education*. London: NMC (http://www.nmc-uk.org).

NMC (2008e) *Your Code of Conduct Applies to your Personal Life*. London: NMC (http://www.nmc-uk.org).

NMC (2008f) *Fitness to Practise Annual Report 2005–2006*. London: NMC (http://www.nmc-uk.org).

NMC (2008g) *Briefing Note for Legal Assessors on Civil Standard of Proof*. London: NMC (http://www.nmc-uk.org).

NMC (2008h) *NMC Advice for Delegation to Non-Regulated Healthcare Staff*. London: NMC (http://www.nmc-uk.org).

NMC (2008i) *Good Health and Good Character: Guidance for educational institutions*. London: NMC (http://www.nmc-uk.org).

NMC (2008j) *What we mean by Good Health and Good Character*. London: NMC (http://www.nmc-uk.org).

NMC (2008k) *Scenarios 4–5: Students on pre-registration programmes*. London: NMC (http://www.nmc-uk.org).

NMC (2008l) *Scenarios 6–7: UK students applying for entry to the register*. London: NMC (http://www.nmc-uk.org).

Pattison, S. (2001) Are nursing codes of practice ethical? *Nursing Ethics* **8** (1), 5–18.

Pearson, A. (2005) Registration, regulation and competence in nursing. *International Journal of Nursing Practice* **11** (5), 191–192.

Porter, R. (1997) *The Greatest Benefit to Mankind; A medical history of humanity from antiquity to the present*. London: Harper Collins.

Sellman, D. (2007) On being of good character: Nurse education and the assessment of good character. *Nurse Education Today* **27** (7), 762–767.

Snelling, P. C. and Lipscomb, M. (2004) Academic freedom, analysis, and the Code of Professional Conduct. *Nurse Education Today* **24** (8), 615–621.

Tadd, W., Clarke, A., Lloyd, L., *et al.* (2006) The value of nurses' codes: European nurses' views. *Nursing Ethics* **13** (4), 376–393.

Tschudin, V. (2006) 30th anniversary commentary on Esterhuizen P. (1996) Is the professional code still the cornerstone of clinical nursing practice? *Journal of Advanced Nursing* **53** (1), 113.

Wainwright, P. and Pattison, S. (2004) What can we expect of professional codes of conduct, practice and ethics? In *Values in Professional Practice*, Pattison, S. and Pill, R. (eds). Oxford: Radcliffe Medical Press, 109–122.

Watson, J. (1999) *Nursing: Human science and human care. A Theory of Nursing.* Boston: Jones and Bartlett.

Wilensky, H. L. (1964) *Industrial Society and Social Welfare: The impact of industrialisation on the supply of social welfare services in the United States.* New York: Russell Sage Foundation.

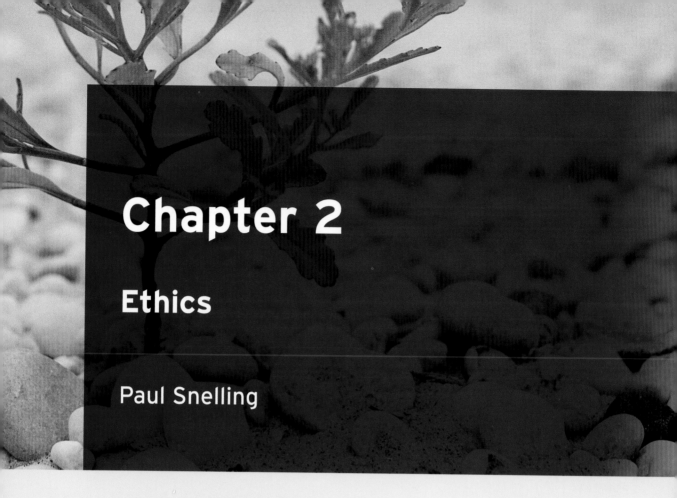

Chapter 2

Ethics

Paul Snelling

Learning outcomes

After reading and reflecting on this chapter, you should be able to:

- Explain the importance of ethics to nursing practice;
- Describe the four principles of bioethics and their application to individual cases;
- Outline critiques of the four principles approach;
- Identify the differences between justice and care orientations to ethics;
- Discuss the importance of both ethical analysis and caring disposition in ethical nursing practice.

Related NMC Standards of Proficiency for Pre-registration Nursing Education (NMC 2004a)

- Ensure the confidentiality and security of written and verbal information acquired in a professional capacity.

- Demonstrate knowledge of contemporary ethical issues and their impact on nursing and health care.

- Manage the complexities arising from ethical and legal dilemmas.

- Maintain, support and acknowledge the rights of individuals or groups in the health care setting.

- Act to ensure that the rights of individuals and groups are not compromised.

- Respect the values, customs and beliefs of individuals and groups.

- Provide care which demonstrates sensitivity to the diversity of patients and clients.

- Identify, collect and evaluate information to justify the effective utilisation of resources to achieve planned outcomes of nursing care.

- Information technology and management – interpret and utilise data and technology, taking account of legal, ethical and safety considerations, in the delivery and enhancement of care.

Introduction

Ethics is central to nursing practice, so much so that ethical and professional practice is one of the four domains of the standards of proficiency for pre-registration nursing. All of us have ideas and feelings about the rightness or wrongness of actions and use them in formulating and discussing our opinions, but ethical nursing practice requires more than unstructured feelings to guide right action. This chapter cannot hope to cover all of the ground of the ethical considerations that confront nurses in their everyday practice, but it is hoped that it will provide an introduction to the topic. Examples taken from current ethical problems and issues are used to illustrate more general points.

The chapter is divided into three parts.

Part 1 will outline the nature of ethics and the reasons why it is so important for nursing practice.

Part 2 will begin to explain ethics further. The four principles approach will be used to discuss some of the most important ethical issues in health care.

Part 3 will explore a number of critiques of the four principles, and alternative and opposing approaches of care ethics will be discussed.

Part 1: Outlining ethics

Case 2.1

Peter, a registered nurse, is working the night duty on a busy medical ward caring for, amongst others, Mr Smith, who was admitted with a chest infection. He is known to be a heavy drinker. During the night he becomes distressed and argumentative with staff who refuse to take him outside so that he can have a cigarette. Peter is reluctant to allow him to go outside unaccompanied because he needs oxygen to maintain his saturation levels. He has been prescribed a sedative by medical staff but he refuses to take it, saying that sedatives make him sleepy the next day. Peter knows that he hasn't taken the prescribed sedative before; it is a new drug known to have very few side effects. He frequently states that he is desperate to go to sleep, and Peter also knows that a good night's sleep will be beneficial for his recovery. As the night progresses he wakes other patients in the bay. He asks for a cup of tea and a colleague suggests that Peter add the liquid preparation of the prescribed sedative. It would solve the problem for Peter and be beneficial for Mr Smith as well as the other patients, some of whom are becoming upset that their needs aren't being met because the nurses are spending a lot of time with Mr Smith. Despite the obvious attractions, Peter hesitates. Is it the right thing to do?

The word ethics is derived from the Greek word *ethos*, meaning custom or convention, the same meaning as the Latin word *mores*, from which the terms moral and morality are derived (Thompson *et al.* 2000). Some texts, for example Thompson *et al.* (2000), attempt to differentiate between the terms ethics and morals. For them, morals refers to standards of behaviour, whilst ethics refers more specifically to the study of morals and morality. Others

(Johnstone 2005, Seedhouse 1998) claim that there is no significant difference in the words and use them interchangeably. There do seem to be conventions in common usage. We speak of 'nursing ethics' rather than 'nursing morals'. There is probably little to be gained from such detailed debates. In simple terms, **ethics**, in theory and practice, is concerned about what is good and right; how we ought to live our lives.

Ethics, in theory and practice, is concerned about what is good and right; how we ought to live our lives.

In a wide sense we can pick up a newspaper or magazine and see ethical elements in many stories, not just obvious ones involving war or crime. Is it right for banks to make huge profits? for schools to exclude unruly pupils? for footballers to be paid such vast sums? for parents to smack their children? or to lie to a friend in order to avoid an unpalatable truth? It has even been claimed that sitting in an armchair is a moral issue in the sense that you could be doing something more worthwhile, and choose not to (Seedhouse 1998).

There is more to professional ethics, especially in the health care professions, than following our common morality which might be relied upon in coffee shop or saloon bar discussions on these questions. There are a number of reasons for this, including:

- In professionally caring for our patients, we are *obliged* to act in certain ways which might be considered *optional* in other settings.
- Patients are generally vulnerable (Sellman 2005) and this has moral significance, for example in the potential for harm.
- Nurses and other health professionals are accountable for their actions, and this requires justified reasons other than 'gut feeling' or unjustified opinion.
- Because of the nature of their work, nurses are faced with many obviously moral problems, more so than would be expected in other walks of life.
- The complexity of problems commonly encountered, for example in developing technologies concerning assisted conception, requires ethical analysis in order to avoid inconsistency.

It is sometimes suggested that there is no right or wrong, and disagreement in moral matters seems justifiable in many cases. In a general sense, for example, there are valid reasons for arguing both in favour and against the legalisation of euthanasia, or the criminalisation of abortion. We cannot appeal to a single, provable (true) law of ethics to help us decide what our opinions should be or what we ought to do in the same way that we can appeal to scientifically verifiable fact (empirical knowledge), or the law (formal knowledge) (Allmark 2005). We *know* that giving a large dose of potassium chloride is likely to kill a person, and we also *know* that it is against the law to administer it with the intention of causing death. Still it does not follow from this that it is wrong for the drug to be administered. We might want to take the view, and many people do, that it is always wrong. Or we might take the view that *sometimes* it would be the right thing to do. These views on morality may in turn influence our views about the legality of the act, whether euthanasia should be legalised, or abortion criminalised. These are opinions, not matters of fact, but saying that opposing viewpoints can both be valid is not the same as saying that everything is right, that we can all do as we feel or think without any attempt at justification. This would lead to inconsistencies and result in patients and colleagues not knowing what they could expect of us or anyone else.

The Nursing and Midwifery Council (NMC) requires that nurses practise within an ethical and legal framework. We can point at the legal framework (see Chapter 3), and also to a professional framework set out in *The Code* (see Chapter 1). However, and despite the recent inclusion of the word 'ethics' in the title, *The Code* does not function as a recognised ethical framework. There is nothing – at least that we can point to as some sort of 'official' ethical framework – that tells nurses, in all cases, what they ought to do and why. There have been attempts to identify decision-making models (Greipp 1992, Seedhouse 1998), but these offer frameworks for analysis of an issue or problem, rather than a prescription for its resolution. Perhaps the most established framework is the four principles approach, and though this is not without its vociferous critics, it is useful in both analysing individual problems and identifying important ethical issues about which there is a deeper consensus. There is also evidence that students find decision-making frameworks helpful (Cameron *et al.* 2001).

Activities

All of the activities in this chapter should ideally be undertaken in small facilitated groups, rather than alone. This is because the nuances of ethical positions are best considered by debate. In this way your positions can be challenged and amended. Having weaknesses or contradictions in your position pointed out, and seeking these in a colleague's position can help to strengthen reasoning. However, caution is required. Often the most interesting and difficult debates concern areas, such as abortion, about which people may have strong feelings and/or personal experience. Rigorous debate needs to take account of these possibilities, and care is needed in expressing opinions.

Activity 2.1

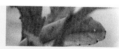

Discuss your initial feelings in groups. Should the medication be given concealed in Mr Smith's tea? What reasons can be given to support your conclusions?

Part 2: Explaining ethics

The four principles approach to ethics

The four principles approach to ethics, known more simply as 'principlism', was popularised by the publication, in 1978, of the book *Principles of Biomedical Ethics*, by two American authors, Tom Beauchamp and James Childress. The

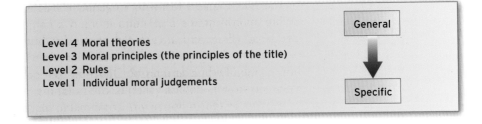

Figure 2.1 Four levels of ethics.

Source: Beauchamp and Childress (2008).

book is now in its sixth edition (2008), and remains highly influential. A more accessible book which retains the systematicity of the original and applies it to nursing practice was published by Steven Edwards in 1996 (Edwards 1996, 2006). The approach highlights four levels of ethics (Figure 2.1).

In a general sense, ethics is concerned with types of actions or situations. Is stealing wrong, and for what reasons? More specifically, the question is whether a certain individual action is right or wrong. Is it right for Mrs Jones to steal a loaf of bread at 5 p.m. in the afternoon in order to feed her hungry children? We might agree that generally speaking stealing is wrong, but that in this case it is acceptable. Perhaps the baker makes excessive profits, or the bread is about to be thrown away at the end of the day, or perhaps the children have not eaten all day. The point here is the relationship, if any, between the view that generally, stealing is wrong (a rule or principle) and the view that in this or that particular case it is acceptable. Morality is more than simply applying general rules to everyday situations. Black and white analyses are easy, but most of life occurs in shades of grey.

Level 1: individual moral judgements

We are often reminded of the moral nature of the situation that we find ourselves in when we understand it in terms of a dilemma. This means that we are unsure about what we should *do* in a particular situation. Two forms of moral dilemma can be identified (Beauchamp and Childress 2001):

1. Where there are good reasons for thinking that an act is both morally right and morally wrong, but where the evidence is inconclusive. The example of a woman grappling with a decision on whether or not to have an abortion is offered as an example of this. It need not be a difficult decision for everybody, however. Many would be quite clear about the resolution of this particular dilemma for themselves and some would seek to impose their opinion on everyone else.
2. Where somebody thinks that two things are morally required but they are mutually exclusive. For example, suppose you have promised to accompany a sick friend to an appointment. You are driving to the hospital, when you come upon an accident. You think that you ought both to keep your promise to your friend and offer assistance to the accident victim. You cannot do both, and your dilemma is which obligation to break. It need not be a difficult dilemma; it would depend on the circumstances.

Case 2.1 (continued)

The case study might be considered a dilemma because the nurse is thinking about *doing* something. Peter is apparently undecided. There are many options open to him, but the one we are discussing is whether or not he should give the prescribed medication covertly. The case study seems to fall within the first category of moral dilemma. Peter feels that there are moral reasons for both giving and not giving the medication. To help him untangle these reasons, and decide between them, Peter refers the dilemma to higher levels.

Level 2: rules

Beauchamp and Childress (2001) 'operate a loose distinction between rules and principles. Both are general norms which guide action' (p. 13). Rules are more specific. Beauchamp and Childress offer the following:

- *Veracity*. This rule requires truth in relationships with patients (Collis 2006, Tuckett 2004).
- *Privacy*. Respecting privacy involves a number of issues concerned with protecting an individual's freedom from interference. These include informational privacy (restricting information), physical privacy (focusing on personal space), decisional privacy (concerning personal choices), and relational privacy (concerning family and other relationships). A nurse who intrudes unnecessarily on a family attempting to come to terms with bad news would breach the rule of privacy.
- *Confidentiality*. There is some overlap between the rules of privacy and confidentiality; keeping a confidence is part of respecting privacy. Breaking a confidence occurs when information is disclosed to a third party. This rule is part of many professional codes – priests must not disclose confessional secrets, and some journalists have gone to prison protecting the identity of their sources. In nursing, keeping confidences is very important in the nurse–patient relationship. The obligation is not absolute, but should only be contemplated in exceptional circumstances (confidentiality is discussed more fully in Chapter 3).
- *Fidelity*. This rule is concerned with the requirement to act in good faith, keeping promises and maintaining relationships (Beauchamp and Childress 2008).

These are prima facie (at first sight) rules, meaning that they are not meant to be followed slavishly. They should inform rather than direct action and can be overruled but only with justification. Nor is the list exhaustive; many further prima facie rules can be contained within them, for example a rule that nurses should not steal from patients is contained within the rule of fidelity. However, the rules cover the wide ground of nurse patient relationships, and a fuller list of derivative rules would be of little value.

Case 2.1 (continued)

Applying these rules to the case study at the beginning of the chapter, we can see that giving the sedative covertly probably breaches the rules of veracity and privacy, but some would claim that this is justified. Applying the rules in this way doesn't seem to help much in this particular dilemma – if it can be resolved by simply invoking a prima facie rule, it cannot have been much of a dilemma.

In order to throw more light on the dilemma and the reasons we might advance for deciding either to give or not give the medication in this way, the dilemma can be analysed with reference to the four principles from which the rules are derived. The principles are:

- Respect for autonomy
- Nonmaleficence
- Beneficence
- Justice.

Level 3: principles

Respect for autonomy.

The principle is that, generally, autonomy should be respected, but there are many problems with this. Autonomy is a complex concept and there is evidence that the term is used in different ways by individual nurses (Aveyard 2000). The word *autonomy* derives from the Greek words for *autos* (self) and *nomos* (rule, governance or law). First understood as the right of a community to self-government, modern accounts see it as relating to personal independence in some way. There are many definitions and nuances in the literature, but simply, **autonomy** is the ability to be able to make decisions for oneself, and respecting autonomy requires that we accept and where possible facilitate the choices of others.

Within the many definitions and accounts of autonomy, two features are common: liberty and agency (Beauchamp and Childress 2008). Liberty means freedom from controlling influences. An extreme example would be a confession extracted under torture, but more subtle controlling influences, based in part on power imbalance in nurse–patient relationships, are possible (Henderson 2003). A decision made by a patient under pressure, either from a nurse or doctor or by an overbearing relative, is not autonomously made. Liberty is part of autonomy but not all of it. Animals can be thought of as free but not as autonomous (Gillon 1985). Nurses should be aware of the potential for influences and take action to minimise them, for example, by enabling discussion of treatment options to take place away from relatives.

Agency means having the capacity to decide. Capacity is reduced in many ways; by illness, learning disability and in childhood. Autonomy is relational in the sense that a capacity to make decisions depends on the nature of the decision being made. For example, a person with a learning disability or a child may lack the capacity to decide whether to undertake chemotherapy, but be perfectly able to decide on meal choices (Taylor 1999). An individual's capacity to decide can also vary in time; a patient who is mildly confused because of infection, or postoperative hypoxia, may not be able to decide whether or not to take medication one day, but be perfectly capable the next.

Respecting autonomy cannot simply be reduced to agreeing with and implementing patients' choices. Respecting autonomy can be analysed in terms of **rights**, which are defined as 'justified claims' (Beauchamp and Childress 2001 p. 357) made upon others and on society. A right to autonomy, like other rights, can be either a **liberty right** or a **claim right**. Liberty, mentioned above

Autonomy is the ability to be able to make decisions for oneself, and respecting autonomy requires that we accept and, where possible, facilitate the choices of others.

A **right** is a justified claim. A **liberty right** requires that the right holder simply be left alone, not interfered with. A **claim right** requires someone to do something for the right holder.

as an almost universally agreed component of autonomy, is associated with negative or passive rights – that is the right not to be prevented from doing something. By contrast, a claim right requires someone else to do something, imposing a duty upon another person – it is a positive, active right.

The distinction can be illustrated by discussing Do Not Attempt Resuscitation (DNAR) orders. Assuming capacity, any patient can refuse treatment, and this includes resuscitation, despite medical nursing or family opinion that resuscitation would be of benefit, and therefore ought to be undertaken. In refusing treatment the patient is claiming a negative right – the right to be left alone. This is a strong claim, and according to the principle of respect for autonomy should be honoured. A different scenario is of a terminally ill patient who asks to be resuscitated despite medical and nursing opinion that invasive and intrusive procedures would not succeed or not be beneficial. In this case, the patient is claiming a positive right, and if accepted, this puts an obligation on someone else to do something, that is it obliges a nurse to initiate resuscitation. This is a weaker claim; health care professionals cannot be required to undertake a procedure which they believe not to be in the patient's interests. In some sensitive areas like DNAR orders it may be justified to accede to the patient's wishes, but this cannot be an obligation (Resuscitation Council 2007).

Some people are obviously unable to make a decision, for example if they are semi-conscious, and health care professionals should not follow wishes expressed whilst in this state. It is not an autonomous decision. A 3-year-old child cannot be expected to make a decision concerning radiation therapy; any more than a severely hypoxic and confused patient can properly decline oxygen therapy. If the patient has sufficient capacity to make a decision, it must be respected. If the patient is not able to make the decision, someone must make it for them. Clearly this is difficult where there is some doubt as to whether the patient is able or not able to make the decision. This judgement is significant because different actions (or inactions) follow directly from it. There must be a robust method of assessing the ability of the patient to make the decision.

This crucial question forms part of the Mental Capacity Act, which is discussed in detail in Chapter 3. It should be noted that the test is not a measure of capacity in itself, but rather a judgement, however crude, of a patient's ability to make a particular decision at a particular time. Following the principle of respecting autonomy, as well as the law, the presumption is in favour of capacity. The legal case which informed the legal test involved a client within a secure hospital diagnosed with paranoid schizophrenia, who was nevertheless assessed by a judge as being capable to decide whether or not his leg should be amputated, illustrating the point that patients who are not fully rational can remain capable of making a major life or death decision. Breeze (1998) suggests that, in relation to mental health patients, autonomy is more likely to be respected when the deciding criterion is capacity rather than rationality.

If the patient has been assessed as not being competent, someone else must make decisions for him. It is sometimes assumed in practice that this duty falls to the next of kin, a position reinforced in the past by the practice of asking next of kin to sign consent forms. Legally, the duty of deciding in the patient's best interests falls to the medical team, led by the consultant (Cornock 2002), though it is becoming more recognised that the senior clinician in certain circumstances may be a suitably qualified nurse (Resuscitation Council 2007). This is not to suggest that relatives should not be consulted or their views dismissed. However, respecting autonomy requires that the *patient's* wishes are considered, and it is not always the case that the patient's wishes are the same as the next of kin's. When discussing decisions with patients' families, as well as being mindful of confidentiality, it should be remembered that asking what the patient would want is not the same question as asking what the relative wants for the patient. There may be tensions. In some cases patients have left detailed instructions about treatment options in certain eventualities – these are known as advance decisions. There are also now legal arrangements for patients to nominate another individual to make decisions on their behalf when incapacitated (see Chapter 3), known as lasting power of attorney (LPA). Both of these new arrangements are justified by the important moral duty to respect autonomy.

Paternalism might be considered as the opposite of respecting autonomy. A nurse acts paternalistically if she does not respect a patient's autonomous decision because she believes it to be against his interests. The word 'paternalism' is based on the concept of 'fatherhood', choosing for one's children in their interest. A distinction has been drawn between weak and strong paternalism (Ikonomidis and Singer 1999). Weak paternalism occurs when an agent (or the state) intervenes on the grounds of beneficence or nonmaleficence on behalf of a person without capacity, even if they are able to express a preference. Strong paternalism occurs where an intervention overrides or disregards the wishes of a person with capacity. Strong paternalism in policy terms has been justified. Certain choices are not available to citizens. Declining to wear a seatbelt is punished by the retrospective levying of fines, and the State acts positively to prevent citizens from using heroin, even when the decision is autonomously made. The justification (Glover 1977) is:

1. That the suffering is very great.
2. That there is very little uncertainty that suffering will occur.
3. That the process of heroin addiction after initial use is not readily reversible, and restricts future freedom of choice.

The most obvious practical manifestation of the principle of respecting autonomy is in requirement for informed consent. This is covered in more detail in Chapter 3.

> **Paternalism** can be considered as the opposite of respecting autonomy. A nurse acts paternalistically if they do not respect a patient's autonomous decision because they believe it to be against the patient's interests.

Case 2.1 (continued)

Mr Smith declined to take the offered sedation. His decision might have been taken on the basis of incomplete information; a major reason for his declining the medication seems to be that sedatives he has taken in the past have made him sleepy, and Peter suspects that the newer ones prescribed will not have this effect. This means that in order to reassess his decision, Mr Smith simply needs more information, it does not affect his capacity to make the decision. Depending on the cause and nature of his agitation, and remembering that the starting presumption is that people are capable of making decisions unless deemed otherwise, Peter assumes that he does have capacity. Respecting his autonomy requires that Mr Smith's refusal to take the sedation be respected.

It might be considered that Mr Smith is being unwise, but to overrule him and give him the medication would be a case of strong paternalism. It might be considered that if he is capable of making the decision, then he is also capable of understanding the consequences of it, not only for himself, but also for the other patients in the ward. Giving the sedation covertly might be justified not in his interests, but in every one else's. In this case it would not be considered paternalistic; perhaps authoritarian would be a more accurate description. Following the principle of respecting autonomy requires you not to give the medication.

Nonmaleficence

The principle of **nonmaleficence** requires that health care professionals should not harm patients.

The principle of **nonmaleficence** requires that health care professionals should not harm patients. On the face of it, this seems straightforward, associated with the maxim (often mistakenly attributed to the Hippocratic Oath): Primum non nocere (first, do no harm). Nurses and others do not require this principle to tell them that they should not punch a patient or steal from them, but the concept of harm is more complex than this, and there are some problems associated with this principle. First is the problem that many health care interventions have harmful as well as beneficial effects. Drugs have side effects; operations require painful incisions. These harms are justified in the pursuit of the overall good, and the need to balance good with harm in this way has led some to argue that the principles of nonmaleficence (avoiding harm) and beneficence (doing good) should be regarded together as a single principle (Beauchamp and Childress 2001).

Second is the problem of defining harm, and the most striking examples of this problem occur at the end of life. Normally, killing would be seen as the most grievous harm that can be visited on a person, resulting in murder being regarded as the most serious of crimes. Yet there have been a number of cases where 'mercy killing' has been treated leniently by the courts.

A powerful argument against euthanasia is that killing a person, even at their express wish, causes them harm. However, for some people near the end of life, the harm, *from their point of view*, lies not in being killed but by remaining alive because their suffering is so great as to be considered, by them, as worse than being dead. Whether or not the idea of death being better than life is accepted, there remains the problem of who decides whether harm has or will be done. Part of the power of the argument in favour of euthanasia derives from the claim that it is for the patient to decide whether harm has occurred; against the principle of respect for autonomy as well as illustrating that the notion of harm is subjective rather than objective.

When the end of life approaches, the focus of health intervention shifts from cure to care. It is recognised that treatments that would be considered beneficial for some patients, such as resuscitation or invasive surgery, would be regarded as harmful for others because of the lack of benefit provided. In addition, dosages of drugs that would normally be considered harmful are routinely given to persons as they approach the end of life, in the knowledge that death may be hastened as a result. This is common practice, considered permissible under the doctrine of double effect.

The doctrine of double effect (DDE) was originally formulated in the Middle Ages by Catholic theologians to describe the circumstances in which evil is permitted in the overall pursuit of good. It allows an 'evil' to occur so long as it is not intended, even though it may be foreseen. The DDE is used to justify the use of very large dosages of opiate analgesia (Kendall 2000) and other drugs (Perkin and Resnik 2002) in terminally ill persons, even though it is known that the side effects of the drugs may shorten life.

Much of the defence for the DDE is based on religious morality, mainly Catholic but also supported by other denominations and religions (Keown and Keown 1995, and see, for example, the joint submission from the Church of England House of Bishops and the Catholic Bishops Conference of England and Wales to the House of Lords Select Committee on Medical Ethics – Appendix 2, Church House Publishing 2000). The DDE has been criticised for its religious roots by Quill *et al.* (1997), who question whether it is right for this tradition to be reflected in the law of multicultural society, in their case, the United States of America. The formulation of the DDE is often merely stated rather than argued. Generally, there are four conditions for an act to be justified using the DDE (Schwarz 2004), and details of how the parts of the doctrine are applied to the case of the administration of large doses of opiate drugs near the end of life are added in italics.

- The act considered separately from its consequences must not be intrinsically wrong. *Giving analgesia near the end of life would be considered morally acceptable, even obligatory.*
- With both a good and a bad effect of a single act, the bad effect must not be intended but simply permitted, even where it is foreseen. *Here the 'bad' effect of the act is the shortening of life. For the DDE to be correctly applied, this must not be an intention. It's an important distinction which separates the use of opiates from (for example) potassium chloride. It would be difficult to argue that there is no intention to end life by giving this drug as it has no analgesic properties.*
- The good effect must be sufficiently desirable to offset permitting the bad effect. *Here the bad of shortening life must be compared with the good of analgesia. In end of life decisions the good of relief from severe pain outweighs the shortening by hours or days of a life of poor quality. It would not outweigh relief from mild pain where life of a reasonable quality was shortened by a longer period.*
- The good effect must not be brought about by the bad effect. *This means for our case that the good effect of painlessness must not be brought about only by the bad effect of shortening life.*

Some formulations of the DDE (for example, Perkin and Resnik 2002) add a fifth criterion, that there should be no other way of producing the intended effect.

Problems with the DDE include difficulties with intention. There is evidence to show that intention is not always as stated (Quill *et al.* 1997). A further difficulty is the notion that we are somehow not responsible for consequences of our actions which are foreseen but can be claimed to be unintentional. It has been described as a 'very dubious and shifty' argument (Warnock 1998 p. 41) and its survival is perhaps a result of its pragmatism rather than its morality (Shaw 2002). Practitioners appear more ready to accept it than philosophers (see Research focus 2.1). UK law enshrines the DDE even if it does not actually state it. It has been described by judges on a number of occasions, notably in the case of R vs Adams, where Dr Adams was acquitted of murdering his patients by giving them increasingly large dosages of opiates. The patients were incurably but not terminally ill. In his summing up the trial judge said that 'the doctor is entitled to relieve pain and suffering even if the measures he takes may incidentally shorten life' (Dimond 2001).

Case 2.1 (continued)

The good effect of giving the sedation could be that he goes to sleep and the bad that his autonomy has been overruled. The bad effect is intended, and it causes the good effect, so the doctrine of double effect could not be applied. Would Mr Smith be harmed by being given a sedative against his wishes? Certainly physical harm would be unlikely. Overriding his wishes might be considered harmful, especially by him, and giving the medication in this way will also probably harm the trust relationship between Mr Smith and the nurses caring for him.

Research focus 2.1

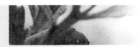

In the study of ethics, definitions of research are not easy (see Chapter 6). Research, including that undertaken in the health environment, is often thought of in terms of the collection of information or data. In universities, there is a wider understanding, with research (perhaps scholarship is a better word) into ethics being concerned with analysis as well as the creation of new data. In a paper published in a nursing journal, Snelling (2004) analyses the current prohibition of euthanasia. It is argued that this position is founded on a duty-based absolutism that allows no consideration of the consequences of an act. Using real and hypothetical cases it is argued that in practice distinctions between ordinary and extraordinary means, acts and omissions, and the doctrine of double effect use considerations of consequences, undermining the consistency of absolute prohibition. The paper is generally sympathetic to euthanasia in certain conditions. Under some definitions of research, this paper cannot be considered as research.

However, data collection in these areas is possible. *Empirical ethics* includes the study of what people think – the word empirical means something that can be measured or seen, and this includes opinions and attitudes. There is surprisingly little research into UK nurses' views on euthanasia. A recent literature review (Berghs *et al.* 2005) included eight studies from the USA, seven from Australia, two each from Japan, Finland, The Netherlands, Canada and Belgium, and one each from Switzerland, Israel and Hungary. No UK studies could be identified for inclusion in the review.

Research by Dickenson (2000) looked at what practising nurses think about the distinctions that Snelling (2004) discussed. A total of 469 UK and hospital and hospice nurses who were students on an Open University course on death and dying completed a questionnaire. Dickenson noted that consequentialist approaches to death and dying have tended to dominate bioethicists' critical analyses, and that a number of distinctions, including the doctrine of double effect had come in for 'demolition'. However, 94 per cent of the nurses in the UK arm of the study agreed or strongly agreed with the statement that 'sometimes it is appropriate to give pain medication to relieve suffering, even if it may hasten a patient's death: 3 per cent of nurses disagreed or strongly disagreed with this statement. Dickenson infers from these figures that the great majority of nurses 'reject the argument (made by the voluntary euthanasia society in the 1994 hearings before the House of Lords Select Committee on Euthanasia) that it is hypocritical to give analgesics in the knowledge that patient's death may result, while claiming only to be concerned with pain'. The study makes no firm conclusions about the numbers of bioethicists' views on the statements provided. Instead it merely states that an overwhelming proportion of practicing nurses find significance in distinctions 'widely disparaged by bioethicists'. It concludes with a reminder of what is known as the naturalistic fallacy – the confusion of *ought* with *is*. This means that it doesn't follow from an observation that a large proportion of nurses *do think* something that they *ought to think* it. Studies in empirical ethics (Dickenson 2000) tell us what nurses do think; analytical (Snelling 2004) or normative ethics tell nurses what they ought to think.

Beneficence

The principle of **beneficence** requires health care professionals to act to promote the general well-being of others. Beauchamp and Childress (2008) discuss two forms of the principle.

First, positive beneficence requires that nurses provide benefits to their patients. Without making claims about the character and motivation of nurses, it is safe to assume that a desire to help people is part of the continuing appeal of nursing and other health care professions, but it is less clear what the nurse is obliged to do for patients, and what they might justifiably do. For example, consider if you were rostered for an early shift, and a number of your colleagues reported sick for the late shift. You might consider that you ought to stay and do a double shift, even if you had tickets to the theatre. If you followed this course of action, you might be considered to have done a good thing, but can you be criticised if you fail to do the double shift? Acting 'above and beyond' the call of duty might be a common occurrence in nursing and other health care provisions, but it cannot be an obligation (Edwards 1996). There are also problems here in balancing the amount of good that you are able to do for one patient when compared with the competing needs of others. This is discussed in the section on justice.

Second, utility requires that nurses balance the good and bad effects of their actions, as discussed in the section on nonmaleficence. Just as harm is difficult to define, so is well-being, and deciding where a person's best interests lie. Even where a nurse overrides the wishes of a patient and coerces treatment, for example in giving a Jehovah's Witness a blood transfusion against their autonomously stated wishes, this is not done out of spite or malice, but in the belief that acting in this way is beneficial. Many of the conflicts between principles occur between beneficence and respect for autonomy, and key to resolving these is understanding that a seemingly obvious and objective benefit, like a life-saving blood transfusion, may not be viewed as such by everyone.

Case 2.1 (continued)

Giving Mr Smith a sedative disguised in tea might be considered a beneficent act, because the resulting rest will be good for him. Perhaps this justification is more attractive to Peter trying to justify giving it this way than to Mr Smith who doesn't want it.

Justice

Justice is a complex concept, but at a simple level, it can be regarded as treating people fairly. This is seen in matters of distribution (distributive justice) and punishment (retributive justice). Justice in health care is largely concerned with the distribution of resources. Newsworthy debates about resource allocation commonly concern the availability or otherwise of drug treatments such as Herceptin for breast cancer, but the same analysis applies to more everyday matters such as a nurse allocating their time. Common to all theories of justice is a minimum formal requirement traditionally attributed to Aristotle: 'Equals must be treated equally, and unequals must be treated unequally'.

It might be suggested that none of us are exactly the same. I have an identical twin brother, and though our genetic material is identical, even we are not *exactly* the same. He is slightly taller and heavier, and wears his hair a little longer. We can point to differences between all of us, men and women, black and white, heterosexual and homosexual, but applying Aristotle's requirement doesn't mean that we should all be treated differently. Justifying treating people differently requires a *morally relevant* difference. Difficulty arises in discussing and deciding what constitutes a morally relevant difference. At this time, almost all would agree that gender, skin colour and sexual orientation are not relevant, though all would have been considered relevant in the not too distant past, and there remains a minority who continue to see the distinction as relevant. There is more debate about whether age is relevant (Shaw 1994), with even a significant minority of older people agreeing that it is right that older people give way to younger people on a heart surgery waiting list (Bowling *et al.* 2002).

There are many ways of attempting fairness in the distributions of health care (Beauchamp and Childress 2008, Cookson and Dolan 2000) including:

- To each person an equal share.
- To each person according to need.
- To each person according to effort.
- To each person according to contribution.
- To each person according to merit.
- To each person according to free market exchanges.

All of these can be challenged, but it is distribution according to need which is nearest to nursing's values and the core principles of the NHS which are summed up in the NHS official website as being 'the provision of quality care that:

- Meets the needs of everyone
- Is free at the point of need
- And is based on a patient's clinical need not their ability to pay.'

(NHS in England 2007)

A challenge to the intuitively attractive requirement that resources should be directed at those who need them is that often those who need treatment most will not benefit from it (Busfield 2000). An alternative understanding of need that addresses this point is need as capacity to benefit. One way in which the needs of different groups and individuals can be compared is by using the quality-adjusted life year (QALY). This is a system whereby quality of life is assessed on a scale from 0 (death) to 1 (normal health). Improvement in health status following treatment can be assessed on the same scale, and the gain in health, multiplied by the length of time for which the improvement remains, gives a QALY score for a particular treatment for a particular condition. This score can then be divided by the cost to give a 'cost per QALY' with the implication that the treatments with the lowest cost per QALY are most cost-effective and therefore prioritised (see Box 2.1).

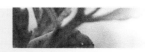

Box 2.1   Quality-adjusted life years

The National Institute for Health and Clinical Excellence (2007) gives the following explanation of how to calcualte QALYs.

Patient × has a serious, life-threatening condition.

If he continues receiving standard treatment he will live for 1 year and his quality of life will be 0.4.

If he receives a new drug he will live for 1 year 3 months (1.25 years), with a quality of life of 0.6.

A new treatment is compared with standard care in terms of the QALYs gained:

Standard treatment: 1 (year's extra life) × 0.4 = 0.4 QALY

New treatment: 1.25 (1 year, 3 months extra life) × 0.6 = 0.75 QALY

Therefore, the new treatment leads to 0.35 additional QALYs (that is: 0.75 − 0.4 QALY = 0.35 QALYs).

The cost of the new drug is assumed to be £10,000, standard treatment costs £3000.

The difference in treatment costs (£7000) is divided by the QALYs gained (0.35) to calculate the cost per QALY. So the new treatment would cost £20,000 per QALY.

A cost of £20,000 per QALY would not generally be considered cost-effective.

National Institute of Health and Clinical Excellence (2007)

There are a number of problems associated with QALYs, not least difficulties in calculating the scores. If the public is involved in setting the scores, the perceived democratising benefit of making resource allocation more visible is offset by the fact that healthy members of the public do not have experience of being ill, and find it difficult to put a value on quality of life for certain conditions, which must be subjective. QALYs seem a rather detached way of assessing priorities, threatening a more caring approach valued by nurses (Hirskyj 2007), and QALYs inevitably disadvantage the old and the chronically sick (Busfield 2000).

A further problem for using need as a criterion for distribution is the difference between needs and wants. For example, when the drug Viagra was introduced offering a treatment for erectile dysfunction, the Government gave guidance about which conditions it could be prescribed for, and also for the number of pills which should be prescribed per week (NHSE 1999). Whether enabling a weekly sex act counts as a need or a want is open for discussion, as are other treatments, for example cosmetic plastic surgery. Does the desire for bigger breasts constitute a shallow capitulation to societal expectations obsessed with appearance, or a treatment to cure pathological insecurity profoundly affecting quality of life? The distinction between needs and wants is of interest both between and within treatments.

There is some appetite amongst the general population for penalising those who are in some way responsible for their health needs (Dolan and Shaw 2003), and so the idea of distribution according to merit requires consideration. In one study 42 per cent of respondents among the general public agreed with the statement that 'People who contribute to their own illness – for example through smoking, obesity or excessive drinking – should have a lower priority for their health care than others' (Bowling 1996). Some have advocated denying smokers treatment for diseases caused by smoking (see Persaud 1995, and Allmark 1995a for fuller discussion on this point). If these attitudes appear to pander to public discrimination, there is also some evidence to show that the public is able to make flexible and thoughtful judgements about these complex issues (Wilmot and Ratcliffe 2002). The NMC code is clear that 'you must not discriminate in any way against those in your care' (NMC 2008).

Case 2.1 (continued)

Some of the other patients in the ward might not regard it as fair that their sleep is being disturbed by Mr Smith, and that their needs are not being attended to as quickly as they would like. It might be considered that he does not need so much care, but that he is choosing to monopolise it by being argumentative. He wants a cigarette, he does not need one. The other patients may feel that it is unjust that Mr Smith is receiving more of a resource (the nurse's time) than he is justly entitled to. It might be considered that in order to redress this unfair distribution, the principle of justice justifies giving the sedative covertly.

Level 4: moral theories

The highest level in the classification is moral theories. Theories provide general methods for resolving problems, and guides for right action (Upton 2003). Beauchamp and Childress (2001) claim that the moral principles they propose are included in most classical theories, and 'the rules and principles shared by various theories seem to serve practical judgement more adequately, at least as starting points, than the theories themselves' (p. 387). If theories agree that their main features are encapsulated within the principles, it might be suggested that there is little point in studying them; much less attempting to apply them to practice-based moral problems. Respecting autonomy is important to two of the most important moral theories, but for different reasons. Why then study moral theory at all?

One answer to this question is that studying moral theories illuminates our reasons for thinking the way we do, and helps us to be clear about the sorts of things which are most important to us. Two important approaches assessing the morality of an act are duty-based and consequence-based moral theories.

Activity 2.2

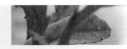

Consider the following scenario.

A passenger plane with 200 passengers on board taking off from Heathrow airport has been hijacked, and it is now flying up the Thames towards Canary Wharf, where 5000 people are working. You have every reason to believe that the hijackers intend to emulate the attacks on the World Trade Center in New York (the 9/11 attacks) by crashing the aeroplane into the building. A fully armed fighter jet is on patrol and can get to the area in time to shoot the airliner down.

It is your decision whether to shoot the airliner down. First, write down your initial reaction. Should you shoot it down? Then take 10 minutes, alone or preferably in small groups, to write down the arguments both for and against shooting the airliner down. Some suggestions are given below.

Duty-based moral theory (deontology)

Deontology is based on the philosophy of Immanuel Kant (1724–1804). Kant argued that intention was all important, and that the good action was the one that followed our duty. In order to determine what our duty is, we should apply the categorical imperative 'I ought never to act except in such a way that I can also will that my maxim become a universal law.'

This means that in the same circumstances, everyone should act in the same way, universally and impartially. This is reformulated as 'One must act to treat every person as an end and never a means only.'

Under this formulation, every person is to be respected and treated with dignity. The details are complex, but amongst the important features of deontology are that it provides absolute rules, and that appeals to the bad consequences of applying the rules simply are not permitted.

Consequence-based moral theory (consequentialism)

The most important figure for consequentialism is John Stuart Mill (1808–1873). There are a number of different versions, of which his Utilitarianism is the most recognised. In consequentialism, it is the consequences of an act which are important. The best thing to do is the thing that gives the best outcomes. This means calculating the probable outcomes for all the different options in any given scenario, and choosing the one that gives the best (or least bad) outcome. There are different versions about the sorts of things that can be included in the calculations, and how the calculations can be made. The important contrasting difference between consequentialism and deontology (sometimes referred to as non-consequentialism) is the consideration of consequences. This can mean that the same act can be allowed or not allowed in different circumstances, depending on the calculations. In the end of life decision discussed earlier, consequentialism sees no difference between giving potassium chloride or giving an opiate at the end of life. The distinction of intention, vital for application of the DDE, is less important for consequentialists. For them the outcomes of giving the two drugs are the same, and so the morality is the same. If it is acceptable to give the opiate, it is also acceptable to give the potassium.

Case 2.1 (continued)

There are so many complications and nuances in the abstract moral theories that simply applying them to complex real-life situations is probably unhelpful for Peter. However, thinking about whether and to what extent we are using consequentialist or non-consequentialist thinking can help in clarifying issues. A deontologist would not give the concealed medication to Mr Smith because it would involve deceit. A consequentialist might give the medication, depending on the details of the case, and the type of consequentialism, but if many other patients were being disturbed, and there was very little risk to Mr Smith, giving the medication concealed in tea could probably be defended on consequentialist grounds.

Returning to Activity 2.2.

Reasons for shooting the airliner down include:

1. Fewer people would be killed – 200 on the airliner against 5000 in the building (c).

2. It would minimise the sense of victory for hijackers, demonstrating the resolve of government (c).

Reasons against shooting the airliner down include:

3. It is wrong to kill innocent passengers (d).
4. It might crash onto another building killing more people (c*).
5. It might not be hijacked at all – it might be a mistake (c*).
6. The passengers might overpower the hijackers (c*).

The obvious consequentialist position is given in point 1, and the deontological position is given as point 3. No amount of arguing for these positions will satisfy the other – the deontologist's position holds even if a million people were in the building, and an appeal to the fact that the passengers would die anyway is met with the response that it is the hijackers that would be killing them, not the fighter pilot. It is not so simple to say that consequentialists would shoot down the plane, and deontologists would not – the reasons marked (c*) are appeals for more information. If there was a good chance that there were only 300 in the building, but that the only place to shoot down the aeroplane would result in 1000 deaths, the consequentialist would not shoot. In classroom discussion of this problem, shooting the airliner down is by far the most popular action, and yet this is an intuitively difficult position. Appeals for more information seem to stem from reluctance to fire on the airliner, but the appeals remain consequentialist in nature; people are attempting to make the calculation more accurate. If opposition to firing on the airliner was the result of a deontological view that it is wrong, appeals to likely consequences are simply not relevant. Apart from valuable dissection and discussion of a pressing moral problem, the value of the exercise lies in identifying the different approaches, helping us to understand why we think in the way that we do.

Applying the principles to the case study

Not all of the principles have equal prominence when applied to individual scenarios. However, applying the principles in Mr Smith's case gives the following reasons for giving or not giving the sedative (Figure 2.2).

In real-life scenarios similar to this, there may be other factors to consider. For example, Mr Smith may tell you that if you do not accompany him for a cigarette he will have one by the bedside, and you may feel that this constitutes a fire hazard because of his use of oxygen. There may also be other options outside the 'give or do not give' dilemma. You may feel that the best thing all round for Mr Smith (and the other patients) might be to take him for a cigarette after all; it would depend on the level of his agitation and his need for oxygen, and in taking him you might also want to consider some other issues such as a nurse facilitating a habit known to be harmful to health. The application of the principles can be amended according to the changed circumstances; the devil is always in the detail. Applying the principles of respect for autonomy and nonmaleficence to a decision about taking a patient with respiratory impairment for a cigarette could provide some interesting and contrasting views.

Applying the four principles has given some insight into the sorts of things that are seen as valuable, and also helped deconstruct the dilemma presented so that it is easier to see which elements are important. What it does not do is tell you what you should do, and this lack of action guidance is one of the critiques of the approach, which will be considered in Part 3.

	Give the sedative	Do not give the sedative
Respect autonomy		Respect for autonomy requires that Mr Smith is not given the sedative covertly because it overrides his autonomous choice not to take it.
Nonmaleficence		Harm to the professional relationship might follow if the sedative is given covertly.
Beneficence	A good night's sleep will benefit Mr Smith. He will feel much better for having the sleep rather than being agitated all night.	
Justice	Justice is served because all of the other patients will get a better night's sleep if Mr Smith is sedated. It is unfair for them to be kept awake when he could be asleep.	

Figure 2.2 Applying the four principles to Mr Smith.

Professional issues

It was noted in Chapter 1 that there is considerable overlap between ethical and professional considerations of practice issues. Peter may have his views about whether giving the medication disguised in the tea is right or wrong, but he should also consider the professional implications. There is an advice sheet available concerning covert administration of medicines from the NMC (2007), and this gives a detailed analysis of the ethical and legal implications.

Activity 2.3

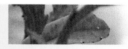

Download the advice sheet on covert administration of medicines from the NMC website, and discuss in groups whether the advice contained in the sheet applies to Mr Smith's case. How does the ethical consideration of this case compare with the professional advice?

Part 3: Exploring ethics

Critiques of principlism

There are a number of critiques of principlism. These can broadly be categorised in three headings:

1. The insufficient philosophy critique.
2. Procedural critiques.
3. The critique from agent-centred ethics.

The insufficient philosophy critique

This critique highlights the fundamental differences in approach that will be discussed shortly. In a famous paper from the *Journal of Medicine and Philosophy* it is argued that the principles do not constitute a coherent moral theory, but rather are 'tantamount to using two three or four conflicting moral theories to decide a case' (Clouser and Gert 1990 p. 221). In applying the principles, 'the agent is unwittingly using several diverse and conflicting accounts rather than simply applying a well developed unified theory (1990 p. 223)'. One problem here is that moral theories tend to be regarded as a 'historical relic' (1990 p. 233), rather than an 'ongoing attempt to explain and justify our common moral intuitions' (1990 p. 233).

The rigid application of Kant and Mill to modern health care problems both lead to some implausible positions, but it doesn't follow from this that moral theory in itself, or the attempt to formulate one, is unhelpful. A problem with the absence of an underlying theory is that a moral agent does not know why he is doing the things that the principles tell him he should do. We might agree that respecting and promoting autonomy is important, even that it is the most important principle, but simply following the principle does not tell us *why* it is important. A similar critique could be levelled at other principle or rules-based systems, even *The Code*. Principlism operates at the level of a useful checklist, a function about which most of its critics seem to agree upon (for example, Harris 2003). Beauchamp and Childress (2008) acknowledge and discuss these critiques in later editions for their work, and a comprehensive overview of the debate is provided by Davis (1995).

Procedural critiques

A number of 'procedural' critiques have been grouped into this section, and there is some overlap between them:

- Principlism does not tell you what to do. Beauchamp and Childress (2001) do not give any indication about which principle should have precedence where there is a conflict, though other supporters of principlism are more specific, holding that respect for autonomy is the most important (Gillon 2003), and that therefore it trumps the rest. The autonomy-weighted version has been referred to as an immodest version, with Beauchamp and Childress's (2008) version being described as modest because it doesn't weight the principles (Edwards 2006). The former version has more action guiding properties, but as we have seen, autonomy can be a difficult concept and the requirement to respect it is clearest where a capable person refuses treatment.
- Following on from this, it is suggested that autonomy is overvalued, representing a predominantly individualised (Callahan 2003) and Western view of the good. In the presented case study, for example, privileging the application of the principle of respect for autonomy seems a little unfair; respecting Mr Smith's autonomy comes at a price paid by other patients. Other moral theories and other cultures take a wider view of moral action.

- It has been criticised as being both too simple and too complex. Too simple because it is difficult to reduce complex moral issues to four principles (Edwards 1996), or even whether ethical principles apply at all (Johnstone 2005). Too complex because of the use of jargon, a point often made by students trying to pronounce and spell the principles.

The critique from agent-centred ethics

However, the major critique is not against the principles themselves so much as against the whole idea that the correct way to decide on the morally good is to analyse it from the question, what should I do? This is the starting point for the act-centred moral theories (deontology and consequentialism) introduced earlier. These theories, also known as 'the ethics of justice', assume that the best way to resolve a moral dilemma is to have a good think about the problem, using reason and calculation, seeing the problem from outside. However, if we try to conjure up an image of a really good person, it is unlikely to be one who focuses right action solely on the ability to reason and calculate. We are more likely to think of someone who has some element of goodness within them, as part of their character, reflecting an ancient way of looking at morality, set out most importantly by Aristotle. In describing virtue ethics, Aristotle concentrated not on what people should do, but how they should be. The differences in approaches are summarised in Figure 2.3.

Virtue ethics

Virtue ethics emphasises the character of the agent – who the person is as well as what they do. It is an *agent*-centred approach to ethics. Good people do good things (as opposed to the possibility of bad people doing good things) because they possess virtues, traits of character or disposition. Courage, compassion and generosity are all virtues. After a long period in decline, the popularity of virtue ethics has increased in recent years. Many nurses are attracted to an account of virtue ethics (Armstrong 2007, Sellman 1997) largely because a description of the good nurse as one who simply calculates what her duty is, or what the consequences would be, coldly and dispassionately offers only an impoverished account. It seems to matter that nurses be caring, compassionate people rather than calculating automatons. Of course this is not to suggest that there is a crude dichotomy between act- and agent-centred ethical approaches; a complete account includes both character and action (Paley 2006). The desirability of good character is recognised by the NMC. Before students can register with the NMC having completed an approved course, a signed declaration of good character is required (NMC 2004b). This does not mean that nurses are required to be compassionate or kind, however important these virtues are in understanding the features of a good nurse, as opposed to a minimally adequate nurse. Instead, the regulatory as opposed to philosophical view of good character involves declaring that no crimes have been committed (NMC 2008, Sellman 2007). The word 'kindly' appears for the first time in the new NMC Code, reinforcing the idea that character is important.

Care and the ethics of care

The concepts of care and caring are central to nursing. Tschudin (2003) starts her book *Ethics in Nursing: the caring relationship* with the observation that

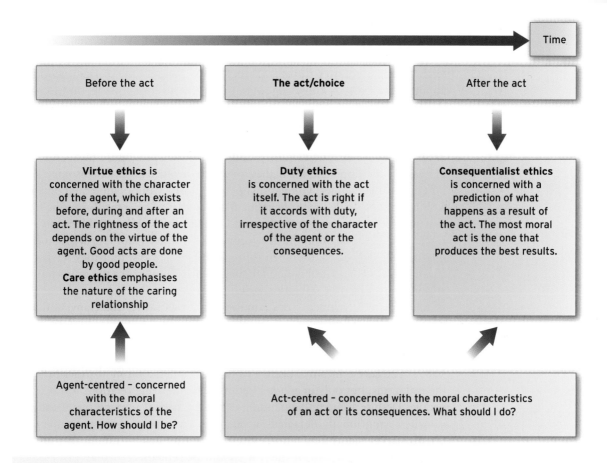

Figure 2.3 Diagram showing different types of moral theory.

'Caring is not unique to nursing, but it is unique in nursing' (p. 1). Other professions 'look after' or 'treat' patients, but only the profession of nursing has care and caring at its core. One problem in understanding the concepts involved is that the word 'care' is used in a number of different ways. We care *for* all sorts of things in nursing; the word can be used to describe everything that we do. A book chapter might describe the care of a person undergoing myocardial infarction, and it would describe the sorts of things that need to be undertaken in caring for the patient. They might need reassurance, information, assistance with hygiene, and certain technical tasks to be performed. In this sense we are describing, as much as anything, technical competence. A different sense of the word is deployed in caring *about*, which implies an emotional component or attachment to something or some person.

There is some debate about whether or not care can be considered a virtue (Allmark 1998). However, unlike virtue, and despite its centrality in the vocabulary and understanding of good nursing, care in this sense defies easy definition or even description (Mackintosh 2000). In an important critique of the body of research which attempts to define the meaning of care, Paley (2001) points out that many studies attempting to discern what nurses understand by caring simply produce a list of synonyms, including empathy, compassion and kindness. This list is virtually indistinguishable from the lists of synonyms to be found in any thesaurus, leading him to call this 'thesaurus knowledge' (Paley 2001 p. 191). The paper is unusual in that it elicited a full paper in response the following year (Deary *et al.* 2002), followed by a slightly tetchy series of shorter ripostes thereafter. As an example of rigorous debate about what counts as knowledge about a central tenet of nursing, this exchange is highly recommended.

Understanding of care as the basis for ethical action has its root in the debates between Kohlberg (1981) and Gilligan (1982). In studying the moral development of children, Kohlberg claimed that they progressed through a series of stages of development, the highest of which involved abstract reasoning based on universal principles. Gilligan, who was a former pupil and collaborator of Kohlberg's, responded with the influential book *In a Different Voice*. She found that women's values were at the middle stages of Kohlberg's hierarchy, and rather than accepting that the development of women's morality was somehow inferior, she argued that women think in different ways, that they have a different moral understanding and language which emphasises the importance of relationships and care (Hugman 2005).

The debate developed from empirical findings rather than any notion of arguments about how people *ought* to be or behave. The feminist ethics of care grew from this debate, and it found an eager home within nursing ethics which was attempting to move on from its place as a subset of medical ethics (Fry 1989). The care ethics perspective cannot be understood in abstract or hypothetical terms, but only in actions stemming from caring relationships between people. Despite some understanding of a professional nursing relationship as somehow emotionally detached, a care ethics perspective must include emotional aspects (Scott 2000) and even love. If this sounds rather aspirational, perhaps beyond the call of duty, it should be remembered that TLC (tender loving care) is a term used by many nurses, usually to communicate that medical treatment has been withdrawn from the patient as they approach the end of life (Kendrick and Robinson 2002). Walker (1998) referred to the different views of ethics of justice and the ethics of care more descriptively as 'theoretical-juridical', and 'expressive-collaborative'. Some differences between the approaches are set out in Figure 2.4.

Ethics of justice tend to be . . .	Ethics of care tend to be . . .
Theoretical-juridical	Expressive-collaborative
Impartial, detached	Partial, based on relationships
Top-down	Bottom-up
Generalisable	Contextual
Objective	Subjective
Male	Female
Rational	Emotional
Reductionist	Holistic
Medical	Nursing

Figure 2.4 Differences between ethics of care and ethics of justice.

Figure 2.4 is illustrative rather than definitive. It is not suggested that the justice orientation is exclusive to male doctors, nor that the care approach to ethics is restricted to female nurses. In medicine, at least as far as numbers are concerned, there is a more equal mix of genders, and though nursing remains predominantly female, males are more heavily represented in certain areas. The distinctions are more than mere stereotype – there is some evidence that nurses and doctors think differently about moral matters (Elder *et al.* 2003, Oberle and Hughes 2001).

Case 2.1 (continued)

Peter has analysed the issue of Mr Smith's medication using the four principles approach, but he feels that it is inadequate to help him decide. He spent a considerable amount of time the previous night getting to know him. Mr Smith explained how exhausted he was with his social circumstances and how desperate he was for a good rest. Mr Smith complimented Peter on how he alone of the nursing staff seemed to make time to listen to him and to understand him. Peter felt that he could understand what Mr Smith really wanted was some sleep and was beginning to consider that covert medication could be the most caring way to help him.

There are problems for both sides of this illustrative dichotomy. Whilst a reliance on abstract deductive reasoning to resolve ethical issues dispassionately does not capture the essence of nursing, relying only on an emotional, contextual and individual way of seeing ethical practice also seems problematic. Its critics suggest that that the ethics of care is 'hopelessly vague' (Allmark 1995b p. 19), but this lack of consistency is accepted by Nel Noddings (2003), an influential feminist philosopher:

> *Clearly I do not intend to advocate arbitrary and capricious behaviour . . . such an ethics [of care] does not attempt to reduce the need for human judgement with a series of 'thou shalts' and 'thou shalt nots.' Rather it recognises and calls forth human judgement across a wide range of fact and feeling and it allows for situations and conditions in which judgement (in the impersonal, logical sense) may properly be put aside in favour of faith and commitment (p. 25).*

An account of nursing ethics that sees the good nurse as someone who cares about the patients and is also able to analyse and justify decisions, taking account of both sides of this rather crude binary analysis (Kuhse 1997). Indeed, most people use both orientations at the same time, in varying degrees (Flanagan and Jackson 1987). An accessible review of the contrast is provided by Botes (2000).

Research focus 2.2

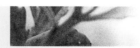

In research undertaken at an ethics conference in the United States, Smith and Godfrey (2002) asked 53 registered nurses to answer two open-ended questions. (1) A good nurse is one who . . . and (2) how does a nurse go about doing the right thing? The two questions are posed from the positions of describing the characteristics of the good nurse (agent-centred – question 1) and describing how a nurse might go about doing the right thing (act-centred – question 2). After analysis of the answers, and to the researchers' surprise, the responses to the two questions fell into the same seven categories. These are:

1. *Personal characteristics*
2. *Professional characteristics*
3. *Knowledge base*
4. *Patient centeredness*
5. *Advocacy*
6. *Critical thinking*
7. *Patient care*

The researchers conclude that 'this finding supports the position that the traditional justice or care dichotomy for explaining nurses' ethical decision-making is far too confining' (p. 309). Many empirical studies of this sort are undertaken in the US, where the health care environment is very different, but there are also enough similarities in, for example, professional roles to make this finding supportive of the intuitive understanding that the binary distinction is insufficiently explanatory.

Lastly, the dichotomy poses a problem for nursing education. The analytical approach to ethics can be taught and learnt in much the same way as any other form of knowledge; it is a subject to know and understand, much like anatomy or physiology. However, possession of knowledge and understanding of moral theory does not in itself mean that the possessor of such knowledge will act in a good way, or be a good person. A pressing question for educators and students is how to facilitate the development of character so that student nurses become moral, sensitive and perceptive carers. These things cannot be taught by lectures and seminars, but they may be developed, largely in practice, by discussion, reflection, communication and observation of experienced nurses and mentors, and by practising ethical nursing; that is, by having the will to become a good nurse (Begley 2006).

Conclusion

The analysis using the four principles approach should help identify some important issues for consideration, helping you weigh them up in arriving at a decision about right action. However, the principles cannot help you come to a view on how your decision will be enacted. This will require a willingness to engage with Mr Smith as a person, with perception and sensitivity to see the whole person with desires, concerns, wishes and feelings; an attempt to empathise with him; to communicate effectively; to understand why he is behaving the way that he is. In short, to care for him, and all the other patients in your care.

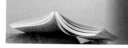

Suggested further reading

Recommended journals:

- *Nursing Ethics*
- *Journal of Advanced Nursing*
- *Nursing Philosophy*
- *Journal of Medical Ethics*
- *Nursing Inquiry*

Textbooks

Beauchamp, T. L. and Childress, J. F. (2008) *Principles of Biomedical Ethics* (6th ed.), Oxford: Oxford University Press. This book is medically and philosophically orientated, and American in origin, but it is very comprehensive.

Davis, A. J., Tschudin, V. and de Raeve, L. (eds) (2006) *Essentials of Teaching and Learning in Nursing Ethics*, Edinburgh: Churchill Livingstone. This book is recently published, containing chapters by different eminent authors. It does not cover issues (such as euthanasia) as such, but rather approaches to ethics.

Edwards, S. D. (1996) *Nursing Ethics: A principle-based approach*, Basingstoke: Macmillan. This is a shorter and simpler to understand application of the four principles approach. A second edition is in preparation for publication in 2009.

Johnstone, M.-J. (2005) *Bioethics: A nursing perspective* (4th ed.) Sydney: Churchill Livingstone. This Australian textbook is comprehensive and well written.

Kuhse, H. (1997) *Caring: Nurses, women and ethics*, Oxford: Blackwell. This book is among the best, in my view. It's not about ethics in the general sense, but it explores the role of women in caring and nursing, and is very good on the care–justice debate.

The following website contains useful material and links elsewhere:

http://www.ethics-network.org.uk/

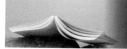

References

Allmark, P. (1995a) Smoking and health: is discrimination fair? *Professional Nurse* **10** (12), 811–813.

Allmark, P. (1995b) Can there be an ethics of care? *Journal of Medical Ethics* **21** (1), 19–24.

Allmark, P. (1998) Is caring a virtue? *Journal of Advanced Nursing* **28** (3), 466–472.

Allmark, P. (2005) Can the study of ethics enhance nursing practice? *Journal of Advanced Nursing* **51** (6), 618–624.

Armstrong, A. (2007) *Nursing Ethics: A virtue-based approach*. Basingstsoke: Palgrave Macmillan.

Aveyard, H. (2000) Is there a concept of autonomy that can usefully inform nursing practice? *Journal of Advanced Nursing* **32** (2), 352–358.

Beauchamp, T. L. and Childress, J. F. (2001) *Principles of Biomedical Ethics* (5th ed.). Oxford: Oxford University Press.

Beauchamp, T. L. and Childress, J. F. (2008) *Principles of Biomedical Ethics* (6th ed.). Oxford: Oxford University Press.

Begley, A. M. (2006) Facilitating the development of moral insight in practice: teaching ethics and teaching virtue. *Nursing Philosophy* **7** (4), 257–265.

Berghs, M., Dierckx de Casterle, B. and Gastermans, C. (2005) The complexity of nurses' attitudes toward euthanasia: a review of the literature. *Journal of Medical Ethics* **31** (8), 441–446.

Botes, A. (2000) A comparison between the ethics of justice and the ethics of care. *Journal of Advanced Nursing* **32** (5), 1071–1075.

Bowling, A. (1996) Health care rationing: the public's debate. *British Medical Journal* **312** (7032), 670–674.

Bowling, A., Mariotto, A. and Evans, O. (2002) Are older people willing to give up their place in the queue for cardiac surgery to a younger person? *Age and Aging* **31** (3), 187–192.

Breeze, J. N. (1998) Can paternalism be justified in mental health care? *Journal of Advanced Nursing* **28** (2), 260–265.

Busfield, J. (2000) *Health and Health Care in Modern Britain*. Oxford: Oxford University Press.

Callahan, D. (2003) Principlism and communitarianism. *Journal of Medical Ethics* **29**, 287–291.

Cameron, M. E., Schaffer, M. and Park, A-E. (2001) Nursing students' experience of ethical problems and use of ethical decision-making models. *Nursing Ethics* **8** (5), 432–447.

Church House Publishing (2000) *On Dying Well. A contribution to the euthanasia debate.* London: Church House Publishing.

Clouser, K. D. and Gert, B. (1990) A critique of principlism. *The Journal of Medicine and Philosophy* **15** (2), 219–236.

Collis, S. P. (2006) The importance of truth telling in health care. *Nursing Standard* **20** (17), 41–45.

Cookson, R. and Dolan, P. (2000) Principles of justice in health care rationing. *Journal of Medical Ethics* **26** (5), 323–329.

Cornock, M. (2002) Legal basis of decision-making in critical care. *Nursing in Critical Care* **7** (5), 235–240.

Davis, R. B. (1995) The principlism debate: a critical overview. *The Journal of Medicine and Philosophy* **20** (1), 85–105.

Deary, V., Deary, I. J., Mckenna, H. P., *et al.* (2002) Elisions in the field of caring. *Journal of Advanced Nursing* **39** (1), 96–102.

Dickenson, D. L. (2000) Are medical ethicists out of touch? Practitioner attitudes in the US and UK towards decisions at the end of life. *Journal of Medical Ethics* **26** (4), 254–260.

Dimond, B. (2001) Legal aspects of consent 18: issues relating to euthanasia. *British Journal of Nursing* **10** (22), 1479–1481.

Dolan, P. and Shaw, R. (2003) A note on the relative importance that people attach to different factors when setting priorities in health care. *Health Expectations* **6** (1), 53–59.

Edwards, S. D. (1996) *Nursing Ethics: A principle-based approach.* Basingstoke: Macmillan.

Edwards, S. D. (2006) A principle-based approach to nursing ethics. In *Essentials of Teaching and Learning in Nursing Ethics*, Davis, A. J., Tschudin, V. and de Raeve, L. (eds). Edinburgh: Churchill Livingstone, 55–66.

Elder, R., Price, J. and Williams, G. (2003) Differences in ethical attitudes between registered nurses and medical students. *Nursing Ethics* **10** (2), 149–164.

Flanagan, O. and Jackson, K. (1987) Justice, care and gender: the Kohlberg-Gilligan debate revisited. *Ethics* **97** (3), 622–637.

Fry, S. T. (1989) The role of caring in a theory of nursing ethics. *Hypatia* **4** (2), 88–103.

Gilligan, C. (1982) *In a Different Voice. Psychological theory and women's development*. Cambridge, MA: Harvard University Press.

Gillon, R. (1985) *Philosophical Medical Ethics*. Chichester: John Wiley & Sons.

Gillon, R. (2003) Ethics needs principles – four can encompass the rest – and respect for autonomy should be 'first among equals'. *Journal of Medical Ethics* **29** (5), 307–312.

Glover, J. (1977) *Causing Death and Saving Lives*. London: Penguin.

Greipp, M. E. (1992) Greipp's model of ethical decision making. *Journal of Advanced Nursing* **17** (6), 734–738.

Harris, J. (2003) In praise of unprincipled ethics. *Journal of Medical Ethics* **29** (5), 303–306.

Henderson, S. (2003) Power imbalances between nurses and patients: a potential inhibitor of partnership in care. *Journal of Clinical Nursing* **12** (4), 501–508.

Hirskyj, P. (2007) QALY: an ethical issue that dare not speak its name. *Nursing Ethics* **14** (1), 72–82.

Hugman, R. (2005) *New Approaches in Ethics for the Caring Professions*. Basingstoke: Palgrave Macmillan.

Ikonomidis, S. and Singer, P. A. (1999) Autonomy, liberalism and advance care planning. *Journal of Medical Ethics* **25** (6), 522–527.

Johnstone, M.J. (2005) *Bioethics. A nursing perspective* (4th ed.). Sydney: Churchill Livingstone.

Kendall, C. E. (2000) A double dose of double effect. *Journal of Medical Ethics* **26** (3), 204–206.

Kendrick, K. D. and Robinson, S. (2002) 'Tender loving care' as a relational ethic in nursing practice. *Nursing Ethics* **9** (3), 291–300.

Keown, D. and Keown, J. (1995) Killing, karma and caring: euthanasia in Buddhism and Christianity. *Journal of Medical Ethics* **21** (5), 265–269.

Kohlberg, L. (1981) *Essays in Moral Development: Volume I, the psychology of moral development*. San Francisco: Harper & Row.

Kuhse, H. (1997) *Caring: Nurses, women and ethics*. Oxford: Blackwell.

Mackintosh, C. (2000) Is there a place for care within nursing? *International Journal of Nursing Studies* **37** (4), 321–327.

NHSE (National Health Service Executive) (1999) *Treatment for Impotence*. Health Service Circular 1999/148. London: DH (http://www.dh.gov.uk).

National Health Service in England (2007) *NHS Core Principles*. London: Department of Health (http://www.nhs.uk).

National Institute for Health and Clinical Excellence. (2007) *Measuring Effectiveness and Cost Effectiveness: the QALY*. London: NICE (http://www.nice.org.uk).

Noddings, N. (2003) *Caring; A feminine approach to ethics and moral education* (2nd ed.). Berkeley, CA: University of California Press.

NMC (Nursing and Midwifery Council) (2004a) *Standards of Proficiency for Pre-registration Nursing Education*. London: NMC.

NMC (2004b) *NMC Guidance on Good Health and Good Character*. London: NMC (http://www.nmc-uk.org).

NMC (2007) *Covert Administration of Medicines – Disguising Medicines in Food and Drink*. London: NMC (http://www.nmc-uk.org).

NMC (2008) *The Code: Standards of conduct performance and ethics for nurses and midwives*. London: NMC (http://www.nmc-uk.org).

Oberle, K. and Hughes, D. (2001) Doctors' and nurses' perceptions of ethical problems in end-of-life decisions. *Journal of Advanced Nursing* 33 (6), 707–715.

Paley, J. (2001) An archaeology of caring knowledge. *Journal of Advanced Nursing* 36 (2), 188–198.

Paley, J. (2006) Past caring. The limitations of one to one ethics. In *Essentials of Teaching and Learning in Nursing Ethics*, Davis, A. J., Tschudin, V. and de Raeve, L. (eds). Edinburgh: Churchill Livingstone, 149–164.

Perkin, R. M. and Resnik, D. B. (2002) The agony of agonal respiration: is the last gasp really necessary? *Journal of Medical Ethics* 28 (3), 164–169.

Persaud, R. (1995) Smokers rights to health care. *Journal of Medical Ethics* 21 (5), 281–287.

Quill, T.E., Dresser, R. and Brock, D.W. (1997) The rule of double effect – a critique of its role in end-of-life decision-making. *The New England Journal of Medicine* 337 (24), 1768–1771.

Resuscitation Council (2007) *Decisions Relating to Cardiopulmonary Resuscitation. A Joint Statement from the British Medical Association, the Resuscitation Council (UK) and the Royal College of Nursing*. (http://www.resus.org.uk).

Schwarz, J. K. (2004) The rule of double effect and its role in facilitating good end of life palliative care; a help or a hindrance? *Journal of Hospice and Palliative Nursing* 6 (2), 125–133.

Scott, P. A. (2000) Emotion, moral perception, and nursing practice. *Nursing Philosophy* 1 (2), 123–133.

Seedhouse, D. (1998) *Ethics: the heart of healthcare* (2nd ed.). Chichester: John Wiley & Sons.

Sellman, D. (1997) The virtues in the moral education of nurses: Florence Nightingale revisited. *Nursing Ethics* 4 (1), 3–11.

Sellman, D. (2005) Towards an understanding of nursing as a response to human vulnerability. *Nursing Philosophy* 6 (1), 2–10.

Sellman, D. (2007) On being of good character: nurse education and the assessment of character. *Nurse Education Today* 27 (7), 762–767.

Shaw, A. B. (1994) In defence of ageism. *Journal of Medical Ethics* 20 (3), 188–191, 194.

Shaw, A. B. (2002) Two challenges to the double effect doctrine: euthanasia and abortion. *Journal of Medical Ethics* 28 (2), 102–105.

Smith, K. V. and Godfrey, N. S. (2002) Being a good nurse and doing the right thing: a qualitative study. *Nursing Ethics* 9 (3), 301–311.

Snelling, P. C. (2004) Consequences count; against absolutism at the end of life. *Journal of Advanced Nursing* 46 (4), 350–357.

Taylor, B. (1999) Parental autonomy and consent to treatment. *Journal of Advanced Nursing* 29 (3), 570–576.

Thompson, I., Melia, K. M. and Boyd, K. M. (2000) *Nursing Ethics* (4th ed.). Edinburgh: Churchill Livingstone.

Tschudin, V. (2003) *Ethics in Nursing: the caring relationship*. Edinburgh: Butterworth Heinemann.

Tuckett, A. (2004) Truth-telling in clinical practice and the arguments for and against: a review of the literature. *Nursing Ethics* 11 (5), 500–513.

Upton, H. (2003) Ethical theories and practical problems. *Nursing Philosophy* **4** (2), 170–172.

Walker, M. U. (1998) *Moral Understandings; A feminist study in ethics.* New York: Routledge.

Warnock, M. (1998) *An Intelligent Person's Guide to Ethics.* London: Duckworth.

Wilmot, S. and Ratcliffe, J. (2002) Principles of distributive justice used by members of the general public in the allocation of donor liver grafts for transplantation: a qualitative study. *Health Expectations* **5** (3), 199–209.

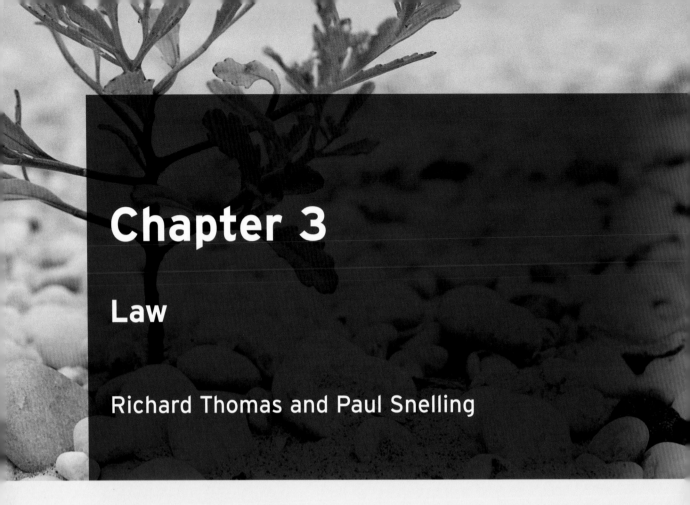

Chapter 3

Law

Richard Thomas and Paul Snelling

Learning outcomes

After reading and reflecting on this chapter, you should be able to:

- Trace the fundamental basis of law in England and Wales;
- Outline the notion of reasonableness, reasonable practice and duty of care;
- Discuss the principles involved in consent to treatment and how these are manifest in acceptable clinical practice;
- Consider The Mental Capacity Act (2005) and its role in clarifying the duty of care owed in nursing practice;
- Outline confidential relationships and discuss their application to patient care;
- Consider how Human Rights legislation applies to nursing and how issues such as withholding and withdrawing treatment and euthanasia are influenced by this legislation;
- State the principles of negligence and discuss these principles in relation to clinical practice.

Related NMC Standards of Proficiency for Pre-registration Nursing Education (NMC 2004)

- Demonstrate knowledge of legislation and health and social policy relevant to nursing practice.

- Ensure the confidentiality and security of written and verbal information acquired in a professional capacity.

- Manage the complexities arising from ethical and legal dilemmas.

- Maintain, support and acknowledge the rights of individuals or groups in the health care setting.

- Act to ensure that the rights of individuals and groups are not compromised.

- Information technology and management - interpret and utilise data and technology, taking account of legal ethical and safety considerations, in the delivery and enhancement of care.

Introduction

The Code (NMC 2008a) makes it clear that nurses must have knowledge of the law for their practice. To remain within the law nurses need to understand what is required, justified and forbidden within their practice. However, it could be argued that the law only provides support and guidance and expects nurses to exercise discretion within a logical, defensible approach. It is therefore important to consider how the law judges qualified nurses as to what is reasonable and as to what is an acceptable standard of practice.

The chapter is divided into three parts.

In Part 1, we outline the fundamentals of law, how it is made and administered, and emphasise the importance of good record-keeping.

In Part 2, we explain some of the legislation that governs nursing practice. A chapter of this size cannot hope to cover all of the ground, but important aspects are explained, including consent to treatment and the Mental Capacity Act (2005), confidentiality, and the Human Rights Act (1998).

In Part 3, we discuss negligence and explore the issues that courts would take into account if an action in negligence is brought by a patient or relative.

Part 1: Outlining the law

Case 3.1

Rhiannon is a student nurse working on a surgical ward. Mr Adams, a widower aged 83, is admitted because of bleeding from a gastric ulcer which he has had for some years. In addition to his ulcer he has arthritis and heart failure, and describes his health as very poor. Major surgery is planned to repair the ulcer and the surgical registrar comes hurriedly to the ward to 'consent him'. Mr Adams' daughter is present while the registrar tells Mr Adams that he has got to have the operation to 'fix his tummy'. During the consultation, she asks questions and interrupts her father when he says that he just 'wants to be left alone'. Mr Adams tires and mumbles during the consultation and his daughter signs the consent form on his behalf. Rhiannon is asked to take Mr Adams to the theatre for the operation, but as she approaches his bed, he tells her clearly that he doesn't want an operation, that he has 'had enough' and wants to be left alone. He says that 'you can't take me to theatre.' The consent form is signed, and the operating theatre is waiting. Without the operation, he will probably die, but Rhiannon feels very uneasy as she accompanies him down the corridor. Have the legal processes been properly followed?

The fundamental basis of law in England and Wales

The law and legal processes in the UK have evolved over hundreds of years and the right of the Sovereign to make and administer the law has been split into two, Parliament and the Judiciary with, in general, Parliament predominant. The two types of law are:

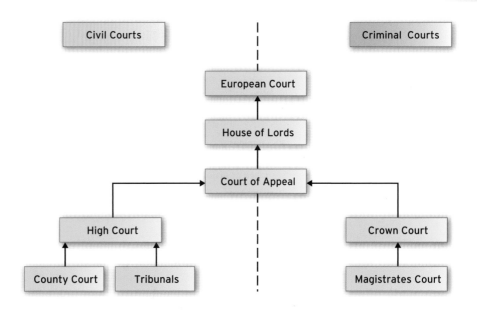

Figure 3.1 Simplified structure of court hierarchy in England and Wales.

1. *Statute law* follows from Acts of Parliament and statutory instruments (enacted from the power of Parliament), including European Community laws. These are known as statutory sources and take precedence over other laws.
2. *Common law*, known also as judge-made law or case law.

Statute, set down in Acts of Parliament, is supreme and overrides any uncertainty or conflict in common law, but it is impossible for legislators to cover every eventuality in the laws enacted through Parliament. Common law sets out areas of law not covered by Acts of Parliament, and interprets the statutes in individual cases. 'Judge-made law' as it is also called sets precedents that are followed by subsequent judgments. Hence previous case law decisions will guide opinion and a Judge will rely in part on previous judgments in arriving at their opinion, applying them to the particular case in question and completing the opinion with final weighing up and legal argument.

Courts in England and Wales are hierarchical (see Figure 3.1).

Under certain circumstances appeals can be made to courts higher in the hierarchy, and lower courts must be guided by decisions made in higher ones. Important decisions of the courts are reported, recorded and published in resources such as the *All England Law Reports* available via Internet databases (e.g. http://www.lexisnexis.co.uk and http://www.westlaw.com) making them available for students and for subsequent court guidance and rulings. The law is administered in civil and criminal courts. The differences between civil and criminal law (summarised in Figure 3.2) include the following:

- *Origin*. Both criminal and civil law can be derived from Acts of Parliament. Judges interpret the law and develop it as common law.
- *Names*. A civil 'wrong' is a tort. A criminal 'wrong' is a crime.
- *Parties*. Cases under civil law involve a dispute between two or more parties, a common example being divorce. Criminal law involves the state, acting on

	Civil	Criminal
Origin	Act of Parliament and common law	Act of Parliament and common law
Names	Tort	Crime
Parties	Two or more parties	The state and an individual or (rarely) organisation
Who decides	Most often judges. Rarely juries.	Juries for verdict Judge for sentence
Standard of proof	Balance of probabilities	Beyond reasonable doubt
'Punishment'	Damages	Fines, imprisonment, community service

Figure 3.2 Comparison of civil and criminal law.

behalf of the Monarch and the people, prosecuting an individual for wrong-doing, or for an offence against the state.

- *Who decides*. Most civil cases are decided by a judge or judges, though juries are employed in certain circumstances. Criminal cases above magistrates' courts are heard before a jury normally of 12 people, who decide on the facts of the case, that is, whether the accused is guilty or not guilty. If guilty, the judge decides on the punishment guided by a tariff of sentencing.
- *Standard*. The standards of proof required are different. In civil law, cases are decided on the 'balance of probabilities'; that is what is most likely to have occurred. Conviction in the criminal courts requires a higher standard. The jury must believe 'beyond reasonable doubt' (or so that they are sure) that the accused is guilty.
- *Punishment*. In civil cases, orders can be granted and damages levied, paid by the loser to the winner. In criminal cases, fines can be levied, community service imposed and in serious cases, people can be sent to prison.

Reasonableness

A significant principle governing legal aspects of clinical practice is that of reasonableness. The word 'reasonable' is used extensively throughout law: for example, a person may use reasonable force in self-defence, and the Disability Discrimination Act (DDA) requires educational institutions (in some circumstances) to make reasonable adjustments. However, despite its importance there is no clear definition of what 'reasonable' means, because it is a subjective adjective. A dictionary definition includes the following 'having sound judgement, sensible, not asking too much' (*Oxford English Dictionary* 2008). So in the case of the DDA, an institution would be expected to do more than install a cursory temporary ramp, but less than a complete rebuilding of a lecture theatre. What counts as reasonable can ultimately be decided on in court, and this is of necessity retrospective, of little help to a nurse attempting to decide on what a reasonable decision is. To put it another way, an action may be compared to what a 'reasonable' person would have done, this person being, in the famous phrase, 'the man on the Clapham omnibus', a metaphor for an average person.

Perhaps a better way of deciding what is reasonable, and where there is no clear case law, is simply to ask how defensible the decision is. There is no compulsion for everyone to do the same thing, but what was done in the circumstances must be reasonable, and considered acceptable by colleagues, employers and regulatory bodies. Authority for decisions can be derived from evidence (hence evidence-based practice) which can be in the form of policy, protocol, directives or guidelines allied with perhaps evidence in the form of research or other sources. It could be argued that it is possible and lawful to be wrong in a given situation as long as the nurse is reasonably wrong, and could not reasonably be expected to have done differently, that is, what was wrong was not obviously wrong.

Activity 3.1

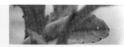

Reflect upon one or two clinical decisions you have seen made in practice. Can these decisions withstand a rigorous critique and examination?

Record-keeping

It is sometimes asserted that health records are legal documents. In fact, all documents are legal documents, insofar as they can be presented as evidence in court. However, when there is a patient complaint or legal action, investigation will start with health records. For this reason (and for many others) keeping good records is an essential part of nursing, although it is sometimes regarded as a chore (McGeehan 2007). The NMC guidance on record-keeping (NMC 2007) points out that courts of law tend to the view that 'if it is not recorded it has not been done' and requires that records should:

- Be factual, consistent and accurate, written in such a way that the meaning is clear.
- Be recorded as soon as possible after an event has occurred, providing current information on the care and condition of the patient/client.
- Be recorded clearly and in such a manner that the text cannot be erased or deleted without a record of change.
- Be recorded in such a manner that any justifiable alterations or additions are dated, timed and signed or clearly attributed to a named person in an identifiable role in such a way that the original entry can still be read clearly.
- Be accurately dated, timed and signed with the signature printed against the first entry where this is a written record, and attributed to a named person in an identifiable role for electronic records.
- Not include abbreviations, jargon, meaningless phrases, irrelevant speculation, offensive or subjective statements.
- Be readable when photocopied or scanned.

A **material fact** is one that if it were withdrawn would make a difference.

Records fulfilling the above criteria are able to represent what was done, and why it was done, showing that acts and omissions were reasonable in their context. In law it is necessary to consider what is material and how **material facts** can be considered in health care decisions. An example of a material fact is that a policy or protocol exists. Professional nurses, utilising and relying upon a body of opinion, are empowered and required to exercise discretion and judgement, but this must normally be within policy, and so nurses should be aware what policies exist. Decisions by nurses must be based on and supported by NMC Standards and Guidance and can also include national, regional and local policy and other relevant codes and requirements, including legal obligations. Any action or omission outside the policy must be defended as reasonable. An investigation (legal or otherwise) will attempt to discover the truth and to determine responsibility, and health records are very important in evidencing what care was given.

Part 2: Explaining the law

In many cases the practice of nurses and other health care professionals is directly governed by law. The law informs the individuals and institutions what they are:

- *Required to do*. For example, nurses are required to report certain illnesses – this means that they are at fault if they do not do this.
- *Justified or allowed to do*. For example nurses with prescribing powers are allowed to prescribe, according to their clinical judgement. It is also lawful in certain circumstances to withhold treatment 'in the patients' best interests'.
- *Forbidden to do*. For example, nurses (and all others) are forbidden to give drugs at the end of life with the intention of shortening the life.

A chapter of this length cannot deal with all areas of health care law. However, the following areas of law are very important, and are covered in more detail:

- Consent to treatment – including the Mental Capacity Act (2005).
- The Mental Health Act (1983 and 2007).
- Confidentiality, including the Data Protection Act (1998) and the Freedom of Information Act (2000).
- Human Rights Act (1998).

Consent to treatment

Consent is giving permission for somebody to do something. To be valid, consent must be given voluntarily by a person who has capacity and sufficient information.

It is a fundamental ethical, legal and professional principle that valid **consent** must be obtained before starting any treatment, investigation or even giving care to a patient. In ethics this is the most obvious manifestation of the principle of respect for autonomy, requiring that nurses and other health care professionals recognise the right of individuals to determine as far as possible what happens to their own bodies. Without consent, touching a patient can amount to the crime of assault and the tort of battery, and if this seems extreme and unlikely, performing a procedure without consent, or deliberately misleading the patient has resulted in legal action. Brazier and Cave (2007) report the

Canadian case of Allan v Mount Sinai Hospital [1980] where a woman expressed a wish to be injected in her right arm. The doctor injected her left, and lost the case in battery. The days of patients passively acquiescing in treatment and care decided for them by health care professionals are thankfully long gone. The giving of valid consent is an expression of the partnership between professional and patient. The Department of Health (DH) has published a series of guides about consent, including an excellent reference guide (DH 2001a). This can be downloaded as a pdf file, or ordered free as a hard copy, and should be considered required reading. This document starts with the following sentence:

> *For consent to be valid it must be given voluntarily by an appropriately informed person who has the capacity to consent to the intervention in question. Acquiescence where the person does not know what the intervention entails is not 'consent'.*

> (DH 2001a p. 4)

From this definition, the following necessary features of valid consent can be identified:

- It must be voluntary
- The patient must be appropriately informed
- The patient must have the capacity to consent.

Each of these will be discussed and related to Case 3.1, which was presented at the beginning of the chapter.

It must be voluntary

Nurses must be aware of the potential for coercion and the way that this can influence a person's decisions. Historically, the clichéd manifestation of this was the powerful doctor, retinue in tow, who would merely decide a course of treatment and assume that the patient would agree. Today, perhaps, influences are more subtle. Overbearing relatives might attempt to influence a treatment, or a choice of home care, and nurses who suspect that this is the case should consider discussing options with the patient in private. Nurses also wield a considerable amount of power (Henderson 2003), and need to be aware of this; when we or the colleagues that we are supervising offer to wash a patient, can we really be sure that he is not merely acquiescing because he can see that we are busy? Or perhaps this busy ness has resulted in us applying a subtle pressure to the patient to agree?

Case 3.1 (continued)

There are a number of issues which may have resulted in Mr Adams feeling pressurised. His daughter interrupts him constantly, and in fact signs the consent form for him. The doctor's explanations are hurried, and this may apply pressure for Mr Adams to make up his mind quickly. In these circumstances, it seems unlikely that initial consent is voluntarily given, and Rhiannon is right to feel uneasy.

The patient must be appropriately informed

A patient must be provided with sufficient information to be able to make a decision about treatment or care. For routine care decisions this does not seem to be difficult, but as decisions increase in their complexity, more information is required, and the interpretation of relevant information and the evidence base for the treatment needs to be presented in a manner appropriate for each individual patient. Written material explaining operations and procedures is often available and can help patients understand what is being proposed. Many of the complex decisions will be about medical treatment and the responsibility here lies with the medical team or senior nurses. However, the principles are the same for all decisions.

The law does not tell us exactly what patients must be told. Instead there have been a number of cases where patients have sued for negligence and these rulings set precedents detailing the amount of information considered reasonable for patients to expect. These cases often result from the occurrence of a known complication of a procedure, where patients sue on the grounds that they would not have consented to the procedure had they known the risks of the complication occurring. In a case heard in 1999, Mrs Pearce was two weeks overdue on delivering her sixth child, and discussed the risks of induction or Caesarean section. She was not told of the small risk (1 in 1000) of stillbirth associated with waiting for a vaginal delivery. The child was stillborn. Mrs Pearce sued and subsequently lost her case. The Judge said that the doctor should inform the patient of 'a significant risk which would affect the judgement of a reasonable patient' (Brazier and Cave 2007, DH 2001a). Mrs Pearce was distressed at the time, and it was judged reasonable not to disclose this risk. By contrast, in an Australian case [Rogers v Whittaker 1992], a patient won a case for negligence because she was not informed of a 1 in 14,000 chance of blindness following surgery, despite voicing her concerns about losing her sight. So it is not possible to specify that risks above a certain likelihood must be disclosed. The law is currently evolving in this area, but, consistent with law and policy in other areas of practice, the discretion of the health care professional to decide what is best for the patient, including how much to tell them about their treatment, is diminishing.

The consent form in use in the UK, downloadable from the Department of Health website, requires the doctor, or whoever is seeking consent, to sign to say that they have explained the intended benefits, serious or frequently occurring risks, and any extra procedures which may become necessary during the procedure, including blood transfusion. On the face of it, detailed information is a good thing although there is some evidence that these complex forms can conflict with patients' needs for personal communication and advocacy (Akkad *et al.* 2004).

Case 3.1 (continued)

There is little detail in the case study about exactly what information was given, and as in all cases, much depends on the detail. However, the operation appears to be life-saving and Mr Adams would need to understand this, and also the risks of the anaesthetic and the likely outcome of the operation, for example, whether a stoma is likely. Telling Mr Adams that the operation is necessary to 'fix his tummy' does not appear to satisfy the minimum requirement for information.

Good and lawful practice includes:

- Giving sufficient information for the patient to understand in broad terms the nature of a procedure (DH 2001a), and other options, including doing nothing.
- Giving information about anaesthesia if appropriate.
- Disclosing details of any 'material' or 'significant' risks.
- Disclosing whether students will be participating in care or treatment.
- Answering questions fully and honestly.
- Making records about what has been discussed. This is also important when patients do not want to know the details of their treatment.

Activity 3.2

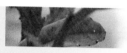

Download the consent form for adults with capacity from the Department of Health website (http://www.dh.gov.uk), using the word consent in their internal search engine. From your experience of observing or participating in the gaining of consent, has the form always been correctly completed?

The patient must have the capacity to consent

Seeking consent for treatment is the cornerstone of the partnership between patient and health professional, but a difficulty arises where a patient is unable to make a decision about their treatment. It is clear that the law absolutely allows people to make decisions that health care professionals may think unwise or even irrational, but this only applies when the patient is able to make the decision. **Mental capacity** 'is the ability to make a decision' (Ministry of Justice 2007 p. 41). This definition refers to having the *cognitive* ability to make decisions and communicate them, rather than the absence of any other restrictions, for example the power relationships discussed earlier. Capacity can be restricted for a number of reasons, including physical and mental illness and cognitive impairment. Examples include:

Mental capacity is the ability to make a decision.

- Stroke or other brain injury.
- A mental health problem.
- Dementia.
- A learning disability.
- Confusion or drowsiness.
- Substance misuse (including alcohol).

The issue of capacity often arises where there is disagreement about treatment options, where, for example, the nurse thinks that a patient needs oxygen therapy, and the patient says he does not want it. After hearing an explanation of the reasons why the nurse thinks that oxygen therapy is necessary, a patient declining to have the therapy may be making a considered judgement based on the information given, or be confused by hypoxia or sedatives, such that pushing away the oxygen mask is not a meaningful act, but just a reflex action. In the former case a patient with capacity has made what might be considered an unwise decision, which must be respected. In the latter, an incapable patient is not able to make a decision at all, and to respect this 'refusal' would be to put the patient at risk of harm. The nurse must look after the patient's best interests and these cannot be served by allowing the refusal of oxygen therapy. Instead the nurse is obliged to make all reasonable attempts at finding an alternative way of giving the therapy which the patient will tolerate, even to the point, perhaps, of sitting with them and holding the mask so that they are unable to push it away.

What this example illustrates most of all is that lawful action depends largely on the issue of whether or not a patient is considered to have capacity, and this applies to all decisions. Since the issue of capacity will frequently arise in heath care, there is a need for a clear process of assessing whether a person has capacity or not, and a clear legal framework of what should be done when a person is considered to lack capacity. These frameworks are provided by the Mental Capacity Act 2005 (MCA), which came into force during 2007. There are excellent, easy to read guides about the MCA, and these can be downloaded free from the Ministry of Justice website. Guide number 3 (Office of the Public Guardian 2007) in particular should be considered essential reading. A full code of practice is also available free to download (Ministry of Justice 2007). The requirement to be aware of legislation regarding mental capacity is stated in *The Code* (NMC 2008a). The five principles of the MCA are:

1. *A presumption of capacity.* Every adult has the right to make his or her own decisions and must be assumed to have the capacity to do so unless it is proved otherwise.
2. *Individuals being supported to make their own decisions.* A person must be given all practicable help before anyone treats them as not being able to make their own decisions.
3. *Unwise decisions.* Just because an individual makes what might be seen as an unwise decision, they should not be treated as lacking the capacity to make the decision.
4. *Best interests.* An act done or a decision made under the Act for or on behalf of a person who lacks capacity must be done in their best interests.
5. *Least restrictive option.* Anything done for or on behalf of a person who lacks capacity should be the least restrictive of their basic rights and freedoms.

Assessing capacity

The presumption is always in favour of the view that the person has capacity. The patient does not have to show that they have capacity, the health care professional must assume that this is the case, unless it can be shown that they do not. It cannot be assumed that just because someone has a particular condition, for example dementia, they can never make any decisions, and neither can assumptions be made about capacity based on age, appearance, or eccentricities of a person's behaviour. The assessment of capacity is always about a particular decision to be taken at a particular time, not made in the general sense for all decisions at all times. Some people are able to make simple decisions but not complex ones, and some people's ability to make decisions fluctuates so that they may have capacity one day and not the next.

The MCA puts into statute a test for capacity which has been in use since 1994, deriving from the case of Re C. In this case, a 68-year-old man who was detained in a psychiatric hospital because of paranoid schizophrenia developed serious leg problems. Doctors treating his leg considered him to have a 15 per cent chance of survival without an amputation, but he refused consent, and sought an injunction to prevent doctors from performing the amputation without his consent. Despite the fact that he was seriously mentally ill, suffering from delusions, the Judge found that he was nevertheless able to make this particular decision (Brazier and Cave 2007). The test for capacity arising from that case is now contained within the MCA (2005), as a two-stage test. The first stage is to decide whether there is an impairment of, or disturbance in the functioning of, the patient's mind or brain. If an impairment is present, the second stage considers whether it results in the person being able to make a specific decision when they need to. A person is unable to make a decision if they cannot:

1. Understand information about the decision to be made (the Act calls this 'relevant information')
2. Retain that information in their mind
3. Use or weigh that information as part of the decision-making process, or
4. Communicate their decision (by talking, using sign language or any other means).

(Ministry of Justice 2007 p. 45)

If the application of this process concludes that the patient does have capacity, then refusal of treatment must be accepted, however unwise it seems to health care professionals. On rare occasions this might even lead to a patient's death, and the refusal of Jehovah's Witnesses to consent to a blood transfusion is a commonly cited example of this (McInroy 2005). Re S and Re T are relevant legal cases. The more serious the decision to be taken, the more formal the application of this test needs to be, and the greater the requirement for sound documentation.

If the patient is not capable of making the decision, then clearly this falls to someone else, normally the doctor, nurse or social worker. It is sometimes assumed that in the absence of capacity that the next of kin has legal responsibility, but in the absence of a lasting power of attorney this is not the case. Decisions must be made 'in the best interests' of the patient. This is not as simple as it may seem, and the code of practice (Ministry of Justice 2007) gives detailed advice on what factors should be taken into consideration. In making the decision, the decision-maker should (see Figure 3.3):

- Encourage participation.
- Identify all relevant circumstances.
- Attempt to find out the patient's views.
- Avoid discrimination.
- Assess whether the patient might regain capacity.
- Not be motivated by a desire to bring about the patient's death.
- Consult others.
- Avoid restricting the patient's rights.

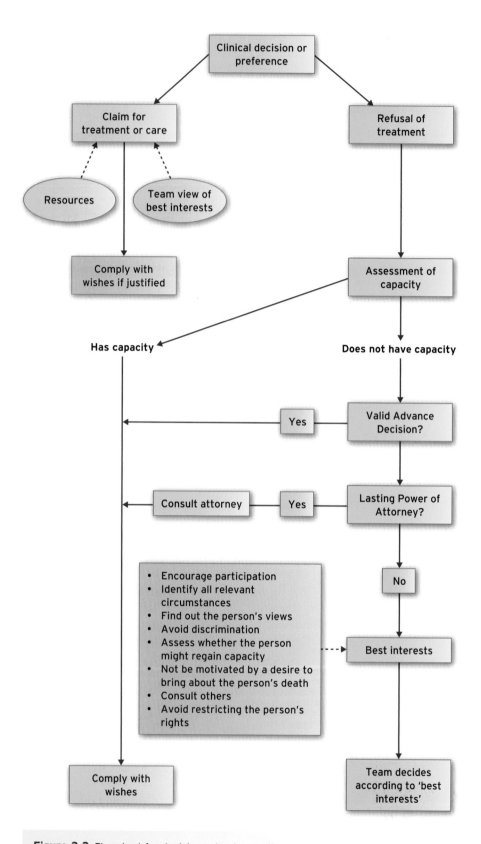

Figure 3.3 Flowchart for decisions about capacity.

Case 3.1 (continued)

The case study shows that a number of errors have been made in consenting Mr Adams for his operation. There seems to have been no assessment of his capacity, it appears to have been assumed that he lacks capacity since his daughter has signed the consent form unlawfully. The details are important, but there does not seem to have been any consideration at all of his views, nor was it apparently considered that Mr Adams' capacity to make the decision may improve with more conservative treatment after, for example, he has had some fluid, oxygen and analgesia. When Rhiannon went to Mr Adams to take him to theatre and he told her he didn't want to have the operation, at the very least this is an indication for an assessment of his capacity, which may have improved since the consent form was (unlawfully) signed. If it cannot be shown that Mr Adams does not have capacity, then his wishes not to have the operation must be respected. An operation undertaken in these circumstances is probably unlawful.

Lasting Power of Attorney and advance decisions

Lasting Power of Attorney allows a person to appoint somebody else to make health and welfare decisions on their behalf should they lose their capacity in the future.

An **advance decision** is a mechanism whereby a person can specify in advance that they do not want certain treatment at a future time when they lack capacity to make the decision.

There are two other areas of the Act which enable decisions to be made for those lacking capacity. First, **Lasting Power of Attorney** (LPA) allows a person to appoint somebody else to make health and welfare decisions on their behalf should they lose capacity in the future. There are specific processes that must be followed to give these appointments legal force, including registration with the Office of the Public Guardian. Second, the Act clarifies the arrangements for **advance decisions** that previously derived their legal status from common law. An advance decision is a mechanism whereby a person can specify in advance that they do not want certain treatment, ensuring that a person's wishes are adhered to at a future point when they are no longer able to make or communicate decisions. This is important when it can be predicted that the person will lose capacity. Again, there are specific rules attached to their operation, and there are further details in the MCA Code of Practice.

- The advance decision must be valid – the person must not have withdrawn it, made a LPA, or acted in a way inconsistent with the advance decision.

- It must be applicable to the treatment in question, explaining the circumstances which the refusal applies to.

- Advance decisions do not apply where people are lawfully detained under the Mental Health Act.

- People cannot ask for their life to be ended.

- People cannot use advance decision to ask for treatment, only to refuse it. This is a very important distinction.

Advance decisions, properly made, are legally binding on health professionals. They do not have to be written in a certain way, or on a certain form, to be binding, though many charities, for example, MIND (2008) and the Huntingdon Disease Association (2008), provide useful templates. However, where the decision refuses life-sustaining treatment, it must be in writing, signed and witnessed, and specifically state that the decision is to be applied even if life is at risk. Some have taken extreme measures to communicate their wishes, for example a woman who had her instructions tattooed on her chest. Though apparently unambiguous and demonstrating a feisty determination to make her wishes known, these tattoos in themselves would not constitute a valid advance decision, because it is not signed or witnessed and does not specify the circumstances in which it applies. The woman in question did have a valid advance decision in her notes and had made her wishes known to the local hospital (Lawn and Bassi 2008).

Documenting consent

Most nurses will be familiar with the signing of consent forms prior to procedures, and this is an obvious manifestation of the process of gaining consent. However, valid consent does not require a signature on a form, though this is considered best practice for many procedures. Valid consent can be obtained without a signature, and where a signature is present, it does not of itself demonstrate that the consent was valid. Consent can also be given orally or by implication. **Implied consent** is when a patient's actions imply that they have consented to what is being proposed, for example by rolling up a sleeve at the approach of a nurse with a sphygmomanometer. Implied consent can be regarded as an 'integral component of the nurse–patient relationship, taking account of the on-going relationship between both parties and the nature of nursing care' (Aveyard 2002 p. 202). There is a danger in confusing implied consent with acquiescence, and Aveyard (2002) suggests that verbal consent should be obtained prior to a nursing care procedure.

Implied consent is when a patient demonstrates by their actions that they consent to treatment, for example, rolling up a sleeve and putting their arm out when they see a nurse approaching with a sphygmomanometer.

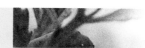

Research focus 3.1

The law and its application to nursing practice do not seem to present many opportunities for undertaking research. A question concerning what is lawful and what is not can only be settled by referral to the appropriate legal processes, not by undertaking or consulting empirical research. However, research can illuminate other concerning aspects of practice which may have legal implications.

One of the groups of practitioners who are frequently required to decide on capacity are those staff working in emergency departments, so it is to be hoped that their level of knowledge supports good and lawful practice. Evans *et al.* (2007) gave a short questionnaire about capacity and consent to 86 doctors, nurses and paramedics working in an accident department in Birmingham. The first question asked; 'what three points would you look for in assessing one's capacity to give valid consent?' (The correct answers are (1) To take in and retain information, (2) believe it, and (3) to weigh the information, balancing risks and needs). Questionnaires which gave two out of three correct responses were deemed correct, but despite this, 33 per cent of the doctors, 90 per cent of the nurses and 100 per cent of the ambulance staff gave incorrect or incomplete answers. The responses to the closed questions that completed the short questionnaire were more promising, but remember that the only available responses were yes/no/don't know. The first question asked 'If a competent adult refuses treatment, can you still treat them under common law? (correct answer = NO): 90 per cent of the doctors, 67 per cent of the nurses, and 91 per cent of the ambulance staff answered correctly. Some of the nurses were untrained, but even allowing for this, 5 registered nurses from the 19 answering the questionnaire (26 per cent) were wrong about this fundamental tenet of the legal system, which is also clearly articulated in the version of the Code of Professional Conduct current at the time of the research. The research was conducted prior to the implementation of the Mental Capacity Act (2005), and noted that the implementation of the Act was not accompanied by any strategy to train those who should be using it. However, this research demonstrates a worrying lack of knowledge of basic legal processes.

Consent and young people

Words are important in describing people under 18. The Children Act (1989), and the law in general, refers to a person under 18 as 'a child'. The Mental Capacity Act (2005) refers to an individual under 16 as a 'child' and an individual of ages 16 or 17 as a '**young person**'.

Gillick competence allows a child under the age of 16 to consent to treatment if he or she has sufficient understanding and intelligence to enable him or her to understand fully what is proposed.

The discussion on consent above specifically applies to adults over the age of 18. Different arrangements apply for young people under the age of 18. The Family Law Reform Act 1969 allows **young people** aged 16 or 17 to consent for their own treatment, and as for adults this is only the case where there is capacity. Under common law, children under 16 are also able to consent for treatment where 'the child has sufficient understanding and intelligence to enable him or her to understand fully what is proposed'. This statement has become known as '**Gillick competence**' arising from the famous case of Gillick vs West Norfolk and Wisbech AHA and Department of Health and Social Service (DHSS). Mrs Gillick challenged the lawfulness of a memorandum of guidance from the DHSS that supported the principle that a doctor could lawfully prescribe contraception to a girl under 16 years old without parental consent. Mrs Gillick challenged this on the grounds that the advice contained in the memorandum was:

- wrong and unlawful;

- harmed or potentially harmed the welfare of her children;

- affected her rights as a parent;

- interfered with her duty to care for her children.

Mrs Gillick considered that the principle within the guidelines effectively put her outside of the law and interfered with her ability and duty to protect her children. She was not suggesting that this treatment would never go ahead, but it should require her prior knowledge and consent. Mrs Gillick eventually lost.

It was ruled that in exceptional circumstances it would be lawful to provide contraceptive advice and treatment to a girl under 16 without parental consent. This ruling led to the notion of *Gillick competence* and the detailed ruling concerning contraception is known now as the *Fraser Guidelines* after Lord Fraser, who stated that the exceptional circumstances are:

1. The girl would understand the doctor's advice.
2. The doctor could not persuade her to inform her parents that she was seeking advice and treatment or allow him to do so.
3. The girl was very likely to have sexual intercourse with or without this advice and treatment.
4. Unless she received this contraceptive advice and/or treatment her physical or mental health (or both) were likely to suffer.
5. The girl's best interest requires the doctor to provide contraceptive advice, treatment or both without parental consent.

On the face of it this could be criticised as supporting unlawful sexual activity. Supporting a girl under the age of 16 in this way perhaps needs to be seen as the least bad option in the circumstances, and it must be remembered that not all children have positive relationships with their parents. This aspect of clinical practice can be seen as a human rights issue and it is the right of the child to be assessed as to the suitability for health care or medical treatment, in this case contraceptive advice or treatment.

The test of Gillick competence is applied to all treatment decisions in children under 16. The test is whether the child had sufficient understanding and intelligence to enable them to understand what is proposed. The test is usually applied by doctors, and a more holistic approach has been advocated (Parekh 2006). If the test is passed, then the child's consent to treatment is valid. In applying the test, nurses should be aware that:

- There is no specific age at which a child becomes competent to consent.
- Each child and each procedure must be considered on his/her/its own merits.
- The seriousness and complexity of the proposed procedures may be such that a child may be capable of consenting to some procedures but not to others.
- Attempts should be made to persuade the child to confide in his/her family.

The discussion above concerns childrens' and young peoples' ability to consent to treatment, but not to refuse it. This is a very important distinction, as the legal right of the young person to control what happens to their body is clear only insofar as they *agree* to what is being proposed. A *refusal* of treatment proposed by others can be overridden, leading Brazier and Cave (2007) to conclude that 'adolescent autonomy is little more than a myth' (p. 404). A number of cases support this view, including where refusal of treatment by young people has been challenged in court. The judge in the case of Re E, a 15-year-old Jehovah's Witness who attempted to refuse a blood transfusion, supported by his parents, commented that 'although parents may martyr themselves, the court should be very slow to allow an infant to martyr himself' (Woolley 2005 p. 717). There is no hard and fast guidance, and it is not suggested that a refusal of treatment by a child or young person can *always* legitimately be overruled by a parent, or a health care professional. Refusal of consent by a young person may be overruled by one or both parents, or where the parents agree with the young person, by health care professionals through the courts. Good practice depends on the individual circumstances, which will include the age and ability of the child, and the nature of the treatment under consideration. The Department of Health offers the following guidance as part of the reference guide to consent (DH 2001a), concerning young people and Gillick-competent children:

- No definitive guidance on appropriateness to overrule has been given, but it has been suggested that it should be restricted to where there is 'grave and irreversible mental or physical harm' (p. 17).
- Even where those with parental responsibility wish to overrule refusal, consideration should be given to applying to the court for a ruling prior to treatment.
- A breach of confidentiality allowing information concerning the nature of the decision to be given to parents may be justifiable where there is serious risk to the child.
- Refusal by a competent child and all persons with parental responsibility can be overruled by the court if the welfare of the child requires it.
- Where there is a life-threatening emergency, the courts have stated that doubt should be resolved in favour of preservation of life.

Nurses and other health care professionals wanting a definitive list of what is lawful and what is not will be doomed to continual disappointment; such a list does not and cannot exist. It is impossible to cover every eventuality as the law considers each case on its individual merits. However, considerable guidance is covered by official publications, and this should be sufficient for nurses to be able to make reasoned opinions, and to contribute to multi-professional decisions which can withstand scrutiny as part of professional accountability. Immediate decisions are seldom necessary and legal advice, even court rulings, can be obtained at short notice where necessary.

Consenting for children

Previous discussions on consent apply only to young people and children who are Gillick competent. Where younger children or those not Gillick competent are treated, consent must be obtained from someone with parental authority or by the court. The Children Act (1989) sets out persons who have parental responsibility (DH 2001b), and this includes:

- The child's parents if married to each other at the time of conception or birth.
- The child's mother, but not father if they were not married unless the father has acquired parental responsibility via a court order, a parental responsibility agreement, or jointly registered the child's birth, or the couple subsequently marry.
- Legally appointed guardian.
- A person in whose favour the court has made a residence order.
- A local authority in a care order in respect of the child.
- A local authority or other authorised person who holds an emergency protection order in respect of the child.

In everyday situations consenting for a child is often straightforward, but numerous complexities can arise. The rights of parents to consent and to refuse treatment for their children are limited and can be challenged. Brazier and Cave (2007) point out that many cases show that where the interests of children are concerned, courts tend to favour medical over parental opinion, and in addition the courts have made it clear that certain procedures, for example sterilisation, should not be performed without a court order. Courts can also be asked to decide where there is disagreement between parents.

It has been perhaps assumed so far that the child will comply willingly with the treatment proposed, but nurses and parents reading this chapter will know that this is not always the case. A small child aged three or four may be carried kicking and screaming into the practice nurse's room to have inoculations, but as children get older their views should at least be taken into consideration. This might be considered good lawful practice rather than the dry application of principles and case law, and it is not suggested that objections should be decisive, even of course where there is Gillick competence. The level to which a child objects to a procedure is one factor that has to be weighed up when considering best interests, and treatment performed forcibly requires justification (Brazier and Cave 2007).

Lastly, in this section, the issue of emergency treatment needs clarity. Where a child requires treatment in an emergency, and no-one is available to give consent, the law is clear that it is permissible to proceed with the treatment, on the basis that it is in the child's best interests. Indeed not to give emergency treatment because no-one is available to consent may well be indefensible.

A further Department of Health publication, *Seeking Consent, Working with Children* (DH 2001b) is available free to download from the Department of Health website, and again this should be considered required reading for those whose practice involves caring for children, and to those of us who care for our own children.

The Mental Health Act (1983 and 2007)

The Mental Health Act (1983) (MHA) governs compulsory admission and treatment of certain individuals with a mental disorder, though the majority of patients within the mental health system are not detained under the MHA and will have sought admission or treatment with consent (Dimond 2008). The main purpose of the MHA (2007) is to amend the MHA (1983).

Compulsory detention

A strict process seeks to ensure that only those who appear to be suffering from a mental disorder and are actively seeking to avoid admission to hospital are compulsorily detained (see Box 3.1). In all other circumstances, informal admission under Section 131 of the MHA (1983) is more appropriate (Griffith and Tengnah 2008). The definition of mental disorder from Section 1(2) MHA (1983) is 'any disorder or disability of the mind'. However, a person with learning disability cannot be compulsorily admitted for treatment or guardianship unless their disability is associated with abnormally aggressive or seriously irresponsible conduct (MHA 1983; Section 1(2A)). In itself, dependency upon alcohol or drugs cannot be considered a mental disorder under the MHA.

The use of powers under the MHA is required to be the least restrictive. Three groups of people are primarily involved in the processes:

- The Approved Mental Health Professional (AMHP).
- A registered medical practitioner.
- The patient's nearest relative.

The AMHP can be a nurse or social worker who has a duty to conduct an interview with a person prior to any application for detention. The AMHP is seen as providing protection from the misuse of powers.

The opinions of two medical practitioners must be sought (only one in an emergency). One doctor must be approved and recognised by the Primary Care Trust. The medical opinion must confirm that the person is suffering from a mental disorder of a *nature* or *degree* that indicates compulsory admission. The *nature* is the prognosis, person's past history, previous admissions and compliance with treatments. The *degree* of disorder is its current severity. Only one criterion has to be satisfied (Griffith and Tengnah 2008).

The nearest relative is a 'statutory friend' and is drawn from a hierarchy of relatives (see MHA 1983; Section 26). Since 1 December 2007 this includes civil partners.

The care of the patient will be supervised by an approved clinician. This can be a consultant psychiatrist but under the MHA (2007) reforms, clinical psychologists, consultant nurses and occupational therapists can also be approved clinicians. Clinicians can supervise treatment, grant leave, renew detention orders and discharge patients from hospital.

A code of practice for the MHA is available at the DH website (DH 2008). At 394 pages, it is a lengthy document, though it is easy to navigate.

Box 3.1 Compulsory admission provisions or sections within the MHA

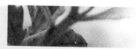

- *Section 2* Ordinary admission to hospital for up to 28 days for assessment. The application made by an Approved Mental Health Practitioner (AMHP) based on two medical recommendations, one of which is from an approved clinician. Not renewable.
- *Section 3* Admission to hospital for up to 6 months for treatment. The application made by an AMHP based on two medical recommendations, one of which is from an approved clinician. Can be renewed for further 6 months, then yearly.
- *Section 4* Admission on an emergency basis for up to 72 hours. The application made by an AMHP or nearest relative founded upon one medical recommendation. Can convert to a Section 2 if a second medical opinion is presented.
- *Section 37* Hospital order by a court for 6 months, renewable for 6 months and then yearly.
- *Section 37* Guardianship order by the court. 6 months, renewable for 6 months then yearly.
- *Section 37/41* Hospital order with restriction. *Without time limit*, with discharge and leave granted by the Home Office.

Holding power of the nurse under Section 5(4) of the MHA (1983)

The nurse must be 'prescribed' under the MHA (1983), meaning that they are trained in mental health or learning disability nursing. Section 5(4) provides for a prescribed nurse to hold a patient for up to 6 hours if they consider the patient to be at risk (Houlihan 2005). This means that the nurse can lawfully prevent an informal patient from leaving the hospital using the minimum force necessary. However:

- The patient must be an inpatient receiving treatment for mental disorder.
- The prescribed nurse must have evidence that the patient is suffering from mental disorder of such a degree that it is necessary for their health or safety or for the protection of others for them to be immediately restrained and prevented from leaving the hospital, and
- It is not possible to immediately secure the attendance of a practitioner who could exercise powers under Section 5(2) of the MHA.

The MHA only applies to care and treatment for mental disorder. If a patient detained under the MHA requires treatment for physical illness valid consent by the patient is required; where capacity is absent, the provisions of the MCA (2005) are applied. The MHA (2007) also amends the MCA (2005). Changes to the MCA (2005) provide for procedures to authorise the deprivation of liberty of a person resident in a hospital or care home who lacks capacity to consent. The MCA (2005) principles of supporting a person to make a decision when possible, and acting at all times in the person's best interests and in the least restrictive manner, will apply to all decision-making in operating the procedures. The changes in relation to the MCA are in response to the 2004 European Court of Human Rights judgment (HL v UK (Application No.45508/99), the 'Bourne-wood judgment') involving an autistic man (HL) who was kept at Bournewood Hospital by doctors against the wishes of his carers. The European Court of Human Rights found that admission to and retention in hospital of HL under the common law of necessity amounted to a breach of Article 5(1) ECHR (deprivation of liberty) and of Article 5(4) (right to have lawfulness of detention reviewed by a court).

Confidentiality

A duty of confidence arises when one person discloses information to another (e.g. patient to clinician) in circumstances where it is reasonable to expect that the information will be held in confidence. Confidentiality is:

- a legal obligation that is derived from case law;
- a requirement established with professional codes of conduct; and
- must be included within NHS employment contracts as a specific requirement linked to disciplinary procedures.

(DH 2003)

The Code (NMC 2008a) requires that:

- You must respect people's right to confidentiality.
- You must ensure people are informed about how and why information is shared by those who will be providing their care.
- You must disclose information if you believe someone may be at risk of harm, in line with the law of the country in which you are practising.

A patient has a right to expect information about them is confidential, and this right is recognised in professional codes of practice and in law. This right places a duty on all professionals and employees to work within the rules of confidentiality and to be aware as to what this duty means for them. Detailed guidance is available from the Nursing and Midwifery Council A-Z of advice and the Department of Health (2003); both are further examples of excellent

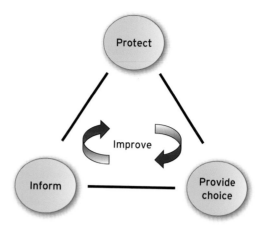

Figure 3.4 Confidentiality model.
Source: DH (2003).

free resources. The Department of Health (2003) proposes a model with four requirements (see Figure 3.4):

1. *Protect* Look after the patient's information.
2. *Inform* Ensure that patients are aware of how their information is used.
3. *Provide choice* Allow patients to decide whether their information can be disclosed or used in particular ways.
4. *Improve* Always look for ways to protect, inform and provide choice.

Confidentiality does not simply cover not discussing confidential details of patients, but also protecting the information. For example if it relates to care and treatment, it is reasonable for nurses to discuss patients between themselves, but care should be taken that these conversations cannot be overheard. Curtain screens around beds are not soundproof. Confidentiality is a duty for many professions, such as journalists, priests and lawyers, and the nature of the duty differs between them. In the area of health care, the duty is not absolute and can legitimately be breached in at least the following circumstances:

1. With the consent of the patient. An example of this is seeking permission from a patient to disclose information to their relatives. It should not be assumed that patients always give consent to allow disclosure to spouses and children about the nature and prognosis of their illnesses, care and treatment.
2. In some cases there is a legal requirement to disclose and failure to do so may result in an offence, or contempt of court. For example, statutory duty to disclose is part of the Road Traffic Act 1988 (as amended) and under terrorism legislation.
3. In the public interest. Public interest is defined by the Department of Health (2003) as:

> *exceptional circumstances that justify overruling the right of an individual to confidentiality in order to serve the broader social interest. Decisions about the public interest are complex and must take account of both the potential harm that disclosure may cause and the interest of society in the continued provision of confidential health services.*

(DH 2003 p. 6)

The Department of Health further notes that:

> *under common law, staff are permitted to disclose personal information in order to prevent and support detection, investigation and punishment of serious crime and/or to prevent abuse or serious harm to others where they judge on a case by case basis that the public good that would be achieved by the disclosure outweighs both the obligation of confidentiality to the individual patient concerned and the broader public interest in the provision of a confidential service.*

(DH 2003 p. 34)

It is worthwhile to quote at length from the NHS code of practice on confidentiality as it illustrates a number of important issues. There seems to be something of a conflict with *The Code* (NMC 2008a), which requires rather than permits disclosure where the nurse believes someone may be at risk of harm (not serious harm), though the relevent paragraph does require action to be 'in line with the law of the country in which you are practising'. Disclosure must be justified on a case by case basis – blanket justification for example in the case of a certain disease is not supported. These decisions can be very complex (Beech 2007), not least in the requirement that health care professionals must also consider wider societal interests of retaining a confidential health service; if patients knew that breaches of confidentiality were made regularly, they might be less likely to divulge information, leading to a detrimental effect on people's health and treatment.

The statement also appears to beg the question of the distinction between crime and serious crime. Like the discussion in Part 1 of this chapter about reasonableness, it must be noted that the adjective 'serious' must be subjectively applied. The Department of Health (2003) suggests that murder, rape, treason, kidnapping and child abuse are all serious, and theft, fraud or damage to property would not generally justify disclosure. It is a further illustration, if one was needed, that exhaustive lists are not possible and nurses must be able to justify their reasonable decisions. The risks of harm to others associated with infection control, for example where a sexual partner is unaware of HIV infection, can also justify disclosure (Dimond 2004). It should be clear that cases are often finely balanced, and a full discussion within the health care team is advisable. Legal advice can also be obtained if necessary.

Activity 3.3

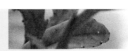

Based on the limited information available, consider how strong the case for disclosure is in the following cases. Imagine that you are involved in a multidisciplinary discussion about whether or not confidentiality should be breached. Giving reasons, what action would you advocate?

- A patient confesses to abusing a child 10 years ago.
- A patient known to have HIV infection has been admitted for treatment of chest infection. It becomes clear that his partner does not know about the HIV infection.
- After being diagnosed with epilepsy, a young woman makes it clear that she will not inform the DVLA of her condition.

Freedom of Information Act (2000)

An individual has the right to apply for access to all types of recorded information held by public authorities regardless of the date of the information. There are 23 exceptions to this right and some of these are based upon a public interest test; that is, the public body must consider if it is in the public interest to withhold the information or to release the information. There are also absolute exemptions where the public interest test does not apply, for example information provided in confidence and personal information where the applicant is the subject, which is covered by the Data Protection Act. Most exemptions fall within the category where the public interest test does apply and this includes personal information and audit functions. Accessible further information can be found on the Ministry of Justice website (Ministry of Justice 2008).

Data Protection Act (1998)

This Act gives right of access to people who have data held about them (data subjects). This includes health records and within this would be nursing records. The Act allows data subjects to:

- Know if personal information is processed.
- To have a description of the data held, purpose of processing and where and to whom it can be disclosed.
- Receive a copy of the information.
- To have details of the source of the information.

The data subject also has the right to have records corrected and apply to the court or information commissioner for an enforcement notice. Data can be corrected, prevented from being released or destroyed, or a true record inserted. The subject can seek compensation if they consider they have been harmed by the incorrect or inaccurate records.

Withholding information under the Data Protection Act

The right of access to information is a conditional rather than absolute right. The Data Protection (Subject Access Modifications) (Health) Order. Statutory Instrument 2000 No.413. makes certain provisions allowing withholding of information:

- If access 'would be likely to cause serious harm to the physical or mental health or condition of the data subject or any other person (which may include a health care professional)'.
- If access is requested by someone other than the subject (perhaps a parent about a child) this access can be denied if the subject expected it not to be disclosed and does not give their permission.
- If giving access to the subject will reveal the identity of another person then access can be denied. If the third party has given their permission then it can be disclosed or if it is reasonable and indicated to comply with the subject's request without the third party consent. Health care professionals are not included in this provision unless it can be shown that they are likely to suffer serious harm to their physical or mental health.

Human Rights Act (1998)

The Human Rights Act (1998) (HRA) made rights from the European Convention on Human Rights enforceable in UK courts (see Box 3.2). The HRA imposes a direct legal obligation on NHS Trusts to ensure they respect European Convention rights in all that they do (McHale *et al.* 2001). This means that NHS Trusts need to consider the human rights implications of all of their policies and practices. Any person who feels that an NHS Trust has breached their human rights may be able to take the Trust to court or use human rights arguments in other processes. The Department of Health (2007) has issued a framework for local action which contains a list of Key things for NHS Trusts to know about human rights:

- They are part of what it means to be a human being.
- They belong to everyone, all of the time – not only certain groups at certain times.
- They cannot be 'given' to us, only claimed or fulfilled.
- They cannot be 'taken away' from us, only limited or restricted in some circumstances.
- They are about how public authorities, such as NHS Trusts, must treat everyone as human beings.
- Sometimes they require NHS Trusts to take steps to protect human rights when they are put at risk by organisations or other individuals.
- They give expression to a set of core principles including dignity, equality, respect, fairness and autonomy.
- They exist as a way of making these core principles real and meaningful in our lives, public services and in society generally.

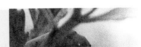

Box 3.2   Articles of the European Convention on Human Rights (ECHR)

Schedule 1 of the Human Rights Act 1998

Article 2 Right to life
Article 3 Prohibition of torture
Article 4 Prohibition of slavery
Article 5 Right to liberty and security
Article 6 Right to a fair trial
Article 7 No punishment without law
Article 8 Right to respect for private and family life
Article 9 Freedom of thought, conscience and religion
Article 10 Freedom of expression
Article 11 Freedom of assembly and association
Article 12 Right to marry
Article 14 Prohibition of discrimination
Article 16 Restrictions upon political activity of aliens
Article 17 Prohibition of abuse of rights
Article 18 Limitation on use of restrictions on rights

An example of a failed attempt to apply the provisions of the HRA is in the case of Mrs Diane Pretty, a 42-year-old woman with motor neurone disease. She wished to take her own life with the assistance of her husband as she was physically incapable of doing it herself. Mrs Pretty was confined to a wheelchair and paralysed from the neck down. Citing articles 2, 3, 8, 9 and 14, she applied for a declaration from the court that her husband would not be prosecuted if he assisted her suicide. In losing the case, the court ruled that, for example, Article 2 (The right to life) did not include the right to die.

This contrasts with the case of Miss B, a 43-year-old former social care professional who was quadriplegic and required artificial ventilation to live. She asked that her ventilation be discontinued in the knowledge that she would die. As an adult with capacity it was ruled that she could insist that treatment be stopped by withdrawing her consent. After a move to another hospital, ventilation was withdrawn and Miss B died. Subsequent debate about the cases of Miss B and Mrs Pretty argued that both women wished to determine their own fate and control their lives, but the differences in outcome did not reflect a moral difference (Singer 2002). Because Miss B required medical treatment to keep her alive and could refuse it, she could exercise her rights. Mrs Pretty could not because she needed assistance to exercise her rights and did not need immediate medical treatment that could be refused and thus withdrawn (McHale and Gallagher 2003).

Part 3: Exploring the law

Registered nurses are accountable in law for their actions and omissions. Student nurses are also accountable, though there has in the past been a misunderstanding that a student is immune in some way from the responsibility associated with mistakes or errors that amount to negligence or recklessness in practice. It is a matter of fact that nurses (student or registered) are accountable in full for all of the things for which they are responsible. The key for all nurses is to work out what they are responsible for. Where there is shared responsibility, each nurse is 100 per cent accountable for their part.

Case 3.2

Mrs Jones, a thin emaciated woman, was admitted to a medical ward one evening. She was considered to be at risk of developing a pressure sore, and an assessment showed that she should be moved to a special pressure-relieving mattress. The special mattress came to the ward at midnight, but Alice, the nurse in charge, decided not to transfer her because she feared that she would wake the other patients. The staff were very busy that night and Mrs Jones did not get turned. In the morning she was turned and it was discovered that a pressure ulcer had formed. She was transferred to the pressure-relieving mattress but the pressure ulcer became infected: it took a long time to heal and caused considerable pain and discomfort. After she finally went home, Mrs Jones sued the hospital for negligence, claiming that she should have been transferred to the special bed when it arrived on the ward.

Accountability under the law can generally be considered as being under the criminal or civil law.

Criminal

Health care staff are rarely charged with criminal offences as a result of their clinical practice, but due to the nature and effect of their practice they might become involved in cases of murder, manslaughter or assault. Criminal law can be seen as a set of rules issued on behalf of the State. These rules act as a deterrent to people who are aware that they will be punished for breaking these rules. It is extremely unlikely that any of the nurses in the scenario will face criminal charges, unless the patient died and it is considered that they intentionally attempted to harm the patient or their acts were grossly reckless.

Civil

Civil law allows individuals redress or remedy against each other when legal rights of the individual have been, or are considered likely to have been, affected. The successful outcome to civil litigation is a court order requiring or preventing an action (an injunction) or an award of money (damages). In clinical negligence claims against a nurse, a patient will seek monetary compensation for any loss suffered. The court's findings will have mainly financial implications, but liability in court can damage a nurse's professional reputation, and their employer and professional body will also be interested in what the courts decide when considering disciplinary or professional action against the nurse.

Clinical negligence

Most claims for clinical negligence never get to court. In the 10 years to 2007, 41 per cent of claims were abandoned by the claimant, 41 per cent were settled out of court, 4 per cent were settled in court, and 14 per cent remained unsettled. However, even if the chances of ending up in court are slim, this is an expensive area for the NHS. In the financial year 2006/7 clinical negligence claims cost the NHS over £600 million (National Health Service Litigation Authority 2007). Clinical negligence is claimed when a patient is dissatisfied by the care received. When people say that they are 'going to sue' it is likely that they will be taking civil action alleging negligence, and seeking damages. For a claim of negligence to succeed the following must be demonstrated:

- There must be a duty of care.
- There is a breach in the duty of care (that is the care is substandard).
- Harm has resulted.

Each of these criteria will be explored in turn in relation to the case involving Mrs Jones.

There must be a duty of care

The claimant must demonstrate that there is a duty of care owed to them personally. In the NHS there will be little difficulty in establishing the duty owed by the hospital to the patients admitted to it (Brazier and Cave 2007). It is more complex in private medicine, where the duty is part of a contract. As far as treatment out of hospital is concerned, there are as yet no laws in the UK that require a nurse to go to someone's aid, unless the victim has an existing professional relationship with the nurse or the nurse caused the situation which resulted in injury. Apart from these circumstances, if harm results from failure to assist a bystander, there can be no negligence because there is no duty of care. If a nurse does go to a bystander's assistance then a duty is accepted, and a claim in negligence is possible. If this seems to discourage nurses from assisting bystanders in peril of their health, it should be remembered that the NMC regard this as a professional if not a legal duty and so a nurse declining assistance unreasonably may find herself professionally accountable (NMC 2008b).

Case 3.2 (continued)

There clearly is a duty of care owed to Mrs Jones as she is a patient in an NHS hospital being cared for by nurses employed by the NHS.

There is a breach in the duty of care

In order to be successful in a claim of negligence, the care must be substandard in some way. In some cases the fact that the care has been substandard is obvious from the facts, for example where a swab has been left inside a patient, or where a patient has been given the wrong tablets. This is known as *res ipsa loquitor* (the thing speaks for itself). In many cases there is room to believe that the care was not substandard, or that it was the best that could be done under the circumstances. In these cases the judge will come to a view about whether or not the care breached the duty. If it did not, the case fails. If it did the case at least has a chance of success. Most judges have limited medical and nursing experience, and cannot decide using their own knowledge. So there are legal tests applied, and in applying these the views of other practitioners are sought. Essentially, there is a process whereby nurses are judged against the actions and standards of their peers. Any legal investigation will seek to compare the facts against what is currently considered adequate practice and from this make a judgement regarding responsibility and blame where there is substandard care.

The Bolam Test is used to determine whether what was done in the circumstances was acceptable and reasonable. Mr Bolam was receiving electroconvulsive therapy (ECT) and there were, in the 1950s, two 'schools of thought' about how patients should be managed and treated during the procedure. One method recommended that relaxant drugs should be used and the other that they should not as there is a risk of fractures to the patient during the treatment. The claimant (Mr Bolam), was not warned of the risk of fractures, had not been given the relaxant drugs, and had not been restrained to prevent injury. He suffered a fractured hip and alleged negligence. In directing the jury (at that time these cases were heard before juries), the Judge said that:

> A doctor is not guilty of negligence if he has acted in accordance with a practice accepted as proper by a responsible body of medical men skilled in that particular act . . . Putting it the other way round, a doctor is not negligent, if he is acting in accordance with such a practice, merely because there is a body of opinion that takes a contrary view.
> Bolam v Friern Hospital Management Committee [1957] 2 All ER 118

Though this case concerned doctors, the same test of comparing a practice claimed to be a breach in the duty of care to practice accepted by a group of practitioners can be applied to nurses and other health care professionals. It has been argued that in the years after the Bolam case was decided in favour of the doctors, the test was used to allow 'judgement by colleagues to substitute for judgement by the courts' (Brazier and Miola 2000 p. 89), forming part of a general deference to doctors by the courts.

The House of Lords has modified or developed understandings of Bolam in the case of Bolitho [1997]. Cases subsequent to *Bolam* used different adjectives to describe the 'body of medical opinion', such as 'responsible', 'reasonable' and 'respectable'. A case in 1997 (though the events took place in 1984) clarified the test. Patrick Bolitho, aged two, was admitted to hospital suffering from respiratory difficulty. He had a collapse, followed by respiratory arrest and subsequently died. The defendant, the paediatric registrar, was summoned but failed to attend the emergency, and admitted that this was a breach of duty. However, negligence was denied on the grounds that even if she had attended she would not have intubated Patrick, and this was required to prevent the subsequent disastrous respiratory arrest. Expert witnesses gave evidence to support both intubation and non-intubation before the collapse, and since a responsible body of medical opinion agreed that she should not have intubated (even if she had attended), then her absence could not have caused the death. So the case failed on lack of causation. On appeal to the House of Lords, their Lordships found that the court does not have to find for the doctor if a responsible body of opinion supports the practice questioned: '. . . the court has to be satisfied that the exponents of the body of opinion relied upon can demonstrate that such opinion has a logical basis'.

Case 3.2 (continued)

In the case of Mrs Jones the question would be whether failure to transfer her to a special bed was a breach of duty. Staff Nurse Smith had decided against because she did not want to disturb Mrs Jones or the rest of the patients. Perhaps witnesses would be called to agree or disagree with this course of action, and the precise details would be very important. It could have been reasonable not to transfer her to the bed if she was turned regularly. Perhaps she was turned regularly, but does the documentation or other evidence support this? Any deviation from normal practice in exceptional circumstances needs to be justified and documented.

Harm has occurred

It is possible that both of the other conditions required for a successful claim for negligence are satisfied, without harm having occurred. So in the case of Mrs Smith, if the nursing staff had acted appallingly by not moving the patient onto the bed because they could not be bothered, but no harm occurred, the case will not succeed and no damages are payable. This does not mean that they would not be held to account in other ways. In other cases for mainly reasons of bad luck, severe harm has been caused. There is a principle within law of 'thin skull', illustrated by the case of Smith v Leech Brain & Co. Ltd, in which a worker was splashed on the lip with molten metal and eventually died. The company admitted liability for the original accident but denied that they were to blame for the unfortunate death from cancer of the victim. The judge in the case ruled that the test in this case was not whether it is foreseeable that the victim would be harmed and that he would die, it was whether the original event was foreseeable. What happens to the victim after this was directly related to the 'constitution of the victim'. The widow was able to win damages. Nurses should be aware that even though they could not see or reasonably predict that serious harm would occur they would be expected to see that their act or omission would cause the initial event (Dimond 2008). Even if the infection in the pressure ulcer was not foreseeable, the fact that a pressure ulcer could form probably was.

The harm has to be reasonably foreseeable. A reasonable person is not expected to predict unknown risks. Unforeseeable risks cannot be anticipated and failing to protect against them would not be negligent. In Roe v. Minister of Health [1954] the claimant (patient) suffered pain and permanent paralysis from the waist down, after being injected with a spinal anaesthesia (nupercaine). This nupercaine had been stored in glass ampoules which had been placed in a phenol solution, a disinfectant. Evidence was produced at the trial that minute and invisible cracks had formed in the glass ampoules, allowing some of the nupercaine to be contaminated by the phenol, which then damaged the patient. It was accepted at the trial that such an occurrence was reasonably unforeseeable and that such a phenomenon had not previously been detected or anticipated. It could not therefore be guarded against and so the defendants escaped liability for negligence. However, the law would expect the health care system to learn from these mistakes and if a similar event were to occur it could be seen as negligence as it should have been anticipated. Safe systems of work need to be introduced so that incidents like this can be reported and disseminated. Risk management is discussed more fully in Chapter 12.

Case 3.2 (continued)

In the case of Mrs Jones, the question would be whether the failure to put her on the bed caused the pressure ulcer. If her position had been changed regularly throughout the night, it may be difficult to demonstrate causation; perhaps the damage had already been done, and transferring her to the special bed would not have made any difference. To succeed in the case, Mrs Jones would have to show that she should have been transferred, *and* that the failure to transfer caused the pressure ulcer. If she can do this, on the balance of probabilities, she could win the case and be awarded damages.

Damages

Legal action can be very expensive, especially if a decision is appealed to a higher court, and damages can be substantial. Nurses are advised by the NMC to have professional indemnity insurance, and this is offered by trades unions and professional bodies. Previously the possibility of having to bear costs may have deterred potential litigants, but in recent years many firms of solicitors have operated a 'no win, no fee' system whereby solicitors' costs are payable only if the case is settled, removing risk but reducing payout, and having at least the potential to increase the numbers of litigants. In some cases claimants

Vicarious liability is when one person, or organisation, is liable for the negligent acts of another person.

can also sue the employer through **vicarious liability**, and so the costs are against the NHS, rather than to individual nurses or their insurers. Vicarious liability arises if certain criteria are satisfied, and if the negligent act occurred during the course of employment. Generally it would be in the interests of the claimant to pursue vicarious liability as, despite their tight financial position, NHS Trusts are better placed to settle claims than individuals.

Employment

As an employee, a nurse has a duty to her employer to obey reasonable and lawful instructions and to take all reasonable care and skill in carrying out duties. This principle is based upon the view of courts, unless proven otherwise, that implied terms exist (conditions or terms that exist even though not explicitly written or discussed) in a contract of employment. Indeed, a job description will usually only reflect a small proportion of duties and responsibilities of the employee; the fine details are implied and relate to the area of practice. It is often argued that it would be impossible to list all duties of an employee and that there is a need for flexibility. This does not, however, give the employer the right to vary terms of employment without consultation.

A nurse will be held personally liable by their employer and subject to disciplinary action, if they fail to take care or fall below a reasonable standard of practice whilst giving care. Under these circumstances the employer has a right to intervene. In fact they might consider this a duty to protect both the public and the nurse. This intervention can range from verbal or written warning through to suspension, compulsory re-training, demotion or possibly dismissal.

Conclusion

Nurses' practice has always been governed and supported by law. In a sense this is self-evident as all citizens are required to follow the law, and are at risk of censure and punishment if it is broken. The standards of proficiency for pre-registration nursing education require that nurses have knowledge of the relevant legislation, and this requirement has been incorporated explicitly in the latest version of *The Code* (NMC 2008a), which refers to the legislation concerning mental capacity. This chapter has given details about some of the important areas of legislation, notably concerning consent to treatment, an area of law which governs practice every time a nurse touches a patient. A common theme running through the chapter is that codified law cannot tell a nurse what to do in every situation, and in this regard at least, legal accountability has similarities to professional accountability. The NMC Code makes it very clear on a number of occasions that the law must be followed in the country in which the nurse is practising, and to do this the nurse must know what that lawful practice requires, and also know the processes that are followed when actions or omissions are challenged. This challenge is the basis of accountability, both legal and professional. Nurses must be able to defend their actions and omissions, and while both legal and professional redress are rarer than many people seem to think, the habit of defending actions to others, to peers, colleagues, in supervision and in audit can only advance practice. As long as a nurse follows the law where it is clear and can defend reasonable actions where it is not, they have nothing to fear from the law.

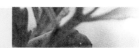

Box 3.3   Cases referred to in the text

These cases are in England unless specifically mentioned otherwise. Other jurisdictions such as Canada and Australia can be quoted in English legal judgments. The numbers and letters refer to where the cases are reported. For example, the case of Bolam v Friern Hospital Management Committee is reported in volume 2 of the 1957 editions of the *All England Law Report* starting at page 118. These references can be used to access a full report of the case, including full judgments, via legal databases.

- Allan v New Mount Sinai Hospital [1980] 109 DLR (3d) 634 (Canadian High Court)
- Bolam v Friern Hospital Management Committee [1957] 2 All ER 118
- Bolitho v City and Hackney Health Authority [1998] AC 232
- Gillick vs West Norfolk and Wisbech AHA and DHSS [1985] 3 All ER 402
- Pearce v United Bristol Healthcare Trust [1991] PIQRP 53
- Pretty v United Kingdom [2002] (Application 2346/02) European Court of Human Rights
- Re C (An Adult: refusal of medical treatment) [1994] 1 All ER 819, (1993) 15 BMLR 77
- Re E (A Minor) (Wardship: Medical treatment) [1993] 1 FLR 386
- Re S (An Adult: refusal of medical treatment) [1992] 4 All ER 671
- Re T (An Adult: refusal of medical treatment) [1992] 4 All ER 649
- Roe v. Minister of Health [1954] 2 QB 66
- Rogers v. Whitaker [1992] 67 ALJR 47 (Australian High Court)
- Smith v Leech Brain & Co. Ltd; QBD [1961] 3 All ER 1159

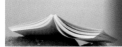

Suggested further reading

There are a number of textbooks covering health care law in general and the law as it affects nurses in particular.

Brazier, M. and Cave, E. (2007) *Medicine, Patients and the Law* (4th ed.), London: Penguin.
Dimond, B. (2008) *Legal Aspects of Nursing* (5th ed.), London: Pearson Longman.
Mason, J. K. and McCall Smith, A. (2005) *Mason and McCall Smith's Law and Medical Ethics*, Oxford, New York: Oxford University Press.

Journals

Journal of Health Politics Policy and Law
Medical Law Review
Medical Law Reports
Medical Law Monitor

Websites

Websites of reputable origin are valuable resources and free. Websites of charities often offer legal resources in their particular field. The value of 'official' websites should not be underestimated, for example, a wide range of resources about the Mental Capacity Act and the Human Rights Act can be found on government websites at the Department of Health and Ministry of Justice, respectively.

References

Akkad, A., Jackson, C., Kenyon, S., *et al.* (2004) Informed consent for elective and emergency surgery: questionnaire study. *British Journal of Obstetrics and Gynaecology* **111** (10), 1133–1138.

Aveyard, H. (2002), Implied consent prior to nursing care procedures. *Journal of Advanced Nursing* **39** (2), 201–207.

Beech, M. (2007) Confidentiality in health care: conflicting legal and ethical principles. *Nursing Standard* **21** (21), 42–46.

Brazier, M. and Miola, J. (2000) Bye-bye Bolam: a medical litigation revolution? *Medical Law Review* **8** (1), 85–114.

Brazier, M. and Cave, E. (2007) *Medicine, Patients and the Law* (4th ed.). London: Penguin.

DH (Department of Health) (2001a) *Reference Guide to Consent for Examination or Treatment*, London: DH (http://www.dh.gov.uk).

DH (2001b) *Seeking Consent: Working with children*. London: DH (http://www.dh.gov.uk).

DH (2003) *Confidentiality. NHS code of practice*. London: DH (http://www.dh.gov.uk).

DH (2007) *Human Rights in Healthcare – A framework for local action*. London: DH (http://www.dh.gov.uk).

DH (2008) *Code of Practice – Mental Health Act*. London: DH (http://www.dh.gov.uk).

Dimond, B. (2004) A patient is told that he is HIV positive and he asks for this to be kept a secret from his wife: what should you do? *Nursing Times* **100** (45), 18.

Dimond, B. (2008) *Legal Aspects of Nursing* (5th ed.). London: Pearson Longman.

Evans, K., Warner, J. and Jackson, E. (2007) How much do emergency workers know about capacity and consent? *Emergency Medicine Journal* **24** (6), 391–393.

Griffith, R. and Tengnah, C. (2008) *Law and Professional Issues in Nursing*. Exeter: Learning Matters Limited.

Henderson, S. (2003) Power imbalances between nurses and patients: a potential inhibitor of partnership in care. *Journal of Clinical Nursing* **12** (4), 501–508.

Houlihan, G. D. (2005) The powers and duties of psychiatric nurses under the Mental Health Act 1983: a review of the statutory provisions in England and Wales. *Journal of Psychiatric and Mental Health Nursing* **12** (3), 317–324.

Huntingdon Disease Association. (2008) *Advance Directive*. (http://www.hda.org.uk).

Lawn, A. and Bassi, D. (2008) An unusual resuscitation request. *Resuscitation* **78** (1), 5–6.

McGeehan, R. (2007) Best practice in record keeping. *Nursing Standard* **21** (17), 51–55.

McHale, J., Gallagher, A. and Mason, I. (2001) The UK Human Rights Act 1998: implications for nurses. *Nursing Ethics* **8** (3), 223–233.

McHale, J. and Gallagher, A. (2003) *Nursing and Human Rights.* London: Butterworth Heinemann.

McInroy, A. (2005) Blood transfusion and Jehovah's Witnesses: the legal and ethical issues. *British Journal of Nursing* **14** (5), 270–274.

MIND (2008) Advance Directive (Personal crisis plan for mental healthcare advance decision-making) (http://www.mind.org.uk).

Ministry of Justice (2007) *Mental Capacity Act Code of Practice.* London: The Stationery Office (http://www.justice.gov.uk).

Ministry of Justice (2008) *Freedom of Information.* (http://www.justice.gov.uk).

National Health Service Litigation Authority (2007) *Report and Accounts 2007.* London: The Stationery Office (http://www.nhlsa.com).

NMC (Nursing and Midwifery Council) (2004) *Standards of Proficiency for Pre-registration Nursing Education.* London: NMC (http://www.nmc-uk.org).

NMC (2007) *Record Keeping.* London: NMC (http://www.nmc-uk.org).

NMC (2008a) *The Code. Standards for conduct, performance and ethics for nurses and midwives.* London: NMC (http://www.nmc-uk.org).

NMC (2008b) *Providing Care in an Emergency Situation Outside the Work Environment.* London: NMC (http://www.nmc-uk.org).

Office of the Public Guardian (2007) *Making Decisions: A guide for people who work in health and social care* (3rd ed.). (http://www.publicguardian.gov.uk).

Oxford English Dictionary (2008) http://dictionary.oed.com/entrance.dtl

Parekh, S. A. (2006) Child consent and the law: an insight and discussion into the law relating to consent and competence. *Child Care, Health and Development* **33** (1), 78–82.

Singer, P. (2002) Ms B and Diane Pretty: a commentary. *Journal of Medical Ethics* **28** (4), 234–235.

Woolley, S. (2005) Children of Jehovah's Witnesses and adolescent Jehovah's Witnesses: What are their rights? *Archives of Disease in Childhood* **90** (7), 715–719.

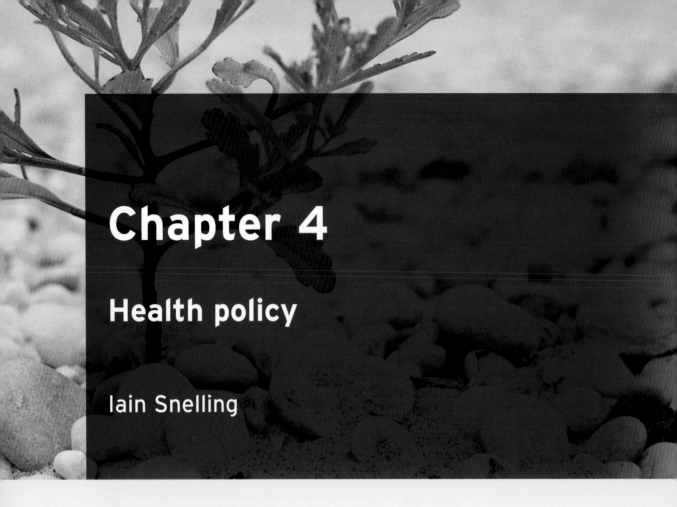

Chapter 4

Health policy

Iain Snelling

Learning outcomes

After reading and reflecting on this chapter, you should be able to:

- Discuss the way in which health care policy is made and implemented;
- Outline the way in which health care policy influences the management of health care services;
- Discuss the relevance of health care policy to nursing practice;
- Explain how you are able to update your knowledge and understanding.

Related NMC Standards of Proficiency for Pre-registration Nursing Education (NMC 2004)

- Demonstrate knowledge of legislation and health and social policy relevant to nursing practice.

Introduction

The establishment and maintenance of the National Health Service (NHS) is rightly considered one of the major achievements of our nation. The intensity of the political debates about the NHS and its future direction is clear evidence of its importance. The NHS is the largest employer in Europe, employing approximately 1.3 million people. Health policy is more than *just* political policy about *just* the NHS. However, NHS spending accounts for the vast majority of all spending on health care, and the way that the NHS is funded and managed are primarily political questions.

The chapter is divided into three parts.

In Part 1, health policy is outlined, the concept of health policy is introduced, and the role of politicians in the running of the NHS is discussed.

In Part 2, the current reforms of the NHS are placed in an historical context. Details about structures of the NHS and how these facilitate reform are explained along with how these put the patient at the centre of the NHS.

In Part 3, the role of research in evaluating and influencing health policy is explored. Recent improvements in performance are discussed and government efforts to look to the medium-term future to produce an NHS for the next generation are introduced.

Part 1: Outlining health policy

Case 4.1

Brian, a recently qualified staff nurse, attended a ward meeting today. The Director of Nursing came to talk about the hospital's application to become a Foundation Trust. She had said that the hospital finances had to be improved. Lengths of stay were too high, and the joint working with community services and GPs could be improved. Some work might be moved out of the hospital. The hospital also had to reduce infections, and make people want to have their treatment there, because otherwise they might go somewhere else. Brian had to leave before the end because there weren't enough nurses on the ward. Brian's colleagues think that they should understand what is driving all these changes so that they can decide how to develop their careers, and help to improve services. Brian is not sure that they shouldn't just try to keep things as they are, and try to get a few more staff.

What is policy and how is it made?

Health policy is the statement of priorities relating to health issues and the broad means through which these priorities will be addressed.

Health policy is determined by the government, principally through the Department of Health (DH) in England, although as far as the availability of resources is concerned, the Treasury will have the major influence.

Government policy is made by ministers who are appointed by the Prime Minister. The senior minister at the DH is the Secretary of State for Health. He or she is a member of the Cabinet which is the highest decision-making body in government, chaired by the Prime Minister, who also appoints all of its members. There are also five junior Ministers in the DH. Ministers of State are a higher rank than Parliamentary Under Secretaries. In December 2008 the junior ministerial posts were:

- Minister of State for Health Services
- Minister of State for Public Health
- Minister of State for Care Services
- Parliamentary Under Secretary of State
- Parliamentary Under Secretary of State for Health Services.

Each minister has a specific portfolio of responsibilities, detailed on the DH website. Ministers have a range of duties but their primary purpose is to be accountable to parliament for the work of the department. Ministers are Members of Parliament either of the House of Commons (hence the initials MP) to which they will have been elected, or the House of Lords. One member of the ministerial team will be a member of the House of Lords representing the whole department there. Accountability means having the responsibility to explain (account for) policies and their implementation, usually through oral and written questions. Where health policy requires a change in the law, ministers present legislation to parliament. Increasingly, accountability has a more public face, with ministers being interviewed through the media to explain policies directly to the population.

Activity 4.1

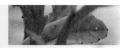

Find out from the Department of Health website who the current health ministers are, and what their duties are.

Each government department has a Permanent Secretary, the highest civil servant in the department, who advises the Secretary of State, and is responsible for the management of the department. There is a clear division in government between making policy, which is the responsibility of ministers, and for carrying it out, which is the responsibility of the civil service. Civil servants remain accountable to the Cabinet Secretary – the head of the civil service – rather than ministers in their own department.

The DH has a Permanent Secretary but it also has a Chief Executive of the NHS who has equal status, reflecting the importance of the NHS in carrying out health policy. There is also a board for the department, and a senior team. One of the members of the senior team is the Chief Nursing Officer. The role of the Chief Nursing Officer is explained on the DH website. The Chief Nursing Officer:

- *provides expert advice on nursing, midwifery and health visiting to government and helps to develop, implement and evaluate government health policy, leading on nursing, midwifery and health visiting policy and strategy in support of the government's objectives*

- *provides professional leadership to the nursing, midwifery and health visiting professions in England, working closely with the professional statutory bodies, professional and staff associations, NHS managers, and the voluntary and independent sectors*
- *ensures an effective UK contribution to nursing and health policy in international fora, including the World Health Organization, the Commonwealth and Europe*
- *contributes to the Department's central task of managing the NHS.*

(DH 2008a)

The Chief Nursing Officer (CNO) has a section on the DH website. A free monthly e-bulletin is issued providing up-to-date information about NHS news and related developments of specific interest to nurses.

Activity 4.2

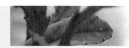

Log on to the CNO website and sign up for the monthly bulletin.

Although a definition of policy has been given, and a distinction has been made between policy-making and implementation, in reality things are more complex. Ham notes that 'although many writers have attempted to define policy, there is little agreement on the meaning of the word' (Ham 2004 p. 113). He makes five points about the study of policy:

1. Policy includes both decisions and actions. We can study formal decisions, and the process through which the decisions were made, but 'what happens in practice may be different from what was intended by the policy-makers' (Ham 2004 p. 113). Understanding how policy is implemented is as important as understanding the policy itself.
2. Policy may not be expressed as a single decision, but as a series of decisions taken by different groups of people. A policy may not have a single clear definition: 'It tends to be defined in terms of a series of decisions which, taken together, comprise a more or less common understanding of what the policy is' (Ham 2004 p. 114).
3. Policy changes evolve over time in a dynamic process rather than a series of discrete steps. An explanation of current policy can be given in terms of how it has evolved through a number of developments, each drawing from the experience of what has gone before. Some of these developments represent discrete changes, while others may involve changes in the pace or style of implementation.
4. Studying how policy is made can ignore the role of maintaining the status quo; 'non decision-making', the political process of resisting change. This may be particularly important when policy is developing quickly, raising the importance of opposition, in terms of both the formal process of decision-making and its implementation. For example in 2001 Dr Richard Taylor, a retired consultant physician, was elected as an independent MP after a local campaign to downgrade the facilities at Kidderminster Hospital. He was re-elected in 2005. This highlights the significance of processes designed to stop change rather than promote it.

5. Finally, policy 'can be seen as actions without decisions' (Ham 2004 p. 114). We normally think of policy as 'top-down' from the government to those who implement it. Policy can also be made 'bottom-up', where the actions of those who deliver services or who lead them, can be said to have made policy. This may become more important as the system of health care provision becomes more diverse and less centrally controlled, one of the key trends highlighted in this chapter.

So, although health policy is at one level a reasonably clear concept, there are complications. It is not as simple as deciding what to do, and then deciding how it should be done. It is a complex evolving process, involving many individuals and groups. Ministers have overall responsibility but they do not simply impose decisions. Many reasons for a particular policy reflect wider changes in society, such as the development of improved information and communication technology, changes in the law (including European law), and the development of consumerism. Learning about health policy is not just about learning what it is. It requires developing understanding of the wider context of health care provision and how it will affect you, your career and your patients.

Policy focus 4.1

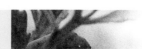

Official Government policy documents

A White Paper is a formal statement of government policy, published 'by command of Her Majesty'. The author of a White Paper is a government minister, who presents it to parliament, hence the author reference is the relevant minister and a command number is included. For example: Secretary of State for Health (2008). *High Quality Care For All*. Cm 7432. London: The Stationery Office. In many cases, a White Paper requires legislation for implementation. White Papers are published by the Stationery Office, and can be downloaded free of charge from DH, although hard copies can only be purchased. These documents tend to be long, but usually have an executive summary.

Green Papers are sometimes presented to Parliament to outline policy options. These are rarer than they used to be, perhaps because there are now many more ways of consulting on policy. An example of a recent Green Paper concerned the future of Social Care for Adults: Secretary of State for Health (2005). *Independence, Well-being and Choice*. Cm 6499. London: The Stationery Office.

Many significant policy papers are published by the DH. For these the author is usually the Department itself. These papers do not require legislation; they usually explain the implementation of policy. These papers can also be downloaded free of charge. An example is: DH (2004) *National Standards, Local Action. Health and social care standards and planning framework*. 2004/5–2007/8.

The DH provides guidance on a number of issues, and its website has a wealth of information. From the home page, there are tabs including 'policy and guidance'. From here there is an A-Z resource, which covers a huge range of policy and guidance, all available to download. Some documents are also available in paper format. One way of finding out which are available in this format is to look at the back page of the electronic version.

Health policy and health care policy

The title of this chapter is Health policy. The learning outcomes relate to 'health care policy'. Health policy, which is concerned with all matters relating to health, is wider than health care policy, which relates to the health care system – how it is financed and delivered. The Department of Health has three departmental strategic objectives, agreed as part of the Government's comprehensive spending review in 2007:

- *To ensure better health and well-being for all: helping you stay healthy and well, empowering you to live independently and tackling health inequalities.*
- *Ensure better care for all: the best possible health and social care when and where you need help giving you choice and control; and*
- *Provide better value for all.*

(Chancellor of the Exchequer 2007 p. 205)

As well as highlighting the distinction between health and health care, these objectives also emphasise the responsibility of the Department of Health for *Social Care*. The relevant standard of proficiency for pre-registration nurse education quoted at the beginning of the chapter also includes social policy, which includes policies relating to a broad range of social issues, including for example wider public services and economic development. It is not possible to include all of these areas in the chapter.

The NHS is the main vehicle through which health care policy is implemented. Over the last decade or so the NHS has gone through significant changes, many of them controversial. A key reference document for understanding current policy and future direction is the White Paper published in June 2008 close to the 60th anniversary of the founding of the NHS on 5 July 1948. *High Quality Care for All* (Secretary of State for Health 2008) is often referred to as the Darzi review, since the work of detailed planning and consultation that preceded it was led by Lord Darzi, a Minister for Health who is also an eminent NHS surgeon. *High Quality Care for All* makes the case for a written constitution for the NHS.

> the NHS must continue to change. But the fundamental purpose and values of the NHS can and must remain constant. Setting this out clearly, along with the rights and responsibilities of patients, the public and staff, will give us all greater confidence to meet the challenges of the future on the basis of a shared understanding and common purpose.

(Secretary of State for Health 2008 p. 77)

A draft constitution was published with the Darzi Review, and after consultation the *NHS Constitution for England* was published in January 2009. It has seven key principles that 'guide the NHS in all it does' (DH 2009, p. 3). The principles are given in Policy focus 4.2, in a briefer form than in the consultation document (DH 2009), and it is intended that the NHS, including independent providers who provide NHS services, will have to take the Constitution into account when making decisions. The principles reflect the aims of policy for the NHS that have been written in various documents over a number of years, but the NHS Constitution will clarify them, giving them an enhanced practical status.

Policy focus 4.2

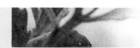

NHS Constitution. Principles that guide the NHS

The NHS provides a comprehensive service, available to all ... (and) it has a wider social duty to promote equality through the services it provides ...

Access to NHS services is based on clinical need, not an individual's ability to pay.

The NHS aspires to the highest standards of excellence and professionalism.

NHS services must reflect the needs and preferences of patients, their families, and their carers.

The NHS works across organisational boundaries and in partnership with other organisations in the interest of patients, local communities and the wider population.

The NHS is committed to providing best value for taxpayers' money and the most effective, fair and sustainable use of finite resources.

The NHS is accountable to the public, communities, and patients that it serves.

(DH 2009)

Activity 4.3

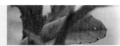

In small groups discuss these principles, and consider the extent to which you think the NHS meets them.

Part 2: Explaining health policy

A brief history of the NHS

Primary Care is given in the community and is something patients themselves choose to access. Secondary care is more specialised, usually based in a local hospital, and requiring a referral. Tertiary care is more specialised still, usually requiring a referral from secondary care, for example specialised surgical services in a regional centre.

A brief history of the NHS may help you understand the context of the changes currently being implemented. The NHS was founded in 1948 as part of the welfare state created after the Second World War. The hospital service, including municipal hospitals run by local authorities, and voluntary hospitals was nationalised. Their employees, including medical staff, became employees of the state, although the right of consultants to maintain private practice was retained. General practitioners (GPs) on the other hand remained independent, contracting to provide services for the NHS. This distinction between **primary care** provided by GPs and hospital care remains substantially in place today.

Reorganisations of the NHS in 1974 and 1982 changed the management structure but left the essential infrastructure intact. In the late 1980s however, there was a series of service crises and bad headlines. A review was followed by publication in 1989 of a White Paper, *Working for Patients* (Secretary of State for Health 1989) which proposed far-reaching changes, much more radical than previous reorganisations and resulting in an 'explosion of opposition' (Klein 2001 p. 163). At the heart of the proposals was the establishment of an internal market, establishing what was known as the purchaser-provider split. The internal market introduced the policy of competition between health care providers for contracts for services that purchasers (mainly District Health Authorities) would manage.

The internal market never really developed into an effective market place. In 1990 John Major replaced Margaret Thatcher as Prime Minister and his approach was less radical. The Major government launched the patients' charter, part of a wider citizens' charter initiative, which gave explicit rights to patients, such as the first maximum waiting time guarantee. However, the reforms of the early 1990s did establish market principles in the NHS.

Development of the NHS was a key area of the 1997 general election with an apparent choice of market principles on the one hand (Conservatives), against the re-establishment of a national, planned service on the other (Labour). Labour won the election and promised to end the internal market. The Labour Party Manifesto promised that 'Our fundamental purpose is simple but hugely important: to restore the NHS as a public service working co-operatively for patients, not a commercial business driven by competition' (New Labour 1997). Since 1997, there have been a number of landmark publications through which the development of health policy can be traced. The first Labour policy statement on the NHS, *The New NHS. Modern. Dependable.* (Secretary of State for Health 1997) announced changes, but also retained the basic structure of the NHS. Over the succeeding years of the Labour Government, the internal market was not abolished but strengthened, although it took many years of development before the structure of the current NHS took shape.

The NHS Plan, published in 2000, (Secretary of State for Health 2000) is widely regarded as a key point for the NHS. The NHS Plan was a start point for recent policy because it developed two themes which have been influential ever since, summed up in its subtitle: 'A plan for investment, A plan for reform'. As well as identifying that additional resources were required, The NHS Plan expressed the firm view that as far as delivering services were concerned the basic model had not really changed since the 1940s. Services were organised from the perspective of the organisations and professions providing them rather than according to the needs and preferences of the people using them. Inefficient appointment systems, waiting lists, poor communication, frequent visits to large impersonal hospitals, and strictly demarcated professional roles were all features of this view. The NHS Plan stated therefore, that the NHS was to be 'redesigned' around the needs and preferences of patients. The NHS Plan contained many targets and pledges designed to improve the patient focus of the NHS. The targets that had the highest profile and caused the most difficulty were waiting time targets, which have subsequently been made tougher still. The reforms evolved into new directions not envisaged at the time, such as changes to the organisational structure of the NHS, but every new policy initiative has had, as a central aim, improving the patient focus of the NHS, not just through structural changes but more importantly through changing the culture.

A significant policy initiative was launched in 2006: *Our Health, Our Care, Our Say* (Secretary of State for Health 2006). This White Paper was subtitled 'A new direction for community services'. Previously the emphasis had been on improving hospital services – for example through reducing waiting lists for services, and improving quality. The new strategic direction emphasised the development of services in the community:

> *Our longer-term aim is to bring about a sustained realignment of the whole health and social care system. Far more services will be delivered - safely and effectively – in settings closer to home; people will have real choices in both primary care and social care; and services will be integrated and built round the needs of individuals and not service providers. Year on year, as NHS budgets rise, we will see higher growth in prevention, primary and community care than in secondary care, and also resources will shift from the latter to the former.*
>
> (Secretary of State for Health 2006 p. 17)

Specifically, the White Paper set out four goals:

1. Better prevention services with earlier intervention.
2. More choice and a louder voice.
3. Do more on tackling inequalities and improving access to community services.
4. More support for people with long-term needs.

This brings us almost up to date – the Darzi review is the most recent key reference point for policy development. Before we get to that though, some of the important themes in health care policy will be identified; the Darzi review is not about new targets or structures but about making the structure we have work better for patients.

Funding health services

The organisation of health services is a key issue for health policy, but perhaps the biggest issue is how health services are funded, and how much spending is devoted to them. Throughout the lifetime of the NHS, it has always been funded predominantly by general taxation.

Activity 4.4

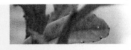

Jot down your answers (or guesses!) to the following questions. If you do this quick exercise in a group, discuss the reasons for your individual answers.

- How much money does the government spend annually on health? How does health expenditure compare with other areas of public spending such as defence and education?
- How does the UK differ from other countries in terms of the percentage of total national expenditure that goes on health and the percentage of spending that comes from the government?

The answers are given at the end of this section.

The answers to these questions sum up important top level health policy issues for government. They are expressed here in financial terms but really they are wider issues. For example, what balance should there be between individual and governmental responsibility for providing health services? How should health care relate to other government expenditure priorities, many of which will affect health – for example, housing and employment? There is a wide consensus in the UK that health care should continue to be funded mainly through taxation, with most services free at the point of use. However, there are other methods of funding, and most countries, including the UK, use a mix of methods. Though the NHS is mainly funded through general taxation, some charges are levied, for example for prescriptions (in England) and dentistry. There is also a small private sector, funded mainly from insurance. Robinson (2006) identifies that funding methods include:

1. Private insurance. This is optional insurance, taken out by individuals, or companies on behalf of their employees.
2. Social insurance. This is a form of compulsory insurance, paid by individuals or employers.
3. Taxation. Funding health services through taxation also has a number of different possibilities since there are many ways of governments raising funds through taxation, for example income tax and VAT.
4. Charges and co-payments. Sometimes this is known as 'out of pocket' charges to distinguish it from insurance.

In recent years there has been a significant increase in health expenditure, starting with the *The NHS Plan* which recognised that underfunding was a major problem in the NHS, and committed to a real terms increase (i.e., after the effects of inflation have been taken into account) of one-third over 5 years. In 2002, the Treasury published a report by Derek Wanless (2002) which considered the resources required for the NHS over two decades, taking into account developments in a number of factors, such as changing expectations and health care needs, and the possibilities offered by medical advances. A conclusion of the review was that health care spending needed to increase substantially over the period considered (up until 2023), particularly in the early years to 'catch up'; a real terms increase in excess of 7 per cent per annum for 5 years was recommended. This was implemented but the period of 'catch up' ended in 2008, and growth in NHS expenditure will return to more traditional levels, still giving a significant real growth in resources each year, 4 per cent for the next three years (DH 2008c). At the time of writing (March 2009) it is not known how the current credit crunch will affect NHS funding.

Answers to questions in Activity 4.4

- The Chancellor's budget in 2008 outlined that the plan for health spending in 2008/9 is likely to be £111 billion (HM Treasury 2008). Other major areas of spending include social protection, which is made up of payments to individuals, such as pensions and benefits (£169 billion), education (£82 billion), defence (£33 billion) and personal social services, which includes publicly funded social care (£27 billion). Total planned Government expenditure in 2008/9 is £618 billion, so NHS expenditure accounts for around 18 per cent.

% of GDP

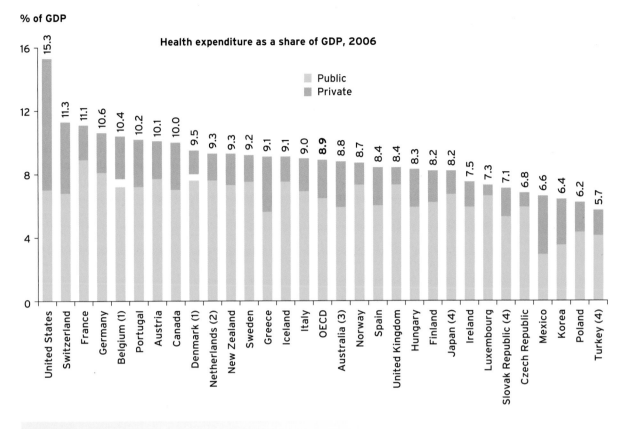

Figure 4.1 Public and private health expenditure for selected OECD countries 2006.
Source: http://www.oecd.org/document/27/0,3343,en_2649_34631_40902299_1_1_1,00.html#.

- The Organisation for Economic Co-operation and Development (OECD) is a group of 30 member countries committed to democracy and market economies. It provides a range of statistical services to support policy development. Its figures for 2006 show that health expenditure as a percentage of GDP (Gross Domestic Product – the total national income) in the UK was 8.4 per cent (OECD 2008). Figure 4.1 shows public and private health expenditure in OECD countries. Overall the UK still spends slightly less in terms of per cent GDP than the OECD average, but with a higher proportion of public spending.

Revenue expenditure pays for day-to-day running of NHS services.

Capital expenditure pays for investments, for example in equipment and buildings.

Capital and revenue expenditure

Expenditure in the NHS is divided into two sorts – revenue and capital. **Revenue expenditure** pays for the day-to-day running, and **capital expenditure** is for major investments, not only new hospitals costing millions of pounds, but items such as medical equipment and maintenance. If more investment is required it is not easy to reduce day-to-day funding in order to pay for it. On the other hand, if more day-to-day spending is required it is easier to reduce investment.

A way of increasing investment without a big increase in public expenditure is to ask the private sector to fund the development which is then paid for over a long-term arrangement, through the NHS leasing back the facilities. This policy, which began in the early 1990s, across a wide range of government departments, is known as the Private Finance Initiative (PFI), or more recently Public/Private Partnerships. As well as increasing investment without increasing public expenditure, the policy was designed to improve planning by making sure that investment could be afforded in the long term.

Critics of PFI schemes (Pollock 2004) point out that the private investment is paid back over a long time and costs more than it would have cost to pay from public funds. Although controversial, new hospitals have recently been almost entirely funded through PFI, and the scheme has helped to achieve a major modernisation of health care facilities.

Current health policy

In summarising current policy, a distinction can be made between:

System reform is the way in which the NHS is organised, funded and regulated.

Service reform is the way in which improvements in services are supported.

- **System reform** – the way in which the NHS is organised, funded and regulated.
- **Service reform** – the way in which improvements in services are supported.

These are not independent areas; systems reforms are designed to provide a structure in which innovation and change flourish. Service reforms will be considered in more depth in Chapter 12. In this chapter we will consider systems reforms, and how they are managed within the structure of the NHS.

Systems reform

Systems reforms are considered in six sections:

1. Financial flows.
2. The NHS as a commissioning organisation.
3. Developing providers and patient choice.
4. Regulation.
5. Patient and public involvement.
6. Workforce development.

Figure 4.2 shows the structure of the NHS in England. You may find it useful to refer to the diagram as you are reading the following sections.

The structure of the NHS in England

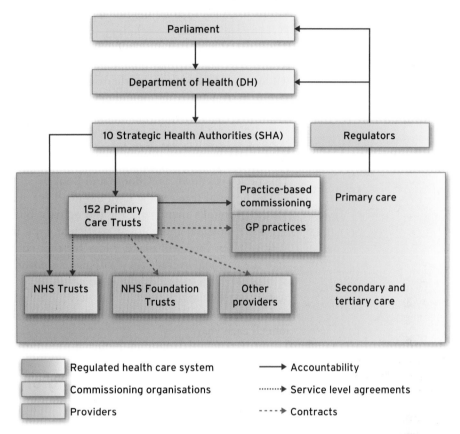

Note: PCTs control around 80 per cent of NHS resources, and they use these resources to fund NHS services. They do provide some services themselves, mainly community services, but only a limited amount. Most services are provided through 'commissioning' services from other providers, including GP practices, different types of NHS hospitals, and the private sector.

Strategic Health Authorities (SHAs) manage the NHS locally, particularly through PCTs. NHS Trusts that have not become NHS Foundation Trusts are also accountable to Strategic Health Authorities.

Figure 4.2 The structure of the NHS in England.

Financial flows

Primary Care Trusts (PCTs) are allocated money by the DH, based on the size of their population adjusted according to indicators of need, such as social deprivation. They spend most of their money in buying (commissioning) services from primary care, hospitals and other health care providers. Commissioning is explained in the next section. The way that hospitals receive most of their money is through **payment by results**. There are detailed issues in implementing payment by results, but the key principle is that a hospital gets paid for

Payments by results is the system whereby hospitals are largely paid according to how much activity they undertake.

every episode of care it delivers, for example admission, outpatients, day case, A&E attendance. Each year a price list is drawn up by the DH.

The price for each element of service (the national tariff) is the same for all PCTs and all providers (including, in principle, the private sector, although this is sometimes a bit more complicated). The price is adjusted for market factors, so that it is actually different for each hospital, but the idea is that hospitals will not compete with each other on the basis of price, but on quality.

The more activity a hospital does, the more money it gets paid. There are limits to this, such as restrictions in income for increases in emergency admissions. Payment by results facilitates patient choice, because for many referrals the patient chooses where to be treated. Patients can choose to go to any hospital offering NHS treatment, and can usually book an appointment online. This policy is known as 'Choose and Book'.

The hospital receives the national tariff for activity. The tariff is based not on the hospital's own costs for the activity but on the national average. If it costs a hospital more for a particular type of activity than the national average, then they will make a loss for that activity. If their costs are lower than the national average they will make a profit for that activity. So this way of funding NHS hospitals gives incentives to reduce costs as well as increase activity, particularly for elective services. The range of exclusions in this policy include mental health and intensive care, and the policy is being gradually refined each year.

The NHS as a commissioning organisation

Commissioning involves buying services from health care providers which might include primary care and hospitals. It is a process which includes needs assessment, planning and joint working with other agencies.

PCTs are **commissioning** organisations. Although many still provide community services, their role is increasingly to act as commissioners. The term 'commissioning' describes the whole process through which the local health system is managed. There is a key difference here between managing the service, which might mean managing hospitals and community health services, and managing the system. Health care organisations manage their services, and will have a contract or service level agreement with the PCT, which will be explicit about what services should be provided. Agreeing a contract with a provider is an important part of commissioning. The DH shows commissioning as a cycle (DH 2006 annex). Steps include:

- Assessing needs.
- Reviewing service provision.
- Deciding priorities.
- Engaging with patients and the public.
- Shaping the structure of supply.
- Managing demand.
- Managing performance.

This is a difficult role for PCTs, and the commissioning role is relatively new. The DH has set up a programme called World Class Commissioning (DH 2007b) which supports them. It has identified a number of competencies that PCTs need to develop in order to undertake their role effectively (see Policy focus 4.3). Local health systems will develop through the commissioning process.

Policy focus 4.3

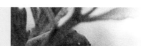

World Class Commissioning requires that commissioners:

1. Are recognised as the local leader of the NHS
2. Work collaboratively with community partners to commission services that optimise health gains and reductions in health inequalities
3. Proactively seek and build continuous and meaningful engagement with the public and patients, to shape services and improve health
4. Lead continuous and meaningful engagement with clinicians to inform strategy, and drive quality, service design and resource utilisation
5. Manage knowledge and undertake robust and regular needs assessments that establish a full understanding of current and future local health needs and requirements
6. Prioritise investment according to local needs, service requirements and the values of the NHS
7. Effectively stimulate the market to meet demand and secure required clinical, and health and well-being outcomes
8. Promote and specify continuous improvements in quality and outcomes through clinical and provider innovation and configuration
9. Secure procurement skills that ensure robust and viable contracts
10. Effectively manage systems and work in partnership with providers to ensure contract compliance and continuous improvements in quality and outcomes
11. Make sound financial investments to ensure sustainable development and value for money.

(DH 2007b p. 4)

A policy which supports the development of local services through commissioning is Practice-based Commissioning, which engages general practitioners in commissioning. PCTs give GP practices information about the cost of services provided to their patients, not just for hospital care, but also for services provided directly by primary care, particularly prescribing. If the practices can make budget savings, they can use a proportion of the savings to develop services locally, subject to the agreement of the PCT. Practices are encouraged to form consortia or groups of practices so that service developments can cover a wider area. GPs can provide some of these new services themselves. An example is the development of GPs with a special interest who treat patients that might otherwise be referred to hospital.

The financial system of payment by results creates powerful incentives for hospitals to increase activity. The same incentives work the other way for the PCTs who pay hospital bills. If they can reduce hospital activity they keep the money saved. If an admission costs £2,000, you don't have to reduce admissions by many to create a significant resource which can be used to develop services in the community, for example to improve services for long-term conditions, reducing the need for hospital care.

Thus far we have been considering the commissioning of secondary services. Primary care, traditionally based around GP practices, accounts for the vast majority of NHS patient contacts. Primary care has been managed differently from hospital care since the NHS was established in 1948. Most GPs are employed by their practice, in which they are usually partners with a personal financial stake. GP practices are businesses which get their income from contracts with the NHS. NHS services provided by dentists, opticians and pharmacists are also provided by independent contractors. PCTs manage contracts with all primary care providers. Contracts with GPs and dentists have recently been renegotiated so there is a greater emphasis on the quality of services provided. The new arrangements are discussed later in the chapter when workforce development is considered.

Developing providers and patient choice

Patient choice is a significant driver for many services. Patient choice has evolved since the 1990s when patients first began to be offered treatment at different hospitals in order to reduce waiting times. From 2004 the new policy of patient choice offered patients a choice of hospital to which they were referred by their GP. Initially, choice was offered from a list of local hospitals, but from 2008, this has been extended to all hospitals which offer the service and meet necessary standards. Patient choice also includes choice of appointment times, so that patients can arrange treatment around other commitments. For patients to exercise choice there must be a range of providers available to choose between. Developing providers has been an important element of systems reform.

Case 4.1 (continued)

Brian was visiting outpatients when a patient who was unhappy because he had to park so far away from the outpatients department told him that he wished he'd chosen to go to the local private hospital for his treatment. It was easier to get to from where he lived and had a better car park. He asked Brian why he should continue to come to the NHS hospital.

NHS foundation trusts are NHS organisations with greater independence and financial freedom. They are accountable to local communities through governors elected by members rather than the Secretary of State. Any local citizen or patient can be a member of a NHS foundation trust.

A key element of this policy was the establishment of **NHS foundation trusts**. These 'operate to NHS standards, be subject to NHS inspection, and abide by NHS principles' (Secretary of State for Health 2002 p. 30) However, they have much greater independence, with accountability to local communities through governors elected by members, rather than to the Secretary of State. They have much greater financial freedoms, for example they are able to borrow money to invest in facilities. In order to become an NHS foundation trust, NHS services have to demonstrate that they are well managed, and meet high performance standards. The decision to grant foundation trust status, under a licence, is made by Monitor, the independent regulator of NHS foundation trusts, discussed in the following section.

The intention is that all NHS Trusts will become NHS foundation trusts, so that the DH will not be directly responsible for delivering NHS services, other than through contracts. Other forms of NHS organisations are also being developed – such as Care Trusts which combine in one organisation services for a particular group of patients or clients that were previously provided by the NHS and by a local authority, for example in mental health services, and Children's Trusts. In the NHS the uniform bureaucracy of hospitals and other services is being replaced by a diversity of providers.

Alongside NHS organisations, there is also a growing role for the independent sector. In 2004, the DH announced that by 2008, up to 15 per cent of NHS procedures would be carried out in the private sector (Secretary of State for Health 2004). Some of this activity will be provided by established private sector hospitals and in addition, the DH have been establishing independent sector treatment centres (ISTCs). These are specialist centres providing elective services in a limited range of specialties. Many ISTCs are run by overseas companies, and recruit from overseas. Contracts were set up through procurement exercises managed by the DH in two phases, starting in 2003. In February 2006 there were 21 ISTCs, with a further 11 opening over the next 18 months. In 2006 they treated around 145,000 patients, with further developments expected to increase that activity to 250,000 (Anderson 2006). The latest phase emphasises diagnostic procedures. Figures for 2007/8 quoted by the Audit Commission (2008b) show that activity in ISTCs accounted for less than 1.8 per cent of elective activity, so even if other private sector activity is included, the maximum of 15 per cent of procedures envisaged is a long way off.

The three principle objectives for the ISTC programme were to:

- increase the capacity available to treat NHS patients,
- offer patients a choice over where they are treated, and
- stimulate innovation in the provision of health care

(Anderson 2006 paragraph 11)

In considering the last of these objectives, Patricia Hewitt, then Secretary of State for Health, made a speech at the King's Fund in February 2007 (DH 2007a). Her theme was commissioning new providers, and this was the example she used to show how competition is improving services.

> *Shepton Mallet Independent Sector Treatment Centre was one of the first wave of ISTCs. At Shepton Mallet, the provider UKSH, whose clinical partner is New York Presbyterian Hospital, see an orthopaedic patient, carry out diagnostic tests and book an operating slot, all in one day – a process that typically would have taken months and at least three appointments in the past.*
>
> *They have also transformed care for a wider group of patients as this example has now been copied by Yeovil NHS Foundation Trust. Managers there say the ISTC made their own clinicians 'sit up and take notice'. As a result, they too have established one-stop outpatient clinics for orthopaedic patients, reorganised the way they use their consultants' time and slashed waiting lists.*

Other forms of NHS provider services are also being developed – for example social enterprises and the voluntary sector. NHS Direct offers patients telephones and web advice and information, and minor injury units have been set up. Both of these initiatives, and others, provide choice for patients.

Taken together the policies of commissioning and developing providers are a good example of how policy is implemented by local initiatives. The following are examples of how services might be developed locally to reduce demand on hospitals:

- Better preventative services, for example in identifying elderly people who are at risk from falling.
- Improved services for people with chronic conditions, like diabetes, so that their conditions can be managed more effectively in the community.
- Responsive social services to reduce admissions for social reasons.
- Specialist services in primary care to provide some outpatient services that would previously have been provided by hospitals, or to provide follow-up care following a hospital consultation.
- Diagnostic services which are usually provided in hospitals, such as imaging or endoscopy.

However, there are potential pitfalls in encouraging a more flexible and dynamic system. The incentives might work in ways which have not been intended, for example:

- Hospitals admitting patients where admission might have been avoided.
- Hospitals following up patients in outpatients unnecessarily.
- Hospitals not doing activity for which they cannot make a profit.
- GPs not referring patients to hospitals when the patient's condition requires it.
- Hospitals keeping service development to themselves giving them a competitive advantage.

One of the ways in which these can be prevented is regulation.

Regulation

Health care **regulation** is the process through which the activities of health care providers (organisations and individuals) are controlled or influenced by organisations with specific authority which were established to achieve specific goals.

Regulation covers both organisations providing health care, and also individual professionals. There has recently been a strengthening of professional regulation (see Chapter 1), but apart from regulation, the motivation and professionalism of individual health care professionals is an important issue in considering how system reforms might change service. For example, the NMC has *The Code* which acts as a set of minimum standards, but the vast majority of nurses and midwives who are covered by the code act professionally from their own motivation and professionalism rather than because it is required of them through *The Code*. This is an important point to note, because many possible unintended consequences of health care are avoided simply because health care professionals do not behave in a way in which incentives might suggest. Health care managers also have a code of conduct (DH 2002), although they are not professionally regulated. They too, in general, have strong values which mean that they generally act in the interests of patients and many have a clinical background.

Health care is regulated by a number of organisations. Perhaps the two most significant are the Care Quality Commission and Monitor (the Independent Regulator for NHS foundation trusts). You may find it useful to browse their websites: www.cqc.org.uk and www.monitor-nhsft.gov.uk. The Care Quality Commission was established on 1 April 2009. It brought together the Healthcare

Commission, the Commission for Social Care Inspection and the Mental Health Act Commission into a single regulator. The Care Quality Commission has new powers to register health care providers, and will take on the roles of its three predecessors. It will be developing its registration processes which will initially concentrate on hygiene standards. We'll consider the Care Quality Commission next in its role as a regulator of health care providers, a role that was previously undertaken by the Healthcare Commission.

Activity 4.5

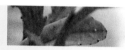

Go to the website of the Care Quality Commission, and familiarise yourself with the new organisation.

The Care Quality Commission

The Care Quality Commission's role is mainly concerned with quality in the NHS. Each year it publishes its Annual Health Check on all NHS organisations (Healthcare Commission 2008a). This gives each provider two ratings on a four point scale: one for quality of services, and one for the use of resources (this will become 'quality of financial management' in 2009). The four point scale is: excellent, good, fair, weak. From 2009, PCTs will be judged separately on their roles as commissioner and service provider.

Case 4.1 (continued)

One morning on the local television news it said that the Care Quality Commission had judged the quality of care at the hospital where Brian worked as only 'fair'. Brian thought that the care his service provided was the best he'd known in his career. On the way to work he wondered whether any patients would ask him whether their care was of poor quality and what he would say to them.

One of the ways in which the Care Quality Commission makes its judgement is through a Trust's compliance with NHS national standards. The standards were published in a document called *National Standards, Local Action* (DH 2004b). There are 24 Core Standards, and 13 Developmental Standards, in 7 domains. Most of the core standards have related developmental standards so the improvement that is required can be clearly seen. All organisations providing NHS care are expected to achieve core standards, and be working towards developmental ones. The seven domains are:

- Safety
- Clinical and cost-effectiveness
- Governance

Domain	Standard
Clinical and cost-effectiveness	C1. Health care organisations protect patients through systems that (a) identify and learn from all patient safety incidents and other reportable incidents, and make improvements in practice based on local and national experience and information derived from the analysis of incidents; and (b) ensure that patient safety notices, alerts and other communications concerning patient safety which require action are acted on within appropriate timescales.
Patient focus	C16. Health care organisations make information available to patients and the public on their services, provide patients with suitable and accessible information on the care and treatment they receive and, where appropriate, inform patients on what to expect during treatment, care, and aftercare.

Figure 4.3 Examples of core standards.

Source: DH (2004b).

- Patient focus
- Accessible and responsive care
- Care environment and amenities
- Public health.

Examples of core standards are given in Figure 4.3.

Each Trust's compliance with the standards is measured mainly through self-assessment. The Care Quality Commission publishes detailed guidance to help them in this task. Trusts submit a return to the Care Quality Commission, which states whether they are compliant with core standards, and the progress being made towards developmental standards. Submissions include comments by Strategic Health Authorities, Local Authority Overview and Scrutiny Committees, Patient and Public Involvement Forums (these are explained in a bit more detail later) and for Foundation Trusts, the Board of Governors. The Care Quality Commission will cross reference a Trust's returns with data that is available such as infection rates, or the patient satisfaction survey. They will inspect a proportion of Trusts to check their self-assessment declarations. Each Trust's declaration is a public document that will be signed off by the Board. In 2009 the Care Quality Commission will visit all Trusts to assess their compliance with the hygiene code.

Activity 4.6

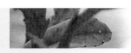

Go to the website of a hospital you know and find their declaration to the Care Quality Commission. You might find it in a 'Publications' section. Is it easily accessible? What does it say about the hospital's performance?

Other information that the Care Quality Commission uses to give its performance assessment is:

- Achievement of targets, including waiting time targets.
- Use of resources, taking information from reviews by the Audit Commission, or for NHS Foundation Trusts, Monitor.
- Improvement reviews, which are considerations of specific clinical areas or for services for a particular client group. These will inform the assurance process rather than the calculation of scores.

The Care Quality Commission is also responsible for investigations where allegations of serious failing in NHS services are made.

Monitor

Monitor is the independent regulator of NHS foundation trusts. Monitor's primary concern is the financial viability of foundation trusts, but it is also concerned with services. When a foundation trust is established, it is granted a licence which sets out the services it should provide. Any changes to the services must be agreed by Monitor, so the regulator acts as a defence against a foundation trust acting only in its financial interests. Monitor has a number of powers it can use when the finances of a Trust are beginning to show signs of weakening. These range from more frequent monitoring to removal of board members or ultimately the removal of the licence of the NHS foundation trust, in which case it would revert to being an NHS Trust accountable to the Secretary of State.

Although a Foundation Trust is regulated by Monitor it is accountable to its members. Any member of the public who lives in the area served by the trust or is a patient of the trust or member of staff can become a member. Members elect governors, who in turn elect directors of the Trust, so there is a mechanism for local involvement in the affairs of the Trust which ensures that the Trust serves the interests of the community.

Other regulators

There are a number of other regulators who have specific roles in influencing organisations providing health care services. All of these regulators have websites, explaining their purpose and the way that they operate. Brief explanations of each organisation's role given below are taken from their website. The regulators have different powers and functions. For example NICE produces 'guidance' but in most areas, the NHS is obliged to provide the funding for the recommended treatments; conforming to guidance forms part of the core standards discussed earlier. Whatever their formal powers, all regulators are influential in determining the activities of the NHS.

- *The National Institute of Health and Clinical Excellence*: http://www.nice.org.uk/ NICE 'is the independent organisation responsible for providing national guidance on the promotion of good health and the prevention and treatment of ill health'.
- *The National Patient Safety Authority*: http://www.npsa.nhs.uk/ The NPSA 'leads and contributes to improved, safe patient care by informing, supporting and influencing the health sector'.

- *The NHS Litigation Authority*: http://www.nhsla.com/ 'The NHSLA is . . . responsible for handling negligence claims made against NHS bodies in England. In addition to dealing with claims when they arise, we have an active risk management programme to help raise standards of care in the NHS and hence reduce the number of incidents leading to claims.'

- *The NHS Institute for Innovation and Improvement*: http://www.institute. nhs.uk/ 'The NHS Institute for Innovation and Improvement supports the NHS to transform health care for patients and the public by rapidly developing and spreading new ways of working, new technology and world-class leadership.' There could be some debate about whether the Institute is a regulator, since it has no specific authority over the NHS. It is, however, very influential.

- *The Mental Health Act Commission*: http://www.mhac.org.uk/ 'The Commission's remit is to keep under review the operation of the Mental Health Act 1983 as it relates to detained patients, and to meet with and interview detained patients in private.' The Mental Health Act 1983 was updated by the Mental Health Act 2007. The functions of the Mental Health Act Commission were taken over by the Care Quality Commission in April 2009.

- *The Human Fertilisation and Embryology Authority*: http://www.hfea.gov.uk/ 'The Human Fertilisation and Embryology Authority is the UK's independent regulator overseeing the use of gametes and embryos in fertility treatment and research.'

As well as these NHS bodies, there are other regulators, including:

- Professional regulatory bodies: the Nursing and Midwifery Council and the General Medical Council. The professional regulatory bodies are overseen by the Council for Healthcare Regulatory Excellence: http://www.chre.org.uk/
- Primary Care Trusts as commissioners of services have a key role in monitoring the services that they commission.
- Local authorities. As discussed below, local authorities have powers of overview and scrutiny over the NHS. They also have a range of powers such as issuing fire and building certificates which will affect the NHS.
- Other regulators, such as the Health and Safety Executive.

An important part of health care policy is to encourage diversity and independence for health care providers, but this is pursued within a strong and evolving framework of regulation.

Patient and public involvement

The policy of patient choice has been discussed above. The payment by results system and the extension in the number and range of providers of NHS services facilitates patient choice. This choice policy is supported by a range of mechanisms to enable 'voice' – the way in which service users and the public are engaged in health issues, either as an individual, or as part of a group. The main object for policy is to produce a culture change in the NHS so that patient choice is viewed as centrally important in the delivery of services. The view expressed in the NHS Plan was that the service was managed for the convenience of the organisations and professionals that delivered the service. The importance of improved patient involvement was a key issue highlighted by the inquiry into poor outcomes achieved in paediatric heart surgery at the Bristol Royal Infirmary, between 1984 and 1995 (Kennedy 2001). The development of clinical governance, which was heavily influenced by the failures at Bristol, had patient involvement as a key area for improvement. Cultural change is promoted by the specific policies that are described below, as well as by general societal changes where, for example, deference to health care professionals is reducing.

Relevant initiatives are:

- *Patient Advice and Liaison Service (PALS)*. Each health care organisation has a PALS. Their role is to provide patients with advice and support and where necessary confidential assistance in resolving issues relating to their health care.
- *The Expert Patient Programme*. There is evidence that enabling patients with chronic diseases to have greater control over their treatment improves outcomes and reduces costs. The DH established an Expert Patient Programme to support changes in service delivery (DH 2001).
- *Foundation Trusts*. All patients, staff, and members of the public in the locality of a Foundation Trust can apply to become a member of the Trust. Members elect governors, who in turn elect directors.
- *Local Involvement Networks*. LINks replace Patient and Public Involvement Forums which were established in each Trust to give a focus to involvement in planning and managing health services. LINks will be organised under the auspices of local authorities to give a focus to involvement across all public services. 'LINks will be established in most areas by the end of 2008. Each local authority (that provides social services) has been given funding and is under a legal duty to make contractual arrangements that enable LINk activities to take place' (DH 2008e).
- *Local Authority Overview and Scrutiny Committees* of local authorities have the right to scrutinise proposals made by health care organisations.

Policy to improve patient and public involvement can be summarised as 'choice and voice'. Choice is driving competition between providers that improves the quality of services. Voice gives a number of ways in which patients and members of the public can become involved in their own care, and health issues generally. The key goal is a culture change through which all staff naturally put the patient at the centre of service delivery.

Workforce development

The *NHS Plan* included specific targets for increasing the NHS workforce. The emphasis now is on changing the way in which NHS staff work. This is driven by the needs of service reform, particularly relating to service redesign, which often requires that staff work more flexibly in the interests of patients. A number of changes have required specific initiatives, such as:

- Re-introducing the role of matron, with an emphasis on being a visible, influential figure who can get things done for patients.
- Allowing professionals other than doctors to prescribe.
- Developing consultant roles in nursing and the allied health professions.

Underpinning specific changes have been reforms to the way in which staff are contracted. The three major reforms have been *Agenda for Change*, the new consultant contract, and the new GMS (General Medical Services) contract for GPs:

1. *Agenda for Change.* New arrangements were agreed in 2004 for all staff in the NHS except senior managers and doctors, changing the system where every staff group had a different set of terms and conditions separately negotiated. The new unified pay scales (and terms and conditions) are based on the evaluation of jobs against a range of criteria. A knowledge and skills framework identifies what level of performance each job requires which helps in professional development. The central idea is that staff are rewarded equally for the job they do, rather than the staff group that they belong to. This is an important objective in its own right, but the new system is also designed to make it easier to create new roles, and a better system for career progression, particularly through reviews and appraisals (DH 2004a).

2. *The new consultant contract.* The changes to the (medical) consultant contract have made the work of consultants much more transparent. In effect consultants become more 'managed', for example in being clear what activities they will undertake and where they will be. Private practice was a key issue in the negotiations. The new contract has a provision that consultants must at least offer additional work over and above the basic contract before they are allowed to undertake private practice. The new contract also included a substantial pay rise.

3. *The new GP contract.* The employment of GPs has always been different from hospital consultants. They have always been contracted to the NHS, rather than employees. Some employed (or salaried) GPs are employed by a PCT or a practice. The new contract with GP practices is designed to focus more on the quality and outcome of services provided, particularly to support development of services in the community.

Evaluations of all three contracts (Buchan and Evans 2007, National Audit Office 2007, 2008) suggest that the costs for all contracts were much higher than expected, and that the benefits have not all been realised.

The DH used Figure 4.4 to summarise the organising framework for health reforms (DH 2006 p. 6). In this chapter we have considered patient choice and commissioning separately, and added the development of the workforce as an element of system reform.

The role of government

The system of a plurality of providers within a strong regulatory environment has been described. In this system, how does the government influence priorities, or set targets? The government can set priorities for commissioners which are then reflected in the contracts agreed between PCTs and providers of services. Achievement of targets is also included in the core standards for the NHS which the Care Quality Commission assess. The DH publishes an operating framework for the NHS each year which identifies priority areas (DH 2008c). A 'Vital Signs' framework has been established for PCTs, with three tiers:

- Tier 1: 'must do' targets which all providers of services must achieve.
- Tier 2: national priorities for local delivery, where action is required across the NHS.

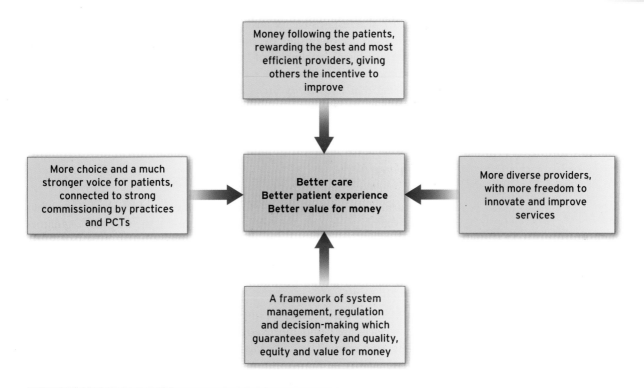

Figure 4.4 Department of Health diagram on system reform.
Source: DH (2006).

- Tier 3: indicators available to PCTs. They can choose where to target effort for local improvement.

Activity 4.7

Find out how your local hospital is performing against its targets to reduce healthcare-associated infection, and other targets. Looking at board papers on their website might be a good place to start.

The 'must do' targets include reductions in healthcare-associated infection and improvements in access to health care including the 18-week target for referral to treatment, improved access to primary care, and specific targets including for cancer treatment. There are also a number of existing commitments such as a maximum 4-hour wait in A&E.

The 18-week target, which applied to all NHS services from December 2008, is the culmination of the reduction in waiting for access that has been a key theme of health policy since the NHS Plan was published in 2000. The 18-week period starts when a patient is referred to a service and ends when the final treatment is started. It includes waits for diagnostic tests before the treatment is decided. Exceptions to the target are made for clinical reasons, or patient choice. When the NHS Plan was published maximum times were typically 6 months for an outpatient appointment, and 18 months for admission with no target for any diagnostic process before the decision to treat was made.

Regulators are also responsible for ensuring that the government's priority areas are addressed. So although the government has set up a system whereby it is losing direct management control of health care providers, it has established a system in its regulatory framework through which it still controls powerful levers ensuring that its priority areas are addressed. Government can decide to change policy, or the emphasis of policy, through the management of the system it has established.

Service reform

Service reform is driven by systems reform. The way in which the money flows round the system, the way that patients exercise choice, the way that regulators require improvements, all combine to make services more responsive and accessible. Workforce development will support service changes. Three areas of service reform which are particularly relevant to the implementation of health care policy are:

- *Service redesign*. This covers a range of initiatives broadly concerned with the way services are being improved locally, primarily through the efforts of staff delivering them. The NHS Modernisation Agency was set up in 2000 to support efforts to change the way that services are delivered, through establishing national programmes, spreading good practice, and providing a number of tools for improvement. It evolved into the NHS Institute for Improvement and Innovation in 2005. Promoting local service user involvement is a key element of service redesign. An example might be redesigning the way a local diabetes service operates. Service redesign might include service reconfiguration which refers to more significant changes in the way that services are delivered, for example changing the services a hospital provides.
- *Clinical Governance*. The establishment of clinical governance was one of the first acts of the labour government in the 1997 White Paper, *The New NHS* (Secretary of State for Health 1997). Clinical governance established a statutory duty on health care providers for the quality of services. Previously the only statutory duty was for financial control. Having limited resources is not an acceptable reason for poor quality. NHS organisations have to ensure that they are implementing systems for ensuring services meet the highest quality standards. Clinical governance is discussed in detail in Chapter 12.
- *Public health and reducing health inequalities*. Public health and reducing health inequalities are now recognised as key areas of policy. NHS bodies are concerned with developing ways of improving the health of the population, rather than only being concerned with providing services that address individuals' illnesses. Public health is considered in more detail in Chapter 10.

Other themes might be identified as significant in their own right rather than covered by these headings, for example interprofessional working.

The Darzi review

When Gordon Brown became Prime Minister in 2007 he announced a review of the NHS, to be led by Lord Darzi, who he had appointed as health minister.

The review was unlike other reviews. It was much more decentralised, with many clinicians being involved in reviews undertaken by Strategic Health Authorities who published their visions before the publication of the final report, timed to coincide with the 60th anniversary of the NHS. The White Paper, *High Quality Care for All* (Secretary of State for Health 2008) announced no new targets or structural reform, but it was no less significant for that. It announced a wide range of new initiatives within the policy direction that has been explained earlier, representing policy development as a dynamic process and placing renewed emphasis on:

- Improving quality. The elements of quality were identified as patient safety, patient experience, and effectiveness of care. New initiatives included the requirement that NHS provider organisations publish 'quality accounts' comparable with financial accounts, to develop the payment by results system and to develop the role and powers of the Care Quality Commission.
- Public health and the development of prevention services. Initiatives include the commissioning by PCTs of well-being and prevention services.
- Empowering patients, through greater choice and better information, including the piloting of personal budgets for some patients so that they can commission their own services, building on similar schemes in social care.
- Continuing to develop primary and community care. The DH published a comprehensive vision for primary and community care (DH 2008d) giving more detail about initiatives which include personalised care plans for people with long-term conditions, and extending patient choice across primary and secondary care. This will include the development of GP-led health centres that 'offer walk-in services and bookable appointments from 8a.m.–8p.m. each day of the week. These services will be available to any member of the public, in addition to the service they receive from their local GP practice' (DH 2008d p. 28). These so-called 'polyclinics' attracted some controversy after the Darzi report was published.
- The importance of the leadership role of clinicians and local managers, and supporting staff. The title of Chapter 5 is 'Freedom to focus on quality. Putting frontline staff in control'. Initiatives include extending the freedoms from central control enjoyed by Foundation Trusts to community providers, improved management and leadership development opportunities, and the 're-invigoration' of practice-based commissioning (Secretary of State for Health 2008 p. 65), which as was discussed earlier is a vehicle for clinical leadership in commissioning services.
- The NHS Constitution.

In the Operating Framework for the NHS in 2009/2010, David Nicholson, the Chief Executive of the NHS explained that:

> *'High Quality Care for All' moves us into the third stage of the reform journey that began with the NHS Plan in 2000. The first stage was about increasing capacity and investment across the NHS. The second stage was about introducing levers to enable reform: choice; contestability; more freedom for providers; and better financial systems. And the third stage . . . is about using the additional capacity and the reform levers to transform services to deliver high quality care for patients and value for money for the taxpayer.*

(DH 2008c p. 3)

The Darzi review is significant for some new initiatives, but also for continuity with the system that has been developed over a number of years. It seems that the policy direction for the next few years at least will be based on continuous improvement of the existing system rather than major new policy change.

Case 4.1 (continued)

Brian was beginning to think about what continuing professional development opportunities might be available to him to develop his career. Initially he thought he would always work in hospitals, and go into management. Perhaps he'd now have a chance to influence the way that services were being provided without leaving his clinical role. He thought that new clinical opportunities may be available in the future, perhaps outside traditional NHS facilities. He decided to find out a lot more about how the service might change before making his mind up.

Regional differences in the UK

One of the issues that Labour addressed in its first term was devolution, quickly implementing its election pledge in establishing a Parliament in Scotland and a Legislative Assembly in Wales. One of the effects of these changes was that health policy in Scotland and Wales became the responsibility of devolved administrations. Northern Ireland has a longer tradition of devolved administration, but because of the political problems of recent years, the development of domestic policy in the province or through the Northern Ireland Office in the UK Government has been slow. The central tenets of the NHS remain across the UK but significant differences in priorities have emerged, so that there are now divergences in health policy in the UK.

Broadly, each of the health systems has an aim to move hospital services into community settings (Smith and Babbington 2006). There are detailed and high-profile differences in policy, reflecting different political decision-making processes. For example in Scotland, personal social care is paid for from public taxation, whereas in England only the nursing element of care is paid for before means testing. In Wales prescription charges have been abolished. England has had considerably more success in reducing waiting times.

A major difference concerns structures that have been put in place to manage the health care system. In England development of a health care market based on patient choice and commissioning was described earlier in some detail. In Scotland, the system has gone in a completely different direction. Here services are integrated rather than fragmented. There is a much stronger emphasis on professional consensus. There is no purchaser/provider split. Instead the NHS in Scotland is organised through 14 Health Boards responsible for managing the whole system of care. Wales initially maintained the purchaser/provider split, but is now reorganising the NHS around regional health delivery bodies. Northern Ireland, alone of the four health systems, has integration of health and social care.

Health policy evolves rather than develops in discrete steps based on thorough evaluation. However, if policy divergences between the four systems in the UK continue, there will be an opportunity to evaluate differences more thoroughly, for example in the degree of success in changing the dominance of hospitals in health care delivery, and the effect of specific differences such as in the funding of personal social care. Whether evaluations are influential in producing more evidence-based policy making is likely to depend on the political policy-making process.

Part 3: Exploring health policy

What evidence is there to support health policies described in this chapter? The requirement for evidence-based practice by health care professionals is well understood, but should we expect policy makers to apply similar principles? For example, what evidence is there for expecting that practice-based commissioning will support the development of community-based services, or that independent regulators will be able to ensure standards in diverse providers?

A number of difficulties can be identified in developing an evidence base for the development and implementation of policy. A key issue is that 'there is usually more room for disagreement about outcomes in policy making than in medicine. In medicine, randomised control trials can (sometimes) clinch arguments about outcomes. This never happens in policy making' (Cookson 2005 p. 119). Context is important in developing an evidence base. This is particularly important when considering evidence from other countries, who have implemented similar policies. The social and political context cannot be controlled in the comparison. Policy depends 'crucially upon people's decision-making behaviour' (Cookson 2005 p. 119). Whether a policy succeeds in achieving its aims is important, but it is also important to understand how it works, and this will depend on many peoples' decisions.

Policy-making is essentially a political activity which seeks to achieve a balance between various perspectives. What balance, for example, should be struck between the rights of professionals to autonomy and the rights of patients to a service which achieves reasonably standard outcomes? In the UK context, the constant demand on policy makers for improvements in health services means that time for researching effects of policy before changes are demanded is rarely available. Politicians who make key decisions are also likely to have strong beliefs that lead to a specific point of view.

Barriers to using research include the lack of personal contact between researchers and policy makers, the lack of timeliness or relevance of research, and mistrust between policy makers and researchers (Innvaer *et al.* 2002).

This is not to say that evidence is not important in making policy, but compared with evidence-based clinical practice a different model of what constitutes evidence and how it is used is needed (Dobrow *et al.* 2004). The evidence for example may be unpublished evaluations supporting the development of policy through implementation, or stakeholder perceptions of policy outcomes. In some areas, evidence comes from high-profile public enquiries, as was the case in the development of clinical governance (Kennedy 2001).

'Mounting pressures for transparency, accountability and efficiency in all areas of public policy continue to increase the demand for evidence' (Cookson 2005 p. 118). Improvements in information and communication technology increase both the volume of evidence available, and its communication.

Are the recent NHS funding and systems reform working?

Earlier in the chapter we noted the influence of a report by Derek Wanless which considered the resources required for the NHS over the next two decades. The report (Wanless 2002) concluded that resources required over the next 20 years depended crucially on whether the public engaged in relation to their health, for example by pursuing healthy lifestyles, and whether the NHS becomes more responsive and efficient, for example in developing information and communication technology (ICT), and becoming more efficient. Wanless identified three scenarios:

- Slow uptake – there is no change in the level of public engagement: life expectancy rises by the lowest amount in all three scenarios and the health status of the population is constant or deteriorates. The health service is relatively unresponsive with low rates of technology uptake and low productivity.
- Solid progress – people become more engaged in relation to their health: life expectancy rises considerably, health status improves and people have confidence in the primary care system and use it appropriately. The health service is responsive with high rates of technology uptake and a more efficient use of resources.
- Fully engaged – levels of public engagement in relation to their health are high: life expectancy increases go beyond current forecasts, health status improves dramatically and people are confident in the health system and demand high-quality care. The health service is responsive with high rates of technology uptake, particularly in relation to disease prevention. Use of resources is more efficient.

The 'fully engaged' scenario envisaged a situation in 2022 where expenditure was £30 billion less than would be required under the 'slow uptake' scenario. In the 'fully engaged' scenario, the health status would also be better – for example life expectancy at birth in 2022 was estimated to be 78.7 years for men under the slow uptake scenario, and 81.6 under the fully engaged scenario. The respective figures for women were 83.0 and 85.5. The 'fully engaged' scenario: better health outcomes for considerably less resources is clearly worth pursuing. Wanless was subsequently asked to consider the achievement of the fully engaged scenario and his second report, published in 2004, set the scene for the development of public health policy (Wanless 2004).

The key issue for Wanless was resources. The 'catch up' he recommended has been achieved. His projections went forward until 2022/23. In the 'solid progress' scenario (the middle one) he estimated that by then we will need to spend 11.1 per cent of GDP on health, which will give a budget of £161 billion at 2002/3 prices, compared with £68 billion in 2002/3. In 20 years, health spending, in real terms, will more than double if Wanless's estimates are reasonable, and if the political make up of the health system stays the same, which was a basic assumption of the review. These increases could be achieved by increasing health spending at between 4.7 per cent and 2.7 per cent above inflation each year.

Wanless identified a number of factors which will determine how much money will be required for the health service:

- Technology and medical advance. The UK has been 'a late and slow adopter of medical technology' (Wanless 2002 p. 52). Some technologies reduce expenditure, for example, through reducing lengths of stay for minimally invasive surgery. However, many increase expenditure, for example new drug treatments.
- Information and communication technology. Increased use of ICT could give significant benefits. There have been significant problems with implementing IT systems, but nevertheless the review considered that IT can make significant improvements in services if well implemented.
- Health Service workforce. The review set out a vision of the NHS workforce, which included:
  1. More nurses and other health care professionals working in community settings.
  2. Health care assistants undertaking 'a large part of the routine work' (Wanless 2002 p. 58).
  3. GPs focusing on more complex problems, facilitating work moving from secondary to primary care.
  4. More older people being 'supported at home or in community-based facilities.'
  5. Major acute hospitals will focus on providing 24-hour intensive and high-dependency care. They will be centres for excellence for tertiary and high-tech services.
- Productivity. Despite more resources being available to the NHS, it will have to become more efficient, through better use of the workforce, better use of ICT, more self-care by patients, including those with chronic illnesses, and concentrating resources on treatments known to be effective.

Although the era of significant additional resources for the NHS began in 2000 with the publication of *The NHS Plan* (Secretary of State 2000), the Wanless report provided justification for maintaining and extending the increase in resources. In 2007, the King's Fund published a review of NHS funding and performance, led again by Derek Wanless (Wanless *et al.* 2007). The review concluded that the extra resources the 2002 report identified had been made available to the NHS, but that in other areas – outputs, outcomes and determinants of health, and productivity – progress is only on a path between slow uptake and solid progress.

In 2008, the Audit Commission published a report evaluating the policy of payment by results. Although this is only part of the new structure of the NHS it is a key part of systems reform. The conclusions were that there is still 'significant weaknesses in commissioning' (Audit Commission 2008a p. 4), but that World Class Commissioning will address these weaknesses. 'Overall PbR has demonstrated its worth, even if it has yet to have a significant impact on activity and efficiency' (Audit Commission 2008a p. 5).

A later joint report between the Audit Commission and the Care Quality Commission identified that the reform programme had achieved some major benefits, but that there were other areas where change was slower, including moving care out of hospital, or foundation trusts developing 'innovative models of patient care' (Audit Commission 2008b p. 4).

The Healthcare Commission published annual reports on the state of health care. Its 2008 report identified that the NHS has made some 'dramatic progress', and that the NHS 'as a whole is getting better at using and managing its resources, and that it is performing better against the wide range of national targets it has to deliver and the core standards it has to meet' (Healthcare Commission 2008b, p. 6). It also identified challenges including improving commissioning, and the variability of service provision, which the Darzi review also identified.

The balance of evidence suggests that recent policy reforms have had some success but have not yet achieved all their objectives.

Development of policy

In this final section we have discussed in a little more detail some longer-term issues relating to health policy. Because of the difficulty in achieving policy goals, there will always be questions and critiques about whether a particular policy instrument will be effective. For example:

- Will practice-based commissioning be effective in redesigning services?
- Will the new contract arrangements for GPs bring about an improvement in preventative services?
- Will Foundation Trusts develop new ways of improving accountability of health care providers to their local communities?
- Will the regulatory regime be able to strike the right balance between assuring standards and strangling providers in red tape?

A key role for the DH and the range of regulatory bodies that have been established will be to keep the system under review, making amendments where necessary to support the achievement of policy goals.

Conclusion

Health policy is a complex area - it is developing all the time, and a key challenge for many in the NHS is keeping up to date with all the changes. The distinction between health policy and health care policy is important. In this chapter we have mainly dealt with health care policy. Health policy includes a range of initiatives, relating to, for example, public health and inequalities that are wider than the health care system. Social policy and the provision of social care are also very important and have not been considered.

In this chapter current health care policy has been outlined, but when you read it there will have been changes. Recommendations for further reading have been provided, and you will need to consider developments to gain a full and up-to-date understanding. After the next election, if there is a change in Government, there may be more changes in health care policy, although the political differences between the major parties have narrowed since 1997.

There are, however, some key themes that are likely to remain constant for some time. The NHS has had a significant increase in spending, and although the rate of increase has slowed down, further increases are likely. The latest developments, particularly the results of the Darzi review, build on the systems reforms that have been implemented, and emphasise the continuing importance of improving quality, and the patient experience, and the role of clinicians and supporting staff in improving services. The importance of the NHS improving its commissioning functions, the development of organisations providing NHS care within a strong regulatory environment, the development of local health services, and patient choice and empowerment are all likely to be central aims of policy and its implementation.

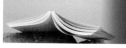

Suggested further reading

A number of books on health policy are cited in the chapter. Unfortunately, because of delays in production, large parts of them are likely to be out of date. This is also the case with this chapter. Keeping up to date with policy developments requires more contemporary resources, and the Internet and other media are key. Tutors will often caution you about your use of the Internet, but for understanding health policy you will need to know your way around some important sites.

- There are a number of professional journals which include news sections and commentaries on contemporary issues, for example the *Nursing Times* and *Nursing Standard*. These are very useful sources of information about policy, although you should be aware that they are often written from a particular perspective. *The Health Service Journal* is an important weekly publication aimed at NHS managers, which gives useful commentaries.
- Because of the enormous public interest in health issues, the media – newspapers, magazines, television, radio and the Internet – are good sources of information, although again you have to be wary of specific perspectives. The 'quality' papers often have in-depth articles, and current affairs programmes on the television and radio often cover health issues. The BBC website has a section on health issues, and also a health section in its news section, which can be very useful. It is so up to date that a week or so after a development, the relevant information is not so easy to find! Other news organisations also provide useful information.
- The DH website (http://www.dh.gov.uk) is a very useful resource. The DH publishes many documents setting out policy and giving guidance for those responsible for its implementation. These documents are often detailed, but they usually include an executive summary which can be helpful in giving an overview and directing more detailed reading. Some particularly helpful documents are produced specifically for the public. DH documents are often available free of charge in printed form. Details of how to order them are on the back cover of the electronic version.
- The devolved administrations in Scotland, Wales and Northern Ireland have their own web resources, with sections related to their health policies and structures:
  i In Scotland, the Scottish Executive: http://www.scotland.gov.uk/Topics/Health
  ii In Wales, the Welsh Assembly Government: http://new.wales.gov.uk/topics/health/?lang=en
  iii In Northern Ireland, the DH, Social Services and Public Safety: http://www.dhsspsni.gov.uk/
- There are many bodies that have been set up to implement health policy. Their websites are often useful sources of information. For example, the Care Quality Commission, and the National Institute for Health and Clinical Excellence.
- Trades unions and professional bodies also produce useful resources, particularly where an issue has specific importance for its membership. For example, the Royal College of Nursing (http://www.rcn.org.uk/) and Unison (http://www.unison.org.uk/) both have useful resources, although you should be aware that they will take a particular perspective on issues.

- There are a number of research organisations and interest groups which consider health issues, and produce resources to support policy debates. Examples include:
  i   The King's Fund (http://www.kingsfund.org.uk/)
  ii The Health Foundation (http://www.health.org.uk/)
  iii The NHS Confederation (http://www.nhsconfed.org/)
  iv The Picker Institute (http://www.pickereurope.org/)

Spending a few hours familiarising yourself with these resources is likely to be very useful.

References

Anderson, K. (2006) *Independent Sector Treatment Centres*. A report from Ken Anderson, Commercial Director, DH, to the Secretary of State for Health. London: DH. (http://www.dh.gov.uk).

Audit Commission (2008a) *The Right Result? Payment by results 2003–07* London: Audit Commission (http://www.audit-commission.gov.uk).

Audit Commission (2008b) *Is the Treatment Working? Progress with the NHS system reform programme.* London: Audit Commission (http://www.audit-commission.gov.uk).

Buchan, J. and Evans, D. (2007) *Realising the Benefits? Assessing the implementation of agenda for change.* London: King's Fund.

Chancellor of the Exchequer (2007) *Meeting the Aspirations of the British People.* Cm 7227. London: The Stationery Office.

Cookson, R. (2005) Evidence-based policy making in health care: what it is and what it isn't. *Journal of Health Services Research and Policy* **10** (2), 118–121.

DH (Department of Health) (2001) *The Expert Patient. A new approach to chronic disease management for the 21st century.* London: DH (http://www.dh.gov.uk).

DH (2002) *Code of Conduct for NHS Managers.* London: DH (http://www.dh.gov.uk).

DH (2004a) *The NHS Knowledge and Skills Framework (NHS KSF) and the Development Review Process,* London: DH. (http://www.dh.gov.uk).

DH (2004b) *National Standards, Local Action. Health and social care standards and planning framework. 2004/5–2007/8.* London: DH. (http://www.dh.gov.uk).

DH (2006) *Health Reform in England. Update and commissioning framework.* London: DH. (http://www.dh.gov.uk).

DH (2007a) *Speech by Rt Hon Patricia Hewitt MP, Secretary of State for Health, 20 February 2007 to the King's Fund: Commissioning new providers.* (http://www.dh.gov.uk).

DH (2007b) *World Class Commissioning. Competencies.* London: DH. (http://www.dh.gov.uk).

DH (2008a) *About the Chief Nursing Officer.* London: DH (http://www.dh.gov.uk).

DH (2008b) *The National Health Service Constitution, a draft for consultation.* London: DH. (http://www.dh.gov.uk).

DH (2008c) *The Operating Framework for 2009/2010 for the NHS in England.* London: DH. (http://www.dh.gov.uk).

DH (2008d) *NHS Next Stage Review. Our vision for primary and community care.* London: DH. (http://www.dh.gov.uk).

DH (2008e) *Local Involvement Networks.* London: DH (http://www.dh.gov.uk).

DH (2009) *The NHS Constitution.* London: DH (http://www.dh.gov.uk)

Dobrow, M. J., Goel, V. and Upshur, R. E. G. (2004) Evidence-based health policy: context and utilisation. *Social Science and Medicine* **204** (58), 207–217.

Ham, C. (2004) *Health Policy in Britain* (5th ed.). London: Palgrave.

Healthcare Commission (2008a) *The Annual Healthcheck in 2008/9*. London: Healthcare Commission (http://www.healthcarecommission.org.uk).

Healthcare Commission (2008b) *State of Healthcare 2008*. London: Healthcare Commission (http://www.healthcarecommission.org.uk).

HM Treasury (2008) *Budget 2008. Where taxpayer's money is spent*. (http://budget.treasury.gov.uk).

Innvaer, S., Vist, G., Trommald, M. and Oxman, A. (2002) Health policy-makers perceptions of their use of evidence: a systematic review. *Journal of Health Services Research and Policy* **7** (4), 239–244.

Kennedy, I. (2001) *Learning from Bristol: the report of the public inquiry into children's heart surgery at the Bristol Royal Infirmary 1984–1995*. Cm 5207. London: The Stationery Office.

Klein, R. (2001) *The New Politics of the NHS* (4th ed.). London: Prentice-Hall.

National Audit Office (2007) *NHS Pay Modernisation: A new contract for NHS consultants in England*. London: National Audit Office. (http://www.nao.org.uk).

National Audit Office (2008) *NHS Pay Modernisation: new contracts for general practice services in England*. London: National Audit Office. (http://www.nao.org.uk).

New Labour (1997) *Because Britain Deserves Better*. (http://www.bbc.co.uk/election97/background/parties/manlab/4labmanecon.html).

NMC (Nursing and Midwifery Council) (2004) *Standards of Proficiency for Pre-registration Nursing Education*. London: NMC. (http://www.nmc-uk.org).

OECD (Organisation for Economic Co-operation and Development) (2008) *Health Data 2008* Paris: OECD (http://www.oecd.org).

Pollock, A. M. (2004) *NHS plc. The privatisation of our health care*. London: Verso.

Robinson, S. (2006) Financing healthcare: funding systems and healthcare costs. In *Healthcare Management*, Walshe, K. and Smith, J. (eds). Maidenhead: Open University Press, 33–52.

Secretary of State for Health (1989) *Working for Patients*. Cm 555. London: HMSO.

Secretary of State for Health (1997) *The New NHS. Modern. Dependable*. Cm 380. London: The Stationery Office.

Secretary of State for Health (2000) *The NHS Plan*. Cm 4818-I. London: The Stationery Office.

Secretary of State for Health (2002) *Delivering the NHS Plan*. Cm 5503. London: The Stationery Office.

Secretary of State for Health (2004) *The NHS Improvement Plan. Putting people at the heart of public servcie*. Cm 6268. London: The Stationery Office.

Secretary of State for Health (2006) *Our Health, Our Care, Our Say. A new direction for community services*. Cm 6737. London: The Stationery Office.

Secretary of State for Health (2008) *High Quality Care for All. NHS next stage review final report*. Cm 7432. London: The Stationery Office.

Smith, T. and Babbington, E. (2006) Devolution: a map of divergence in the NHS. *Health Policy Review, Summer*. London: British Medical Association.

Wanless, D. (2002) *Securing our Future; taking a long term view*. London: H M Treasury.

Wanless, D. (2004) *Securing Good Health for the Whole Population*. London: H M Treasury.

Wanless, D., Appleby, A., Harrison, A. and Patel, D. (2007) *Our Future Health Secured?* London: King's Fund.

Chapter 5

Interprofessional working

Katherine Pollard and Francesca Harris

Learning outcomes

After reading and reflecting on this chapter, you should be able to:

- Identify why interprofessional working is important;
- Acknowledge your responsibilities and obligations as a registered nurse in relation to interprofessional working;
- Outline different types of interprofessional working within nurse practice environments;
- Identify evidence to support interprofessional working;
- Outline the history of interprofessional working in UK health and social care services;
- Discuss the different forms interprofessional working can take;
- Identify factors that enhance or inhibit interprofessional working.

Related NMC Standards of Proficiency for Pre-registration Nursing Education (NMC 2004)

- Establish and maintain collaborative working relationships with members of the health and social care team and others.

- Participate with members of the health and social care team in decision-making concerning patients and clients.

- Review and evaluate care with members of the health and social care team and others.

Introduction

Interprofessional working/collaborative practice is seen to be an essential aspect of the delivery of health and social care in general and nursing care in particular. In this chapter we aim to present a comprehensive overview of the issues you need to consider in order to acquire the necessary understanding and skills to engage in effective interprofessional working.

The chapter is divided into three parts.

In Part 1, we provide an outline of interprofessional working explaining in general terms why it is important, what it looks like, and what sorts of skills and attitudes are needed to make interprofessional working effective.

In Part 2, we further explain the importance for nurses of interprofessional working before looking at how professions in the UK and other countries have interacted in the past. We also investigate specific features of interprofessional working more closely, and examine some of the barriers to effective interprofessional working. Part 2 concludes with an outline of the current evidence base for interprofessional working.

In Part 3, we explore interprofessional working in nursing practice in more depth, and discuss the skills that nurses need to ensure successful interprofessional working. Issues of relationships and communication affecting collaboration are highlighted, as well as nurses' involvement in leadership and co-ordination between different groups of professionals, care sectors and agencies. The chapter concludes with a consideration of the role of the nurse in effective interprofessional collaboration.

Part 1: Outlining interprofessional working

Case 5.1

Involved in the discharge planning arrangements to enable Mrs White, a frail 82-year-old widow, to return home are an occupational therapist, a physiotherapist, the ward manager, a community staff nurse for adults and older people, a social worker, Mrs White's daughter, the hospital consultant and Mrs White's general practitioner. Between them they work out a plan of care which involves, amongst other things, making some minor modifications to Mrs White's house which can be completed before she is ready for transfer home. This also provides sufficient time for appropriate community care to be organised.

Why interprofessional working?

Nurses rarely work in isolation. Typically, as illustrated in the case of Mrs White (Case 5.1), patients will find practitioners from more than one professional group involved in the delivery of their care. Although the range of professionals and practitioners will vary, it is unusual to find health care situations where

Interprofessional working
requires professionals and
others to work collaboratively
for the benefit of patients/
clients/service users.

nurses are not involved. Thus it is a fact of professional life that nurses must work with others in the delivery of care. This recognition is the starting point for effective **interprofessional working** and it is no accident that in both acute and primary care settings, nurses are often ideally placed to take on responsibility for co-ordinating processes and procedures involving other professionals and practitioners.

What is interprofessional working?

The term **collaborative practice** is sometimes preferred to 'interprofessional working' because it is more inclusive and explicitly allows for the contribution of non-professionals to the delivery of care (in particular, the service user or the service user's carers).

Interprofessional working is understood as a particular way of working with others. The essential feature of interprofessional working is collaboration; hence the use of such terms as collaborative working or **collaborative practice**, which involve both professionals and non-professionals in the provision of care. Thus interprofessional working is more than merely having contact with other professionals involved in the care of a given individual. It requires the recognition that no one professional or practitioner can meet all the needs of any one client. This being so, nurses need to develop the skills and attitudes that foster collaborative ways of working in order to minimise the fragmentation of care that **patients** might otherwise experience.

Patient, client, or service user?
Nurses from different areas of care are likely to have a preferred term to describe those in receipt of care. In this chapter the terms patient, client and service user are used interchangeably.

What skills and attitudes are needed for effective interprofessional working?

A number of barriers to effective interprofessional working have been identified and some of these will be detailed and explored later in the chapter. For now it is enough to say that a commitment to interprofessional working necessarily involves attempting to overcome obstacles to collaborative practice. Effective interprofessional working does not just happen; it requires an active contribution from each member of the interprofessional team as well as an environment that provides the opportunity for all members to participate in discussion and decision-making.

To engage with interprofessional working it is necessary for individuals to have, amongst other things:

- A knowledge and understanding of the roles and responsibilities of other care providers.
- A willingness to identify personal strengths and weaknesses together with a willingness to accept the need for personal and professional development.
- A willingness to trust, respect and value the contributions of all involved in the delivery of care.

Part 2: Explaining interprofessional working

Why interprofessional working is important for nurses

Interprofessional working is seen as a way of minimising the fragmentation of services that often accompanies the delivery of health care when two or more professional groups are involved (and arguably, there is always more than one professional group involved in the care of any one particular service user).

There are obvious dangers inherent in a system in which different professional groups organise themselves in different ways and specialise in particular aspects of care delivery. The most common dangers are the failure to collaborate and the failure to communicate. Sometimes these problems lead directly to tragic outcomes, as reported in the enquiries into a number of high-profile cases (see, for example, DH 1994a, Kennedy 2001, Laming 2003). One of the key consequences of these enquiries was the recognition that no profession or agency has a monopoly on care. Interprofessional working, with an emphasis on collaborative working and effective communication, is seen to be one way of preventing such failures.

The ideal of interprofessional working is that different professionals work together in an attempt to reduce the fragmentation of care as experienced by service users. For example, accurate assessment of a service user's condition or situation is important for the subsequent delivery of appropriate care. The common information available from a single systematic and structured assessment ought to be able to serve as a basis for subsequent profession-specific assessments without the need for a patient to respond to the same questions from three or four different professionals. Yet traditionally professional groups have perceived a need for profession-specific assessment processes. Arguably **the best interests of the patient** trying to rest in a hospital bed are not served by a succession of visits from, for example, a nurse, a phlebotomist, a pharmacist, another nurse, an occupational therapist, a social worker as well as a ward round of doctors all within the space of a single morning. Attempts to reduce this sort of fragmentation are not new and the idea of seamless care, integrated care pathways and the single assessment process are consistent with and, in some cases, pre-date the move towards interprofessional working. These processes all require professionals to orientate their work in terms of patient benefit rather than on the basis of professional identity and/or boundaries.

The best interests of the patient: the crux of interprofessional working is that it focuses on patient-centred care delivery.

How have professions in the UK interacted in the past?

In the UK the work of health and social care practitioners is highly institutionalised. Acts of Parliament have established professional and statutory bodies for the registration and regulation of different professional groups: the Nursing and Midwifery Council (NMC) for nurses, midwives and health visitors; the

General Medical Council (GMC) for medical practitioners; the General Social Care Council (GSCC) for social care workers; and the Health Professional Council (HPC) for allied health professionals (including, among others, radiographers, physiotherapists and occupational therapists). Although similar arrangements exist in most developed industrialised countries, this is by no means a global phenomenon. In some developing countries, such as Haiti, there is no organised health or social care system (St Boniface Haiti Foundation 2005).

Even in the UK, the institutionalisation of health care is relatively recent. Health care has been organised and regulated for little over a hundred years, while the organisation and regulation of social care has been even more recent (Taylor and Vatcher 2005). Across the health and social care spectrum, different professions have different histories with different social trajectories. The most powerful of the professions has been, and arguably still is, medicine. The delivery of health care was controlled and directed predominantly by medical professionals during the whole of the twentieth century. Where health and social care practice have intersected, the medical profession has often retained primacy (Hudson 2002). Medical professionals directed the practice of other health professions even more closely, often controlling their establishment and regulation from the outset (Witz 1992). Although nursing skills have been exercised by individuals for centuries, nursing as a distinct profession was only recognised at the end of the nineteenth century; national regulation of nursing (albeit featuring medical control) was only established in the UK in 1923 (Dingwall *et al.* 1988).

The two major developments affecting the organisation of health care in the UK during the twentieth century were the creation in 1948 of the National Health Service (NHS) and of the World Health Organization (WHO). Before the Second World War (1939–1945), health and social care in the UK was provided by a patchwork of civic bodies, charitable institutions and individual professionals in private practice. Collaboration between these various entities occurred only on an ad hoc basis, dependent largely on individual inclination and ability. Recognition that the needs of the population could not be met by such a piecemeal approach resulted in the establishment of the NHS, and the implementation during the 1940s of legislation concerning education and social care for vulnerable groups, including children (Gladstone 1995). However, communication and collaboration between different professions continued to occur in a disjointed manner, often dominated by medical priorities, and still dependent on individual initiative and inclination, rather than on systematic processes (Pollard *et al.* 2005a). It is only in the last two decades that UK governments and health and social care professionals have started to address these issues in a systematic fashion.

Professional interactions beyond the UK

In the wider social context, collaboration between epidemiologists from different European countries has been occurring since the 1920s through the League of Nations Health Organization. The main concern of this body was public health and the incidence and control of communicable diseases across Europe (League of Nations Health Organization 1931). The scope of the organisation expanded after the Second World War, culminating in the establishment of the WHO, whose aim is 'the attainment by all peoples of the highest possible level of health. Health is defined in WHO's Constitution as a state of complete physical, mental and social well-being and not merely the absence of disease or infirmity' (WHO 2006). WHO continues its influential role today, and provides a forum through which health professionals from all over the world are able to share knowledge, opinions and perspectives. In addition, governments of both developed and many developing nations aim to implement WHO recommendations.

A closer look at interprofessional working

Case 5.2

After a fifth incident of self-harm Tracy, 17, and her mother were asked to attend a case conference. Although Tracy's social worker, community psychiatric nurse and general practitioner were present, the consultant psychiatrist did not attend. Nobody had told her the venue had been changed.

Interprofessional working is one of those things that most people agree is a good idea but about which there are multiple understandings. For some, interprofessional working is just a new name for the way nurses have always operated. Looking at the number of different professionals involved in care services for Mrs White (Case 5.1) and for Tracy (Case 5.2) it is easy to imagine a nurse saying something like: 'we have always worked with other professional groups so interprofessional working is nothing new'. While it is possible that this claim may have some basis in truth, there is a good chance that what she or he thinks of as interprofessional working is merely a matter of regular contact with other professionals such as doctors, physiotherapists, social workers and so on.

Effective interprofessional working is more than merely having contact with individuals from other professional groups. Nurses often claim to have different perspectives to those of doctors and interprofessional working assumes nurses can and should make a valuable and valid contribution to patient care. Interprofessional working requires that individuals within an interprofessional team regard each other with mutual respect. A fundamental aspect of collaboration is the recognition that each member has an important contribution to make in meeting the needs of an individual patient or client.

Participation and collaboration

While it is true that during their working day nurses often have contact with other professionals, the current emphasis on interprofessional working suggests that the relationship between nurses and other health care professionals may not always be effective. The interprofessional focus on appropriate care for Mrs White (Case 5.1) only came about after a series of misunderstandings and missed opportunities for collaborative working.

Case 5.1 (continued)

A district nurse visits Mrs White following a brief answer phone message from the general practitioner in which he mentions that she has alluded to an incontinence problem. During the course of the visit, the nurse notices Mrs White has an unsteady gait and uses an old walking stick. The nurse has brought some incontinence pads and leaves a pot for Mrs White, so that a urine specimen can be collected the following day. She assumes that Mrs White's unsteady gait is not a problem, as no one has told her otherwise. As the next day is her day off, she leaves an answer phone message asking a colleague to visit Mrs White regarding her incontinence problem. She forgets, however, to mention that the purpose of the visit is to collect the urine specimen. Thus the second district nurse visits, only to be told by Mrs White that she has already been provided with incontinence pads; Mrs White too has forgotten about the specimen. As a consequence, the second district nurse thinks her visit unnecessary, assumes there has been some miscommunication and discharges Mrs White from her list.

Communication between the general practitioner and the first district nurse, as well as between the first and second district nurse, in the case of Mrs White was clearly less than satisfactory, but perhaps not entirely unusual. You may have come across similar examples of poor communication leading to missed opportunities for collaboration and resulting in fragmentation of care. As it turned out, Mrs White did have a urine infection that contributed to her continence difficulties as well as to her general low mood and feeling of being unwell. This series of negative outcomes could have been dealt with much earlier or even prevented had the professionals involved worked collaboratively. The infection was discovered only when she was admitted to hospital some four weeks later, following a serious fall at home, which resulted directly from her as yet unexplored problem of unsteadiness. Once the urine infection was treated with a course of antibiotics, and complete assessment of her mobility problems was undertaken, Mrs White's mental and physical condition improved dramatically within the space of a few days.

Activity 5.1

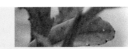

Think about health care settings you have been in and try to identify the sorts of working between different professionals that took place. Make a note of all the professionals or non-professionals involved.

As you will probably have identified from Activity 5.1, working practices between professional groups can be undertaken in different ways. The essence of interprofessional working, as it is currently understood, is *participation and collaboration*. There are a number of terms used to describe interprofessional working and they are sometimes used as if they are interchangeable. However, these terms can reflect a range of different understandings about the nature of interprofessional working. Although it is true that interprofessional working can take many forms, and can be described using a variety of terms, what is often referred to as *interprofessional* working might be better described as *multiprofessional* working.

Common terms in use are: *interprofessional*; *multiprofessional*; *interdisciplinary*; *multidisciplinary*; *inter-agency*; and *multi-agency*. A basic **rule of**

Rule of thumb: the prefix *inter* implies active collaboration whereas the prefix *multi* merely suggests there is more than one group or individual involved.

thumb is that the prefix *inter* implies that all individuals engaged in the process will actively contribute to it, and, in particular, communication and decision-making will involve representatives from each profession, discipline or agency concerned: 'practices which respect and utilise the contributions of members of the health and social care team' (NMC 2004 p. 32). By contrast, where the prefix *multi* is used, there is no such implication; for example, a multidisciplinary meeting may mean that individuals from a range of different disciplines are in attendance, but that not all of them will take an active part (Øvretveit 1997, Payne 2000).

In the context of interprofessional health care practice the term *team* is also in common use but is interpreted in different ways. Teams can vary and can range from close-knit groupings of individuals who work alongside one another on a regular basis, to loose networks of individuals from different agencies and services, who collaborate only when a particular situation demands it. Decision-making processes can vary considerably between different types of teams, and may even differ within a single team. A key feature of successful interprofessional working is that all those involved agree about what sort of collaboration is envisaged, and in particular, what sort of communication and decision-making processes are to be established (Øvretveit 1997, Payne 2000).

Interprofessional working does not exclude contributions from non-professional carers

The contribution of support workers to interprofessional working is both invaluable and indispensable – for example, home care assistants, health care assistants and administrative staff.

Although the term *interprofessional working* implies collaboration between qualified professionals, a more flexible interpretation is often needed. In most health and social care settings, the **contribution of support workers**, such as health care assistants and home carers, as well as administrative staff is an integral part of care provision. Some professions have a tradition of involving service users in the planning and delivery of care, for example in social services and mental health services (DH 1994b, Social Care Institute for Excellence 2001). This involvement of the service user is becoming increasingly widespread throughout health care services in the UK. Awareness of the rights of the individual service user has spread among professions, and it is now widely accepted that the service user voice should be heard in the process of service provision (Thomas 2005). So it is generally understood that the term *interprofessional working* implies collaboration between qualified professionals, support workers, administrative staff and/or service users, in various combinations. For these reasons and because it more accurately describes the kind of working envisaged, there are some who use *collaborative practice*, *collaborative working* or *partnership working* in preference to the term *interprofessional working*.

What gets in the way of effective interprofessional working?

When asked whether interprofessional collaboration is a good idea, most health or social care professionals are likely to answer in the affirmative. However, getting individuals to work well together can be problematic. Possible barriers to effective interprofessional collaboration include:

- different professional priorities and boundaries
- lack of understanding of others' roles and obligations
- hierarchical structures
- communication mechanisms
- poor interpersonal skills.
  (see Barrett and Keeping 2005; Bliss *et al.* 2000; Hornby and Atkins 2000)

Different professional priorities and boundaries

When considering the needs of service users, individual professionals are likely to prioritise their own professional perspectives. For example, and broadly speaking, social workers are likely to focus on issues of social support, medical staff will probably remain primarily interested in physical symptoms or disease progression, and occupational therapists will be concerned with the provision of an environment conducive to promoting a person's ability to perform daily activities. In some circumstances the values of different professional groups may be at odds with one another: for example, there may be significant disagreements about issues such as the extent of service user representation or consultation in decision-making. In some contexts, it may not be possible for some professionals to get **their own point of view** taken as seriously by colleagues either as they would wish or as they would consider appropriate.

Effective interprofessional working demands that individual practitioners transcend **their own point of view**, in order to appreciate those of other individuals involved.

Activity 5.2

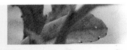

Think about all the professions involved in arranging care for Mrs White to be able to return home (see Case 5.1). How important do you think it is that consideration is given to each of the different professional perspectives?

Despite differing perspectives, there is often significant overlap between different professionals' spheres of practice, and this can lead to conflict. For example, it has been reported that physiotherapists sometimes feel their territory is encroached upon by occupational therapists, and vice versa (Booth and Hewison 2002); doctors may have reservations about nurse prescribing as this has traditionally been an exclusively medical responsibility (Moller and Begg 2005); and health visitors and midwives may disagree on what advice to give to new mothers about infant feeding (Farquhar *et al.* 1998). These situations can lead to individuals feeling they need to defend what they perceive as their uniprofessional territory, rather than engaging constructively with colleagues from other professions.

Lack of understanding of others' roles and obligations

Of course, all professional perspectives are important, and should be borne in mind: however, it is sometimes difficult for individual professionals to appreciate one another's concerns, particularly if they have little knowledge of each others' roles. There is some evidence that individual professionals appear unwilling to admit they do not know what their colleagues do: in two independent studies, all the professionals surveyed claimed to understand the roles and responsibilities of other professional groups, while believing their own roles and responsibilities to be misunderstood (Pellatt 2005, Pollard *et al.* 2003). The likelihood is that most professionals have some idea of what their colleagues do, but over- or under-estimate the scope and extent of their spheres of practice and professional responsibility. Indeed some individuals may not even have a full understanding of their own professional responsibilities and obligations (Pollard 2003).

Activity 5.3

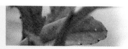

Find out how much you really know about the roles and responsibilities of other health and social care professionals by selecting and reading a chapter from *Interprofessional Working in Health and Social Care* by Barrett *et al.* (2005) (see Suggested further reading).
   After reading the chapter try to identify:

1. The differences between the role and responsibilities of nurses and those of whichever other professional group you chose to read about.
2. Any areas of overlap that might lead either to conflicts or duplication of effort.

Hierarchical structures

In many health care settings, there is a hierarchy which determines who is authorised to make decisions. Traditionally, the medical profession has domin-ated this hierarchy, while other professions have jostled for position on the lower rungs (Witz 1992). Egalitarian approaches to planning and delivering care can be severely hampered by hierarchical structures. When representatives of one profession are used to having overall authority, and are operating within systems that reinforce the status quo, it can be difficult for individuals from that profession to step back and enable others to air their views and contribute to decision-making. Conversely, those unused to making decisions can find it intimidating and stressful when they are expected to do so. This situation can be detrimental for service users, as important issues may be missed or neglected, or managed inappropriately. For individual professionals this may lead to feelings of frustration and/or disempowerment, especially if they believe their professional perspectives go unheard or unvalued, or both.

Case 5.2 (continued)

The case conference involving Tracy was organised by the social worker who decided it should take place in the hospital. That he made this decision reflects the position consultants are often believed to have in the health care hierarchy relative to other professional groups and to service users. Tracy did not, however, want to return to the hospital and it was only after the intervention of the community psychiatric nurse that Tracy agreed to meet at all, and then only at a local health centre. Unfortunately, this last minute change of plan did not reach the consultant in time.

Communication mechanisms

There is a considerable variety of mechanisms available for communication between different professionals in different health and social care settings. In some areas of practice, regular meetings are held, attended by all professionals involved in care delivery; in other areas, communication may be haphazard and ad hoc, reliant upon individuals being in the right place at the right time.

Case 5.2 (continued)

Tracy's community psychiatric nurse, Martha, was in the right place at the right time because she and Tracy's social worker, Yusuf, shared a number of clients on their respective case loads. This close working partnership between the professionals meant the necessary change of plan was communicated by a quick telephone call. Yusuf had no direct way of contacting the consultant psychiatrist and a message had been left with his secretary.

Where communication mechanisms between different professions, care sectors and agencies are not streamlined, professionals need to be particularly vigilant about making sure that relevant information is shared with everyone who needs it.

In many acute areas information is relayed between professionals in written form. While the written record may be streamlined and well-organised with each professional writing in a single set of notes for individual service users, it is still common to find information about clients held in a number of different types of records: for example, nurses may write in one set of notes while medical staff write in another; other professionals may or may not write in either. Since professionals will tend to read only the set of notes in which they write this can result in individual professionals not having all the information necessary to meet the needs of the service user; and of course, this problem will be compounded where individuals neglect to write pertinent information anywhere at all.

Many professionals rely on the telephone for conveying information. Community practitioners spend a great deal of time away from their office base, and often rely on answer phone messages. When these messages are not coherent or do not contain sufficient detail, important information can be missed. This is illustrated in the messages left, first by the general practitioner and then by the district nurse in the case of Mrs White (Case 5.1).

Poor interpersonal skills

An examination of the factors listed above supports the conclusion that effective collaboration is fundamentally dependent on both the willingness and the ability of individuals to communicate effectively with others. If any member of an interprofessional working group is not committed to the principles of collaboration problems may ensue, particularly if the member in question holds a relatively powerful position in the organisation. Poor interpersonal skills on the part of any member can lead to misunderstandings and reactions, which may have knock-on effects on the way care is provided. Language itself can be divisive: most professions ascribe meanings to words that may be understood differently by members of other professions and, similarly, professionals frequently use acronyms or jargon when they speak. Hence interprofessional collaboration can be hampered by a lack of awareness of profession-specific meanings for a word and by the unintelligibility of professional acronyms. In addition, some professionals tend to colonise service users when, for example, speaking about 'my patient' or 'my client'. If this is interpreted as one profession claiming exclusive responsibility for the well-being of a service user, other colleagues may become alienated from the process of collaboration (Barrett and Keeping 2005, Hornby and Atkins 2000).

Of course, expressing oneself is only one component of communication. If professionals are unwilling or unaware of the need **to listen** to what colleagues are saying, or to give due consideration to individuals' priorities, then it is unlikely that they are going to be able to work well together (see Chapter 9 for more information on communication and interpersonal skills).

The ability **to listen** is an essential skill for effective interprofessional working.

The evidence base for interprofessional working

In the UK, health professionals are obliged to provide evidence-based care (Parnham 1999) and evidence often takes the form of guidelines, in particular those issued by the National Institute for Health and Clinical Excellence (NICE) targeting specific areas of practice. In 2000, the Health Development Agency (HDA) was established to develop the evidence base for care delivery and to help implement that evidence in practice with the stated aims of improving health and reducing health inequalities. A key strategy for the HDA was to work with organisations such as Local Government Associations (LGA), which represented local authorities at a national level. In 2005, the functions of the HDA were transferred to NICE. While there is no NICE guideline focusing specifically on interprofessional issues, HDA publications provide evidence and support for establishing and maintaining interprofessional collaboration (see, for example, LGA/HDA/NHS 2003).

Support for interprofessional working comes from an assumption that working collaboratively will reduce the fragmentation of care delivery. The conclusions of enquiries into high-profile cases identify, amongst other things, failure of communication between different professionals involved in care as a significant feature contributing to negative patient outcomes, and this lends support to the introduction of systematic interprofessional working. Yet the idea of interprofessional working is not without its critics. There is a view that setting up systems and processes to support interprofessional collaboration may not be cost-effective (Freeth 2001); although many proponents believe that, as well as improving service delivery, effective interprofessional working can conserve resources within organisations by, for example, avoiding duplication of effort (Paul and Peterson 2001).

There is some evidence to suggest that ineffective collaboration between professions increases the risk of poor outcomes for service users. This suggests that service users will benefit from better co-ordination of care and better communication between the professions, as well as from the targeted allocation of resources across different services and agencies. However, the evidence base to support this assumption is not well developed.

One of the reasons for the paucity of evidence concerning the effect of interprofessional collaboration on service user outcomes is that it is a difficult topic to research. Processes that involve communication and joint working between different groups are complex and varied, and involve a number of interdependent factors: these include the effect of individual personalities, differing professional perspectives, the way systems are set up, how decisions are made, and how or whether actions follow those decisions. Other factors that affect care outcomes include service users' conditions or requirements, as well as relevant psychosocial factors such as individuals' social support systems. Because of these and other issues it is almost impossible to isolate and assess the effect of any single factor contributing to this amalgam of conditions and influences.

Carefully planned research can help to build the evidence base supporting inter-professional working in health and social care.

These difficulties notwithstanding, some researchers have attempted to produce evidence to support interprofessional collaboration. Problems conducting research into interprofessional issues can be minimised if settings are chosen where staff turnover is relatively low; where most of the professionals involved in delivering care are located in the same place; and where systems and processes for staff interaction are clearly articulated and understood. Projects that have attempted to assess the link between interprofessional collaboration and outcomes for service users tend to be conducted within dedicated settings where small teams of professionals provide care for specific service users. For example, in studies of acute psychiatric services (Akhavain *et al.* 1999), stroke rehabilitation (Kalra *et al.* 2005), cardiology services (Dykes *et al.* 2005) and neonatal intensive care (Smith 2005) researchers have been able to demonstrate a positive impact of interprofessional collaboration on service user outcomes.

Research focus 5.1

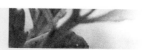

Dykes *et al.* (2005) report a study examining levels of knowledge among different professionals, and compliance with recommendations from the American College of Cardiology/American Heart Association Task Force on Practice Guidelines, before and after the implementation of the HEARTFELT initiative in a community hospital in Connecticut, USA. HEARTFELT incorporates practice guidelines within a clinical pathway, of which a significant component is patient education for self-management (known to improve prognosis after the diagnosis of heart failure). HEARTFELT was planned and implemented by an interprofessional team, comprising doctors, case managers, nurses, dietitians, information systems specialists, a pharmacist and a medical librarian. The team was co-led by a doctor and a nurse. The quasi-experimental study compared treatment records over 6 months for four patient groups. Two groups comprised historical controls, being composed respectively of patients diagnosed with heart failure (n = 90) and stroke (n = 55), treated before HEARTFELT began. The other two groups consisted of patients who were diagnosed with either heart failure (n = 96) or stroke (n = 75) after HEARTFELT started. Stroke patients were included in the study because they share many risk factors and self-management needs with heart failure patients. After the implementation of HEARTFELT, professionals were significantly more likely to record information about self-management issues in patient records (p < 0.001) and to provide patients at discharge with written information concerning self-management (p < 0.001). Adherence to guideline-based medical interventions increased in both groups during HEARTFELT, although these differences were not statistically significant. The authors note that evaluation over a longer period would provide a larger sample and facilitate identification of outcomes related to behaviour change.

There have been attempts to widen the evidence base supporting interprofessional collaboration. While the emphasis on specific service users has remained, some recent studies have shown effective interprofessional working makes a positive contribution to outcomes where care is delivered in more diverse settings, with less clearly defined processes (e.g., Ashburn *et al.* 2004, Cheek *et al.* 2004). Other studies, exploring the views of both service users and staff, have found higher levels of satisfaction (a 'soft' outcome in terms of service delivery) in settings where effective communication and co-ordination of care between professionals has been established (e.g., Akhavain *et al.* 1999, Aston *et al.* 2005, Schulman-Green 2003).

Research focus 5.2

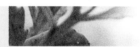

Aston *et al.* (2005) present findings from a qualitative evaluation of regular surgical morning meetings (SMMs) between doctors and nurses on a ward for infants and toddlers at a specialist paediatric hospital in Sydney, Australia. The SMMs were expressly instigated in order to improve interprofessional communication on the ward. Semi-structured interviews were conducted with ten doctors and nine nurses. The interview schedule focused on participants' experiences and views of the SMMs. Thematic analysis of the data identified four broad, interrelated themes: predictability, knowledge/perspectives, relationships/support and desired outcomes. Both nurses and doctors thought that the SMMs created a positive structure for starting the working day, and helped to increase predictability concerning their daily workload. Participants associated this with increased levels of certainty, comfort and feelings of control. Direct and indirect learning about each other's professional roles and perspectives was identified as another benefit of the SMMs, which in turn increased interprofessional understanding and respect among the staff on the ward. The SMMs were felt to be instrumental in breaking down traditional barriers between the two professional groups. Although some exceptions were noted, collegial relationships developed through the SMMs, resulting in generally improved working relationships. Nurses reported enjoying greater confidence, while doctors appreciated gaining a more holistic view of their patients' needs. Participants from both groups indicated that these benefits increased their ability to communicate with patients' parents more effectively, and in a more comprehensive way. This in turn was perceived as decreasing parents' stress levels, and facilitating the provision of appropriate information and care.

The evidence base has been extended further by reviews examining results from collections of small studies. This can result in a reinforcement of the idea that there is insufficient evidence to support the effectiveness of interprofessional collaboration in a particular area (Britton and Russell 2006). However, some of these reviews have helped to show that good working relationships and integrated practice do contribute to improved service user outcomes (Cameron 2005, Maklebust 2005, McCluskey *et al.* 2005, Rapport *et al.* 2004).

Research focus 5.3

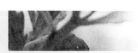

Rapport *et al.* (2004) analysed 30 peer-reviewed research articles underpinning 19 recommended practices in interdisciplinary models of early intervention and early childhood special education. The identification of these practices was part of a wider project, which entailed the development of 240 practices over seven strands. Each practice in the interdisciplinary models strand was developed following input from these 30 articles, scientific experts and/or nine stakeholder groups. For each practice, the authors detail the number of articles whose findings/results support it, identify the stakeholders supporting it, as well as the settings and study participants involved, classify the research approaches, and list the types of disability on which the studies focus. Five practices were supported only by input from either scientific experts or stakeholders, and two were incorporated into the interdisciplinary models strand from another strand in the programme. The remaining 14 practices were supported by findings/results from a number of studies reported in the articles, ranging from one to seven. Stakeholders comprised practitioner groups, and settings included children's homes, segregated and inclusive classes, hospitals and clinics. Typical children and those with disabilities participated in various studies, as did their families and personnel involved in their education and care. Both quantitative and qualitative research approaches were used. Findings/results from the studies recommended that teams comprising practitioners and family members work and make decisions together; that professionals cross disciplinary boundaries where appropriate; that intervention is based on the needs of the individual child, and not on the organisation of the services; and suggested that outcomes are the shared responsibility of all those involved in the child's care and education.

Although it can be argued that many of these studies have not produced results which can be thought of as 'hard science', there is a logic in the assumption that improving interprofessional communication and practice to enhance the quality of care will lead to improved outcomes for service users. Most available research findings support this logic.

Part 3: Exploring interprofessional working

The main rationale for improving interprofessional collaboration is the belief that it will enhance service user outcomes and experience (Øvretveit 1997). So it is crucial to consider factors influencing interprofessional collaboration in terms of the effect on service delivery. It is rare that poor outcomes in health and social services are caused by a single event, it is much more usual to see a cascade of occurrences involving poor relationships, poor communication, poor leadership and/or poor co-ordination.

Activity 5.4

Make a list of all the professionals involved in the care of Mrs White (Case 5.1) and Tracy (Case 5.2). In each case give reasons for who you think should be responsible for ensuring relevant information is passed between the various professionals at different points in time.

One of the things that doing Activity 5.4 should help to illustrate is the complexity of relationships between different professional groups. Although effective communication is a necessary requirement, effective interprofessional working is also dependent on clear understandings about leadership and co-ordination of care.

What does interprofessional working in nursing practice look like?

Nurses contribute to many different types of interprofessional working across a variety of settings. In the acute sector, nurses interact closely and systematically with a range of other health and social care professionals, support workers, administrative staff and service users, particularly in specialist areas such as stroke rehabilitation, neurology and intensive care. Collaborative episodes involving nurses may be more sporadic in other acute settings (such as within general medical wards) but the effectiveness of collaboration in these environments is equally important. In this context, the nurse's awareness of factors impacting on interprofessional collaboration may be particularly significant precisely because it may be infrequent and/or irregular.

Case 5.1 (continued)

Although a number of professionals had noticed Mrs White's unsteadiness no one person had done anything about it. It was the hospital ward manager who instigated the physiotherapy referral for Mrs White that led to collaboration between the ward nurses, the physiotherapist and the occupational therapist. For this crucial aspect of Mrs White's care it was the nurse who took a leadership and co-ordination role.

Care in the community is becoming increasingly common (DH 2002), and developments over recent years have resulted in new patterns of caregiving. For example, there are now integrated health and social care teams whose function is to deliver complete packages of care to service users with learning difficulties (Walker *et al*. 2003). These teams are managed by social services, and typically employ, among others, psychiatrists, psychologists, physiotherapists, occupational therapists, learning disabilities nurses and social workers. In addition to within-team collaboration, team members must also liaise and co-ordinate care with support workers in care homes, as well as with general practitioners and a range of different nursing groups employed by primary care trusts. Other community settings where nurses practise range from health centres to residential units for targeted service users.

An example of how effective interprofessional collaboration in community care can improve outcomes for the service user and those professionals involved can be found in the provision of palliative care. To provide improved palliative care services the *Gold Standards Framework* (GSF) (Thomas and DH 2005) has been designed for primary health care teams and now forms part of the National Health Service End of Life care initiative (DH 2006).

Activity 5.5

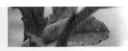

Take a look at the scenarios in Figure 5.1 to see how the GSF can enhance the patient's journey and how much it relies on good communication and awareness of individuals' perspectives and priorities, both within the team and with service users.

Mr B's reactive patient experience without the Gold Standard Framework	Mrs C's proactive patient experience with the Gold Standard Framework
General practitioners and community nurses have ad hoc arrangements – no plan of care discussed or communicated	On supportive care register Home Pack – information given to carer and patient
Problems with symptom control – high anxiety	Regular support, visits, phone calls – proactive care
Crisis call: e.g. out of hours – no management plan, handover form, or drugs available	Assessment of symptoms – referral to specialist – customised care to patient

Figure 5.1 The Gold Standard Framework adapted from the Gold Standards Framework.

Source: Thomas and DH (2005).

As the GSF in Figure 5.1 demonstrates, a key priority for effective care is that it is service user-centred. This means that the processes and implementation of care should be planned and delivered with input from all those involved, with a central focus on what is most appropriate for the service user (as opposed to what is most appropriate for the professionals or the organisation). To this end, there may be a need to develop effective partnerships, not only between different professionals and agencies, but which also include service users and other sectors within the community (DH 2001).

What do nurses need to ensure successful interprofessional working?

Most of the obstacles outlined in Part 2 of this chapter can be overcome if professionals are willing to engage in activities that promote mutual under-standing and respect. Although organisational barriers to collaboration may be difficult to change, individuals can enhance collaboration by ensuring that they have a good understanding of their colleagues' professional roles, as well as an understanding of the scope and limits of their own professional practice. An appreciation and acceptance of the differences between various profes-sional perspectives and values is essential, as is the appropriate involvement of all interested parties, including service users. A key feature of effective inter-professional collaboration is the development and implementation of **decision-making processes** that are acceptable to all those concerned. It should be obvious that effective communication skills, combined with attitudes that encompass trust, respect and the valuing of contributions from all parties, play a pivotal role in determining the quality of interprofessional interaction and collaboration (Barrett and Keeping 2005, Hornby and Atkins 2000).

Mutually agreed **decision-making processes** are crucial for successful interprofessional working.

An important starting point for nurses engaged in interprofessional collaboration is an awareness of the different perspectives, priorities and values of other professional groups. Nurses need to have confidence in the value of the nursing contribution, as well as respect for other professionals' points of view: both components are needed if one professional perspective is not to be eclipsed by another.

Traditionally nurses have been subservient to doctors, and this history is reflected in some of the structures within which nurses practise today (Dingwall *et al.* 1988). You may not be in a position to affect some of the wider factors militating against effective collaboration, for example, the professional hierarchy in the National Health Service. However, by equipping yourself with appropriate skills, you can influence the way in which you work together with your colleagues. For example, learning how and when to use negotiation skills and assertiveness techniques can be useful in preventing inappropriate decisions being made which may result in service users not receiving the most suitable care. A major benefit of developing such skills is that they can help you to avoid difficult interpersonal situations arising from an overly compliant or confrontational stance. Thus it would seem appropriate for nurses to take advantage of the many and varied techniques for developing effective communication skills.

Support may not always be forthcoming for junior nursing staff to contribute constructively to interprofessional interaction. Nursing in the UK has developed from a model drawing on the structures of both the armed forces and domestic service and the hierarchical nature of both remains in evidence (Dingwall *et al.* 1988). It has been found that while senior nurses often communicate and collaborate effectively with colleagues from other professions, nurses in more junior positions are not always included in these processes. In many instances, this situation may simply be a result of habit, rather than any conscious attempt to exclude junior staff from interprofessional interactions. The role of the nurse continues to develop and there is now an expectation that all nurses will embrace professional values, particularly those related to autonomous thinking. If junior staff display appropriate communication skills they will, in many cases, be able to establish themselves as full members of the team.

Nurses are in key positions in many areas, often being well placed to have a clear overview of a service user's requirements (Pollard *et al.* 2005b, Sellman *et al.* 2005). It is therefore essential that nurses engage effectively in interprofessional collaboration, so that these requirements can be clearly stated and considered by colleagues from appropriate disciplines. The antidote to barriers to the nursing contribution resides in individual nurses developing:

- attitudes of confidence in their own perspective and abilities;
- trust and respect for their colleagues from other disciplines;
- appropriate communication skills which enable them to facilitate decision-making in the best interests of service users.

Relationships and communication affecting collaboration

Case 5.1 (continued)

In the case of Mrs White it was her daughter, Ruth, who had the most active involvement with the health care services. It was Ruth in whom Mrs White first confided her problems of unsteadiness and incontinence. It was Ruth who contacted the general practitioner (Dr Robinson) after failing to convince her mother to contact him about these difficulties. Mrs White was upset by her daughter's approach to Dr Robinson and suspected Ruth might be trying to pack her off to an old peoples' home. Her reluctance to go into hospital resulted from the idea that she might not be allowed to return home.

Mrs White and her daughter

Professionals need to remember that carers may play a significant role in interprofessional working.

Relationships among family members can have a powerful influence on collaboration with and between professionals. Carers often feel they need to act on behalf of their relatives, just as Ruth did in seeking to 'champion' her mother's need for care. However, professionals must recognise that carers, even if they think they are acting in their relative's best interests, do not always have the needs of their family member as a priority. Being aware of differing agendas between the carer and the service user is vital to ensure appropriate user-centred care.

While her daughter would have welcomed involvement from medical and social services, Mrs White was afraid that this would spell the end of her independent living. In this case it was clear that Mrs White's ideas about her long-term prospects were different from those of her daughter. The breakdown of communication between mother and daughter caused a tension that effectively drove Mrs White away from seeking the help she needed. The discharge planning provided the opportunity for Ruth to gain insight into the care package and reassured her about some of the worries regarding her mother remaining at home. She felt less burdened once she could share the responsibility for her mother's care. Providing information can minimise stress and clarify the true picture.

Case 5.1 (continued)

After being contacted by Ruth, Dr Robinson felt he could not refer Mrs White to hospital for investigations against her wishes (he had offered to refer her 3 months earlier, during an appointment she had with him in the surgery). Dr Robinson did however feel it was appropriate to request a community nurse visit to assess her continence difficulties.

Mrs White and her general practitioner

Within health and social care, doctors have traditionally taken a dominant role. In society as a whole there has been a perception that doctors are omnipotent within their sphere of influence (Annandale 1998). It is only relatively recently that the balance of power between doctor and service user has started to change towards a more equal partnership style of relationship (Thomas 2005).

Mrs White, however, is of a generation that rarely questions what they perceive as the doctor's all-powerful status. Mrs White believed that Dr Robinson had the power to make decisions about her care without her input. She was particularly keen to avoid a hospital admission for investigations, as she believed this would spell the loss of her independence. However, Dr Robinson appeared to have little awareness of Mrs White's sense of vulnerability about this issue. He offered no other solution to Mrs White's increasing loss of mobility other than to be referred to the hospital for investigations.

The daughter and Dr Robinson

The situation became more confusing as a result of Ruth contacting Dr Robinson without the knowledge or consent of her mother. Dr Robinson was bound by confidentiality issues and so put the needs of the service user (that is, Mrs White) first (GMC 2004). Dr Robinson appeared to respect Mrs White's wish not to enter hospital, but did nothing further. Although this is an understandable response from an overworked professional who perhaps felt unable to negotiate with a patient unwilling to follow his advice, it was in fact inadequate. Ruth's action did, however, provide him with information about Mrs White's incontinence, which enabled him to make a proactive decision in the interests of Mrs White's well-being.

Dr Robinson's lack of action might have been a result of the cultural norms of his profession and the society in which we live, rather than poor practice as such. The concept of the 'expert' is very powerful among both health and social care professionals and the wider public. Despite recent changes in the professional–service user relationship, there remains a widespread assumption that an integral aspect of the professional role is to make decisions regarding the course of action service users should follow, sometimes without engaging them in a consultation process. Some professionals regard this as normal practice, with the consequence that if service users do not wish to follow the recommended course of action, the professional may not know how to proceed and may end up doing nothing. Professionals may also only consider a limited range of options, often excluding possibilities that do not centrally or directly involve their own profession.

Case 5.2 (continued)

As a result of the incident of self-harm, Tracy had been taken to the Accident and Emergency department, where she was seen by the duty psychiatrist and subsequently discharged. It was the Accident and Emergency nurse who stayed on after her shift finished in order to inform Yusuf (Tracy's social worker) about events. After Tracy's discharge, the consultant had written to the general practitioner informing her of this latest episode of self-harm. Yusuf made the decision to hold the case conference at the hospital, knowing that there was more chance of the consultant attending. However, in his decision-making he did not involve the client, Tracy.

Relationships between the professionals involved in Tracy's care

A noticeable feature of Tracy's case was the lack of cohesive relationships among all the professionals needed to ensure that she received the care she required. Despite her history, there appeared to be little awareness of the range of services with which she was involved, and many of the professionals were unknown to each other. It was simply a matter of luck that the community psychiatric nurse, who was so crucial to her continuing care in the community, was known to the social worker, and that their relationship was sufficiently developed for them to engage in appropriate communication with each other.

Interprofessional teams are often made up of diverse groups of practitioners and even those who work in the same setting may see each another infrequently. When individuals are based in different buildings or services, contact can be even less frequent, particularly where formal channels of communication have not been established. Such lack of contact can contribute to a poor grasp of colleagues' roles and responsibilities and to ignorance concerning some details of an individual service user's care, thus compounding problems with interprofessional collaboration and communication.

In Tracy's case there was no formal mechanism for communication between all of the carers involved. The consultant wrote to the general practitioner (the traditional method of communication between hospital- and community-based medical practitioners) while the social worker made use of his informal arrangement with the community psychiatric nurse. However, events in Tracy's case illustrate the point that although there may be a number of different professionals working with a single client, there is not always a sense of collaborative working. As far as Tracy's care was concerned, the consultant psychiatrist, the general practitioner, the social worker and the community psychiatric nurse made up a collection of individual workers rather than an interprofessional team.

Activity 5.6

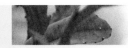

Spend some time thinking about how, if you were the community psychiatric nurse, you might go about helping to establish more collaborative working between the professionals involved in Tracy's care.

The effect of the NHS hierarchy on communication

The role of the consultant psychiatrist is particularly interesting here. Although Tracy was nominally 'her' patient, when considered within the hierarchical system of the health service, she was unaware that the community psychiatric nurse was seeing Tracy regularly in the community. One explanation for this may be that the psychiatrist, as a member of the medical profession, assumed that responsibility for care in the community would be the province of another medical practitioner, that is, the general practitioner, who would arrange and monitor any nurse involvement (which is not the case). The social worker's decision about the case conference venue is also worth reviewing: in our society, it is usual for individuals of inferior status to accommodate those of superior status when negotiation or consultation is required. Given the superior position that medical consultants occupy in the health service hierarchy, it is perfectly understandable that Yusuf assumed any meeting involving other professionals and service users would take place on the consultant's territory, a place more to the consultant's convenience. This assumption contributed to an unsatisfactory outcome and failed to involve Tracy in addressing her needs.

Both cases illustrate the need for professionals to be aware of a number of key factors in relation to communication and relationships if they are to promote effective care delivery for service users. These factors include:

- The need to consult and negotiate with service users.
- The need to understand the roles and possibilities offered by other disciplines and professionals.
- The need to recognise the effect of established systems and methods of working on the way workers in health and social care services relate to one another.
- The need for individual professionals to acquire appropriate interpersonal skills in order to manage conflict and differences of opinion in the work setting.

Nurses' involvement in leadership and co-ordination

Issues of co-ordination and leadership within an interprofessional team are important. A common cause of poor interprofessional working is a lack of clarity regarding roles and responsibilities within the team. A decision about who is best suited to take on the lead role is crucial as this person is ultimately accountable for the plan of care. In addition, for the service user and/or carer it provides a single point of contact. Clear guidelines need to exist for ensuring that one named member of the team takes the lead in co-ordinating care.

Leadership in the community

General practitioners have traditionally been considered gatekeepers in providing medical care in the community, although increasingly, specialist nurses working in collaboration with general practitioners are taking more of a lead role (Sellman *et al.* 2005). In the cases of Mrs White and Tracy, however, there appeared to be a lack of leadership and co-ordination; it is unclear which, if any, of the community health professionals was to take the primary lead.

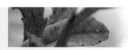

Activity 5.7

Who do you think is the most appropriate professional in the community to take the lead role in providing care to Mrs White or to Tracy? Why? If you were the district nurse caring for Mrs White, or the community psychiatric nurse caring for Tracy, what steps might you take to ensure that an appropriate system for co-ordinating care between all the relevant professionals was in place?

In requesting a home visit, Dr Robinson provided an opportunity for the district nurse to make a holistic assessment of Mrs White's needs. However the message left was ambiguous and the district nurse interpreted the request as a one-off visit. While nurses are becoming increasingly autonomous, cultural traditions and expectations within nursing mean that it is not uncommon to find individuals assuming that another professional (particularly a medical practitioner) is in overall charge or is responsible for care provision (Annandale 1998). This lack of clear parameters or agreement about spheres of responsibility can compound poor practice. The subsequent lack of communication between the nurses together with the lack of a written record compounded the mismanagement of Mrs White's suspected urine infection.

The admission into hospital triggered a more co-ordinated approach to Mrs White's care. Proximity and frequency of interaction have been shown to enhance collaborative working (Miller *et al.* 2001); and with a team working in one place it is often easier to co-ordinate a care team to provide different aspects of therapy. Discrete areas of hospital care delivery, such as rehabilitation, have a relatively established history of promoting effective interprofessional working (e.g., Allen *et al.* 2002, Booth and Hewison 2002, Dalley and Sims 2001, Miller *et al.* 2001). Once admitted to hospital, referrals were made that provided Mrs White with a team of professionals able to respond to her specific health and social needs.

However, Tracy's case shows that poor co-ordination of interprofessional collaboration can also occur within the hospital setting. While the Accident and Emergency nurse appeared to take her role and responsibilities as an interprofessional team member seriously to the extent of not wishing to delegate the responsibility of contacting Tracy's social worker, this was not the case with other members of the team. The duty psychiatrist appeared to assume that 'others' would complete the plan of care once Tracy moved from the hospital back to the community. It is important that individuals within an interprofessional team consider each other as equals, with no one practitioner being any more or less responsible for overall care provision than another.

In addition, there was considerable overlap between the disciplines in Tracy's mental health services, with involvement from the social worker, the community psychiatric nurse and the consultant psychiatrist. As mentioned earlier, such an overlap is sometimes perceived as a threat to one professional's sphere of practice and it is not uncommon for a member of the team to neglect the input of another, believing that they themselves have already addressed that particular element of care. Once again, awareness of the roles and spheres of practice of other professionals is essential for all workers engaged in interprofessional collaboration. Having explicit systems for co-ordinating care can help to minimise the incidence of any one professional's input being ignored or overlooked.

Every individual has to share responsibility for team tasks if interprofessional working is to succeed.

The interface between the acute and primary sectors

A crucial component for improving care delivery is the establishment of effective, functioning systems and relationships between the acute and primary sectors. Although both are staffed and run by health and/or social care professionals, the nature of the environment, the professional role and the relationships with service users vary considerably between them (Allen *et al.* 2002, Miller *et al.* 2001, Sellman *et al.* 2005). Many professionals working in the community will have worked in hospitals at some time during their career; however, because of a greater emphasis on community provision of care, it is no longer unusual to find newly qualified practitioners employed in community posts. Hospital-based staff may never have had any experience of community practice. In particular, nurses working on hospital wards and those working in the community may hold different priorities, expectations and experiences concerning the nature of the nursing role (Sellman *et al.* 2005). Just as it is important for professionals from different disciplines to understand each other's roles, it is equally important that practitioners from the same profession, but who are based in different environments, understand the implications for co-ordination of care delivery when service users move between them.

The cases of Mrs White and Tracy illustrate the need for professionals (including, and perhaps particularly, nurses) to be aware of a number of key factors concerning **leadership and co-ordination** if they are to promote effective care delivery for service users. These factors include:

Appropriate **leadership and co-ordination** are essential components contributing to good interprofessional working.

- The need for clear guidelines for leading and co-ordinating a team successfully.
- The need for all involved to know who is the overall co-ordinator of care.
- The need to ensure clear lines of communication about who is responsible for which particular aspects of care.
- The need to ensure no one professional's input is being ignored or overlooked.
- The need to recognise that different practitioners based in different environments may have different priorities, expectations and experiences of their role, even when they belong to the same profession.
- The need for practitioners based in different environments to understand the implications for co-ordination of care delivery when service users move between them.

It would be unrealistic to assume that all professionals will equip themselves with the requisite skills and knowledge to promote effective interprofessional collaboration so that service users receive the care they need. However, in most health care settings, nurses are well placed to take on co-ordination if not leadership roles within interprofessional teams (Pollard *et al.* 2005b). If nurses take it upon themselves to develop appropriate skills and to practise as part of an integrated interprofessional team, then they can make a real difference to the way that care is co-ordinated and delivered on the ground.

Conclusion

This chapter has attempted to illustrate the importance of interprofessional working and some of the factors that can hinder or help in the development of effective interprofessional care. By reading this chapter we hope that you will have come to recognise that you can influence the quality of care given to patients, clients and service users and that you can contribute to effective interprofessional working by following a relatively simple course of action that includes:

- Involving service users in plans of care.
- Consulting service users about their circumstances and in particular finding out which other professionals they deal with.

- Ensuring all professionals involved with service users remain informed about issues affecting care.
- Providing sufficient detail to colleagues, particularly in areas where you know that assumptions may be operating, for example, the identity of the professional taking the lead in a case, or the possible venue for a meeting.

This may seem to imply that nurses must single-handedly take on the responsibility for improving interprofessional collaboration. This is not so; but if nurses are to fulfil their professional obligations to service users, then they must lead the way and demonstrate an awareness of and capacity for effective interprofessional working.

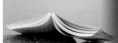

Suggested further reading

Barrett, G., Sellman, D. and Thomas, J. (eds) (2005) *Interprofessional Working in Health and Social Care: Professional perspectives*. Basingstoke: Palgrave Macmillan.

Øvretveit, J., Mathias, P. and Thompson, T. (eds) (1997) *Interprofessional Working for Health and Social Care*. Basingstoke: Palgrave.

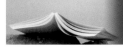

References

Akhavain, P., Amaral, D., Murphy, M., Uehlinger, K. and Cardone, M. (1999) Collaborative practice: a nursing perspective of the psychiatric interdisciplinary treatment team. *Holistic Nursing Practice* **13** (2), 1–11.

Allen, D., Lyne, P. and Griffiths, L. (2002) Studying complex caring interfaces: key issues arising from a study of multi-agency rehabilitative care for people who have suffered a stroke. *Journal of Clinical Nursing* **11** (3), 297–305.

Annandale, E. (1998) *The Sociology of Health and Medicine: A critical introduction*. Cambridge: Polity Press.

Ashburn, A., Jones, D., Plant, R., *et al*. (2004) Physiotherapy for people with Parkinson's disease in the UK: an exploration of practice. *International Journal of Therapy and Rehabilitation* **11** (4), 160–167.

Aston, J., Shi, E., Bullot, H., Galway, R. and Crisp, J. (2005) Qualitative evaluation of regular morning meetings aimed at improving interdisciplinary communication and patient outcomes. *International Journal of Nursing Practice* **11** (5), 206–213.

Barrett, G. and Keeping, C. (2005) The processes required for effective interprofessional working. In *Interprofessional Working in Health and Social Care: Professional perspective*, Barrett, G., Sellman, D. and Thomas, J. (eds). Basingstoke: Palgrave Macmillan, pp. 18–31.

Bliss, J., Cowley, S. and While, A. (2000) Interprofessional working in palliative care in the community: a review of the literature. *Journal of Interprofessional Care* **14** (3), 281–90.

Booth, J. and Hewison, A. (2002) Role overlap between occupational therapy and physiotherapy during in-patient stroke rehabilitation: an exploratory study. *Journal of Interprofessional Care* **16** (1), 31–40.

Britton, A. and Russell, R. (2006) Multidisciplinary team interventions for delirium in patients with chronic cognitive impairment. *Cochrane Library Database* (1): (CD000353).

Cameron, D. (2005) Coordinated multidisciplinary rehabilitation after hip fracture. *Disability and Rehabilitation* **27** (18/19), 1081–1090.

Cheek, J., Gilbert, A., Ballantyne, A. and Penhall, R. (2004) Factors influencing the implementation of quality use of medicines in residential aged care. *Drugs and Aging* **21** (12), 813–824.

Dalley, J. and Sims, J. (2001) Nurses' perceptions of physiotherapists as rehabilitation team members. *Clinical Rehabilitation* **15** (4), 380–389.

DH (Department of Health) (1994a) *The Report of the Enquiry into the Care and Treatment of Christopher Clunis*. London: HMSO.

DH (1994b) *Working in Partnership: A collaborative approach to care. Report of the Mental Health Nursing Review Team*. London: HMSO.

DH (2001) *Making a Difference in Primary Care: The challenge for nurses, midwives and health visitors. Case studies from NHS regional conferences*. London: DH.

DH (2002) *Liberating the Talents. Helping primary care trusts and nurses to deliver the NHS plan*. London: DH.

DH (2006) *End of Life Care Initiative*. (http://www.dh.gov.uk).

Dingwall, R., Rafferty, A. M. and Webster, C. (1988) *An Introduction to the Social History of Nursing*. London: Routledge.

Dykes, P. C., Acevedo, K., Boldrighini, J., *et al.* (2005) Clinical practice guideline adherence before and after implementation of the HEARTFELT (HEART Failure Effectiveness and Leadership Team) intervention. *Journal of Cardiovascular Nursing* **20** (5), 306–314.

Farquhar, M., Camilleri-Ferrante, C. and Todd, C. (1998) Working with team midwifery: health visitors' views of one team midwifery scheme. *Journal of Advanced Nursing* **27** (3), 546–552.

Freeth, D. (2001) Sustaining interprofessional collaboration. *Journal of Interprofessional Care* **15** (1), 37–46.

Gladstone, D. (1995) Individual welfare: locating care in the mixed economy. Introducing the personal social services. In *British Social Welfare: Past, present and future*, Gladstone, D. (ed.). London: UCL Press, pp. 161–170.

GMC (General Medical Council) (2004) *Confidentiality: Protecting and providing information*. London: GMC.

Hornby, S. and Atkins, J. (2000) *Collaborative Care. Interprofessional, interagency and interpersonal* (2nd ed.). Oxford: Blackwell Science.

Hudson, B. (2002) Interprofessionality in health and social care: the Achilles' heel of partnership? *Journal of Interprofessional Care* **16** (1), 7–17.

Kalra, L., Evans, A., Perez, I., *et al.* (2005) A randomised controlled comparison of alternative strategies in stroke care. *Health Technology Assessment* **9** (18), iii–iv, ix–x, 1–79.

Kennedy, I. (2001) *Learning from Bristol: The report of the public inquiry into children's heart surgery at the Bristol Royal Infirmary 1984–1995*. London: The Stationary Office.

Laming, Lord (2003) *Inquiry into the death of Victoria Climbié*. London: The Stationery Office.

League of Nations Health Organization (1931) *League of Nations Health Organization*. Geneva: WHO Information Section.

LGA/HDA/NHS (2003) *Planning with a Purpose. Local authorities and the NHS: planning together to improve health and well-being across the local strategic partnerships*, (http://www.nice.org.uk).

Maklebust, J. (2005) Pressure ulcers: the great insult. *Nursing Clinics of North America* **40** (2), 365–389.

McCluskey, A., Lovarini, M., Bennett, S., *et al.* (2005) What evidence exists for work-related injury prevention and management? Analysis of an occupational therapy evidence database (OTseeker). *British Journal of Occupational Therapy* **68** (10), 447–456.

Miller, C., Freeman, M. and Ross, N. (2001) *Interprofessional Practice in Health and Social Care. Challenging the shared learning agenda*. London: Arnold.

Moller, P. and Begg, E. (2005) Independent nurse prescribing in New Zealand. *New Zealand Medical Journal* **118** (1225), 1724.

NMC (Nursing and Midwifery Council) (2004) *Standards of Proficiency for Pre-registration Nursing Education*. London: NMC.

Øvretveit, J. (1997) How to describe interprofessional working. In *Interprofessional Working for Health and Social Care*, Øvretveit, J., Mathias, P. and Thompson, T. (eds). Basingstoke: Palgrave, pp. 9–33.

Parnham, J. (1999) Clinical governance and evidence-based health care: is there a governance-evidence gap? *MIDIRS Midwifery Digest* **9** (2), 144–146.

Paul, S. and Peterson, Q. (2001) Interprofessional collaboration: issues for practice and research. *Occupational Therapy in Health Care* **15** (3/4), 1–12.

Payne, M. (2000) *Teamwork in Multiprofessional Care*. Basingstoke: MacMillan.

Pellatt, G. C. (2005) Perceptions of interprofessional roles within the spinal cord injury rehabilitation team. *International Journal of Therapy and Rehabilitation* **12** (4), 143–150.

Pollard, K. (2003) Searching for autonomy. *Midwifery* **19** (2), 113–124.

Pollard, K., Ross, K., Means, R. and Thomas, J. (2003) *Transference to Practice (TOP): A study of collaborative working in placement settings (Phase 1 and Phase 2)*. Bristol: University of the West of England. (http://hsc.uwe.ac.uk).

Pollard, K., Sellman, D. and Senior, B. (2005a) The need for interprofessional working. In *Interprofessional Working in Health and Social Care: Professional perspectives*, Barrett, G., Sellman, D. and Thomas, J. (eds). Basingstoke: Palgrave Macmillan, pp. 7–17.

Pollard, K., Ross, K. and Means, R. (2005b) Nursing leadership, interprofessionalism and the modernization agenda. *British Journal of Nursing* **14** (6), 339–344.

Rapport, M. J. K., McWilliam, R. A. and Smith, B. J. (2004) Practices across disciplines in early intervention: the research base. *Infants and Young Children* **17** (1), 32–44.

Schulman-Green, D. J. (2003) Psychosocial issues in palliative care: physicians' self-perceived role and collaboration with hospital staff. *American Journal of Hospice and Palliative Care* **20** (1), 34–40.

Sellman, D., Godsell, M. and Townley, M. (2005) Nursing. In *Interprofessional Working in Health and Social Care: Professional perspectives*. Barrett, G., Sellman, D. and Thomas, J. (eds). Basingstoke: Palgrave Macmillan, pp. 83–99.

Smith, J. R. (2005) Early enteral feeding for the very low birth weight infant: the development and impact of a research-based guideline. *Neonatal Network* **24** (4), 9–19.

Social Care Institute for Excellence (2001) *About SCIE* (http://www.scie.org.uk).

St Boniface Haiti Foundation (2005) *Working Together to Bring Healthcare and Humanitarian Aid to the Poor of Rural Haiti* (http://www.haitihealth.org).

Taylor, P. and Vatcher, A. (2005) Social work. In *Interprofessional Working in Health and Social Care: Professional perspectives*, Barrett, G., Sellman, D. and Thomas, J. (eds). Basingstoke: Palgrave Macmillan, pp. 155–169.

Thomas, J. (2005) Issues for the future. In *Interprofessional Working in Health and Social Care: Professional perspectives*, Barrett, G., Sellman, D. and Thomas, J. (eds). Basingstoke: Palgrave Macmillan, pp. 187–199.

Thomas, K. and DH (2005) *The Gold Standards Framework. A programme for community palliative care. NHS End of Life Care Programme* (http://www.goldstandardsframework.nhs.uk).

Walker, T., Stead, J. and Read, S. G. (2003) Caseload management in community learning disability teams: influences on decision-making. *Journal of Learning* **7** (4), 297–321.

WHO (World Health Organization) (2006) *About WHO* (http://www.who.int/about/en/).

Witz, A. (1992) *Professions and Patriarchy*. London: Routledge.

Chapter 6

Evidence-based practice

Mark Broom and Derek Sellman

Learning outcomes

After reading and reflecting on this chapter, you should be able to:

- Identify the range and scope of evidence;
- Have an awareness of hierarchies of evidence;
- Acknowledge the relevance of evidence to nursing practice;
- Outline some of the difficulties in using evidence in practice.

Related NMC Standards of Proficiency for Pre-registration Nursing Education (NMC 2004)

- Ensure that current research findings and other evidence are incorporated in practice.

- Identify relevant changes in practice or new information and disseminate it to colleagues.

- Engage with, and evaluate, the evidence base that underpins safe nursing practice.

- Use evidence-based knowledge from nursing and related disciplines to select and individualise nursing interventions.

Introduction

There is a great deal written about evidence-based practice and the phrase has come to mean different things to different people. Some suggest that the wholesale adoption of evidence-based practice in nursing is a bad idea, while others believe it to be the best thing since sliced bread. Whatever the reality, evidence-based practice is now considered essential for safe and effective nursing practice. In this chapter we offer some information that we hope will be useful to you in your attempt to practise from an evidence base.

The chapter is divided into three parts and structured around four phases of evidence-based practice: reviewing practice; finding evidence; appraising evidence; and changing practice.

In Part 1, we offer some general ideas about evidence. We note that not all evidence is of equal value, that the evidence of our senses can be wrong and we outline the reasons for the need for nurses to be able to appraise evidence in whatever form it appears.

In Part 2, we say more about the nature of evidence and begin to offer some ideas around the notion and importance of reliability. We offer some examples of how we all use evidence in our everyday and non-nursing situations and we outline some important sources of evidence with a few tips on searching the literature. The focus here is on reviewing practice and finding evidence.

In Part 3, we explore ideas around recognising the value of different forms of evidence before engaging with some issues of critical appraisal. The focus here is on reviewing evidence with a few suggestions about implementing change where that proves to be appropriate.

Part 1: Outlining evidence-based practice

Case 6.1

It is Maurice's first day as a student nurse on Charterhouse Ward. He is surprised to find the 'underarm lift' being used routinely by staff on the ward. When he asks why this discredited lift is still being used when the evidence points to its potential to cause harm to both patients and staff, Kathy, his mentor, says it is because of: pressure of time; busyness of the ward; unavailability of suitable equipment and so on. Finally Kathy admits that the underarm lift shouldn't be used but says 'it is just what we do here'.

Of course, it does not happen like this in all practice areas but in asking the seemingly innocent question 'why do it that way?' Maurice has uncovered the complex nature of the relationship between evidence and practice. Even in cases where the evidence is uncontroversial (such as in relation to the underarm lift) there is no guarantee that nurses will base their practice on that evidence. There are many possible reasons for this and some of these will be explored later in this chapter.

Why evidence-based practice?

As well as '**evidence-based practice**' you are likely to come across terms such as 'evidence-based medicine', 'research-based practice', 'evidence-based health care' and 'evidence-based nursing'. Sometimes these terms are used interchangeably in the literature yet they each mean slightly different things: to use them interchangeably is to confuse medicine with nursing and to confuse evidence with research. For reasons that should become clear as you read this chapter we prefer the term 'evidence-based practice'.

That practice should be based on evidence seems so self-evident that it is hard to understand why anyone would disagree. Yet the continued emphasis on the need for nurses to base practice on evidence suggests not only that some current nursing practice is not evidence-based but also that the idea of **evidence-based practice** is not as straightforward as it might appear.

Yet we all make use of evidence everyday. We use the evidence of our senses to see, hear, smell, taste and feel the things around us. Under normal circumstances we can rely on the evidence of our senses. When we wish to cross a road we interpret the evidence that comes from our eyes to determine the distance and speed of approaching cars. We turn our head to see who is running when we hear the rapid fall of footsteps behind us and we discard the milk that smells bad rather than use it in our coffee. Such everyday decisions are made on the basis of evidence. In these examples the evidence comes from our senses and our senses usually serve us well. Generally speaking we know the evidence of our senses to be reliable although we also know that sometimes it can be unreliable. Some of the things our senses tell us are real we know to be illusory: for example, we know that railway lines do not converge despite the evidence of our eyes and similarly we know that a straight stick looks crooked when partly immersed in a pond.

Thus we already know there is evidence that we can rely on and evidence about which we should be wary. To ignore the evidence about an approaching car when we cross the road would be foolish indeed but it would be equally foolish to walk on railway lines believing that trains cannot travel on tracks that converge. In both situations we make a judgement about the evidence before deciding what action to take. In other words, the evidence does not speak for itself. Rather we make an assessment about which evidence we should pay attention to and which evidence we should ignore. In making such a judgement we demonstrate that not only do we already know not all evidence to be of equal value, but also that we have the ability to appraise evidence; that is, to make judgements about the relative value of different pieces of evidence.

Thus you already have an ability to appraise evidence. You do this everyday in relation to all sorts of decisions you make and actions you take. To appraise evidence for nursing effectively merely requires you to have some knowledge and understanding about the criteria for making judgements about the value of different pieces of evidence. In other words, if you are going to be able to make effective judgements about which evidence you should pay attention to and which evidence you should be wary of as you go about your everyday nursing practice you need to be able to know the relative value of different pieces of evidence. And just as you have previously learned what you know about the dangers of approaching cars and walking on train tracks, so you can learn how to distinguish between weak and strong evidence for nursing practice.

Simply put, evidence-based practice requires nothing more than:

- reviewing practice;
- finding evidence;
- appraising the evidence;
- changing practice where appropriate.

Of course, it is not quite that simple, as each of these activities requires specific knowledge and skills. Reviewing practice requires some form of reflection; finding evidence requires search and retrieval skills; appraising evidence requires knowledge of the criteria against which judgements are made; and changing practice requires, amongst other things, effective interpersonal skills as well as leadership and management skills.

Nevertheless, Maurice has set the ball rolling for evidence-based practice and he and Kathy, his mentor, are about to embark on a steep learning curve in order to discover best manual handling practice and to try to implement it on Charterhouse Ward.

Part 2: Explaining evidence-based practice

Why evidence-based practice is important for nurses

The adoption of evidence-based practice for nursing follows the development of evidence-based medicine that recognised the importance of the need for a systematic appraisal of the evidence on which clinical decisions are made. Evidence-based nursing is seen as attractive because it offers an alternative to the 'sister knows best' or 'this is the way it is done on this ward' approach to the delivery of nursing care. This approach, which had been so pervasive for so long, came in for criticism particularly during the 1980s and was given voice in the book *Nursing Rituals* (Walsh and Ford 1989) in which everyday routine nursing practices (such as pre-operative fasting, the use of saline baths, and the taking of temperature) were scrutinised against the available evidence. What Walsh and Ford found was a dominance of ritual over rational action.

Research focus 6.1
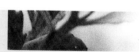

Without rejecting the potential value of the saline bath, Walsh and Ford found that a specific concentration of salt would be required to achieve any therapeutic effect yet routine practice was merely to pour an unspecified amount of table salt into a bath. Thus the possibility of therapeutic action became a matter of chance depending on how much salt any particular nurse put into the bathwater on any particular occasion. If a saline bath is to have a beneficial effect then those responsible for preparing it should at the very least be able to know how to get the correct concentration.

The use of evidence for professional practice

The use of evidence is common among professional groups. For example, we all know that the police need to gather sufficient evidence of wrongdoing before a person can be charged with a crime. We also know that both the prosecution and the defence will use evidence in court in the attempt to persuade a jury of the guilt or innocence of the accused. We like to think that any evidence used during criminal proceedings is sufficiently accurate to ensure the defendant gets a fair trial. If we subsequently find that the evidence used to convict someone turns out to be faulty, or was used in such a way as to give a false impression of guilt or innocence, then we immediately recognise that something has gone wrong. When this happens we know that recompense is required: the trial will be abandoned; the prisoner found guilty as a result of false evidence will be released; and so on.

Generally speaking, we like to think that only the guilty go to prison and we like to think that the evidence on which they are found guilty is definitely true. Yet, as noted in Chapter 3, even in law evidence does not have to be conclusive. In criminal law, the role of evidence is to 'prove' something beyond reasonable doubt, whereas in civil proceedings all that is required is that evidence leads to a conclusion on the balance of probability. In other words, even in an area that we often imagine requires straightforward and well-defined standards of evidence, the evidence can be (and often is) contradictory, contestable, and open to interpretation.

In this respect nursing is no different. The evidence that nurses use to guide their practice can also be (and often is) contradictory, contestable, and open to interpretation; it can also be less or more reliable. The safe and competent nurse is the one who, amongst other things, is able to distinguish between reliable and unreliable evidence; and who can identify contradictions in evidence, understand why some evidence is contestable, and recognise that in some cases different interpretation of the same evidence is possible. Thus while sometimes the evidence for nursing practice is comprehensive and uncontroversial (such as the evidence in relation to the prohibition on the underarm lift) it may be more common to find the evidence either inconclusive or weak. Thus in order to appraise evidence for practice a nurse may need to act not only for the defence and the prosecution but also as judge and jury.

In court it is the job of both the prosecution and defence lawyers to convince the jury of:

1. The strength of the evidence supporting their case.
2. The weakness of the evidence of their opponent.

The questioning and cross-examination of witnesses is designed to test the strength of the evidence on which the jury is asked to make a decision and the role of the judge is to ensure that only relevant and appropriate questions are asked. It is in the asking and answering of the questions that the strengths and weaknesses of the evidence are exposed.

Similarly there is a need to ask relevant and appropriate questions of the evidence on which nursing practice is based or proposed. **Critiquing frameworks**

The ability to successfully analyse or critique research requires knowledge and understanding of the research process and method. **Critiquing frameworks** are tools comprising of a series of focused questions that help you determine the usefulness of the research article in practice. Later in this chapter you will encounter a variety of differing critique approaches.

are merely systematic ways of asking relevant and appropriate questions so that judgements can be made about the strength of evidence.

Thus a critiquing framework is a tool to aid in the appraisal of evidence. We need to know the strength of different pieces of evidence in order to base nursing decisions and actions on the strongest evidence available: where strong evidence exists it would be foolish to rely on weak evidence. We do not walk on train tracks because the evidence of our eyes (in this instance) is weaker than other, stronger evidence telling us that train tracks do not converge.

It might be helpful to think about this in terms of the use of evidence in court. The strongest evidence is that which leaves the jury in no doubt about the guilt or innocence of the accused. If there remains room for doubt, then the next strongest evidence is that which is 'beyond reasonable doubt'. Where there is still reasonable doubt, then the next level of evidence is that which leads to a conclusion on the 'balance of probability'. So we have three levels of evidence here:

1. Evidence about which there is no doubt.
2. Evidence that leads to a conclusion 'beyond reasonable doubt'.
3. Evidence that leads to a conclusion based on the 'balance of probability'.

On this account, 'balance of probability' evidence is the weakest type. Yet in the real world of nursing this is the most likely form of evidence to be readily available. This goes some way to explaining why so much emphasis is placed on the **hierarchy of evidence** and helps to explain why 'beyond reasonable doubt' evidence is given such high value.

> The ability to rank or categorise evidence assists the practitioner when making decisions about the quality of the research article read. **Hierarchies of evidence** are systematic and robust tools used when classifying articles.

Activity 6.1

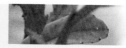

Imagine you are planning to buy a brand new car (if only nurses could afford such a luxury!). Have a go at making a list of the criteria you might use to help you choose which car to buy.

With such an expensive item as a car it is likely you will spend some time browsing through manufacturers' glossy brochures and, perhaps, even reading one or two motoring journals. This will provide you with a range of information (or evidence). Some of this information will be in the form of 'hard' evidence (e.g., statistics on fuel economy or CO_2 emissions) and some will be of the more 'soft' variety (e.g., descriptions of comfort or safety features).

The hard information will include statistics such as the number of miles travelled for each litre of petrol, figures for carbon dioxide emissions, and the passenger safety record. Having information of this type allows you to make judgements about, for example, the relative environmental impact of the cars on your shortlist. However, if each manufacturer is using a different test to calculate carbon dioxide emissions then some cars may appear to be more environmentally friendly than others. This is similar to assuming foods advertised as low fat are healthy options (this is not necessarily true as noted in Chapter 10). It is only possible to make direct comparisons when the figures from all manufacturers are based on standard tests. Thus figures on fuel economy for different cars can only be meaningfully compared if manufacturers adopt standardised testing, and this is exactly what manufacturers are required to do in the UK. So if you think fuel economy is important then you can make a direct comparison between different cars because manufacturers produce data for fuel consumption based on a standard urban cycle.

The type of hard evidence illustrated above can be relied upon precisely because it allows direct comparisons to be made. To return to the law analogy, it represents 'beyond reasonable doubt' type of evidence. Using this kind of evidence you can say with some confidence that, for example, car X performs best in terms of fuel economy, carbon dioxide emissions and passenger safety and that on these grounds it would be the best car to buy. However, you may not choose to buy car X for all sorts of other reasons, some of which are more rational than others, and most of which will be derived from a more soft type of evidence.

Although often crucial, soft information cannot be compared in the same way as hard evidence. There is no point in buying the car with the best environmental record if when you sit in the driving seat your feet do not reach the pedals. So you need to try it out. You need some first-hand information on things such as comfort, all-round visibility and ease of manoeuvrability. It will not matter how persuasive the hard evidence is if you find car X uncomfortable to drive, or if you find you cannot see out of the side windows. In fact, this evidence is not soft at all, but neither is it quantifiable in the way fuel economy is. Nevertheless, it is evidence that is no less important to you than the hard evidence.

When decisions are influenced by our own experience or personal interpretation of that experience then it is deemed to be **subjective**. In contrast, objective decisions are said to be undistorted by these factors and are easier to quantify and be reproduced by others when similar decisions are required.

There is yet more soft information (or evidence) that may influence your choice. You may have a bias against a particular manufacturer (you may have heard people say things like 'you wouldn't see me dead driving one of those'); you may have what advertisers call 'brand loyalty' based on positive previous experience of a manufacturer; or you may have a preference for a particular colour or shape. This information is much more **subjective**, and may well involve your emotions. As such, it is less reliable and may lead you to neglect or ignore relevant evidence. For example, you may simply not consider any car from one manufacturer because they once had a reputation of producing cars that rust; or because a distant uncle had no end of trouble with one in the 70s and no one in the family has ever bought one since.

Activity 6.2

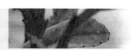

Look again at the criteria you made earlier (Activity 6.1).
Try to work out which of the items on your list are hard evidence and which are soft evidence.

Chances are that your list will contain some hard and some soft types of considerations and both influence the choices we make. If we choose a car purely on soft types of evidence we may be swayed by factors that relate to our feelings or preferences alone; we might choose a car that comes in our favourite colour only to find later that it is much more expensive to run, or that the nearest service centre is 50 miles away. If we choose purely on the rational grounds of hard evidence we would try to consider each make and model on its merits. We would try not to let our feelings (either negative or positive) get in the way of making the best decision. We would rely on current rather than past evidence. We would look for the most recent evidence to see if the 'rust bucket' reputation is still deserved; and we would recognise the possibility that our uncle's experience might not have been as bad as family mythology makes out (he may just have been particularly unlucky).

In using hard evidence as a starting point we not only increase the choices available to us, we also reduce the influence of unreliable evidence on our decision-making. In this sense, at least, evidence-based practice is an attempt to reduce the influence of unreliable evidence on nursing decisions.

The choices nurses make in relation to the delivery of care are subject to the same pressures, biases and irrational feelings that we all share when making other choices in our lives. The difference is that while it is acceptable to allow these things to influence our choice of car (because that is a purely personal choice) it is not acceptable to allow them to dominate choices in relation to nursing care. This is because nursing decisions need to be related to the needs of patients rather than to our own preferences. So while some of the different types of information and evidence illustrated in the buying a car example will be appropriate to decision-making in nursing, other types will be unhelpful and possibly harmful. As a registered nurse, it is important to be able to distinguish between the two. Figure 6.1 illustrates the similarities in evidence used when buying a car and when making choices for nursing practice.

Buying a car	Providing evidence-based care
• Seeking up-to-date advice from the literature by exploring motoring magazines and brochures	• Looking for best practice in academic journals
• Analysis of performance data	• Analysis of statistics/results
• Discussions with friends and family	• Peer discussion on best practice
• Your attitude, the feel and drivability of the car	• Feelings and the lived experience presented by qualitative research
• Past experience of driving and car ownership	• Established nursing practice/how it has always been done

Figure 6.1 Comparison of types of evidence used in buying a car and in providing care.

Reviewing practice

Reviewing practice is a precursor for evidence-based practice. Reviewing practice requires thinking about nursing. This may range from merely wondering if there might be a better way of doing something to undertaking a full-blown structured reflection following a critical incident and using one or other of the established models of reflection (see Chapter 13 for more information on the process of reflection).

If we give Maurice (Case 6.1) the benefit of the doubt we can say that he was merely asking an innocent question because he has received conflicting information about nursing. His tutors (who are not there with him in practice) point him to the evidence about the dangers of the underarm lift, while the nurses with whom he is working use it all the time. Maurice merely wants to know who is right so that he can become a safe practitioner. He finds it hard to imagine that the nurses on Charterhouse Ward would knowingly put themselves and the patients at risk of harm so he thinks they must know something he does not. And he tries to find out what this something is by asking his mentor.

If we also give Kathy (Maurice's mentor and the ward sister) the benefit of the doubt and assume she is not deliberately trying to put the nursing staff or the patients at risk of harm, then we might say that she has to ensure everything gets done within the available time. Hence Kathy has a bigger picture in mind as she allows the practice to continue. She knows the underarm lift is not good practice but since she became ward manager she has had a number of more demanding pressures to deal with and anyway, no one has been injured as far as she can tell. Hence she has just let poor practice continue. However, now Maurice has raised the issue she realises it is time to do something about it. In this sense then, and despite being a first-year student nurse, Maurice has made a difference; he has acted (albeit unintentionally) as an agent of change.

Finding evidence

Case 6.1 (continued)

Most of the patients on Charterhouse Ward need help with mobility. Having been prompted to action by Maurice, Kathy now wants to learn more about best practice in manual handling. As a first step she will need to find the evidence.

Kathy goes in search of the Trust policy on manual handling. She is a little disappointed with what she finds. While it contains some useful information about the need to undertake mobility assessments on individual patients and has some references, it is undated and provides only a few specific recommendations for good practice, although it does reinforce the message that the underarm lift is about as far away from good practice as it is possible to get. Thus Kathy's search for evidence is far from over, and she decides to enlist the help of Maurice with his new-found knowledge gained from the university about evidence-based practice. Unfortunately, Maurice has only just begun to learn about doing a literature search so is not very experienced. They agree to work together to see what they can find.

Finding evidence is a crucial step in evidence-based practice. This much should be obvious, but it needs to be the right sort of evidence; and finding the most appropriate evidence for any particular aspect of nursing practice can be a daunting prospect. While the Internet has undoubtedly made searching for information relatively easy, finding reliable evidence means you need to know something about sources of information, and how authoritative those sources are. Using search engines and online encyclopaedias will certainly help you to access a huge amount of information but that in itself can create difficulties. When there is so much information, it can be difficult to choose between articles; when there is so much information you need some form of **search strategy**.

A little time spent planning your **search strategy** results in a more realistic outcome and in less frustration from a practitioner's perspective. The use of key words, time range, limits on language, type of article (e.g. original research, literature review or full text) will help give focus to your search. Spending time learning how to use databases and search engines effectively will be rewarded in the future in less time spent exploring search results that do not match your original criteria. Thus finding the right sort of information requires an element of computer literacy, avoiding information overload and searching effectively.

Computer literacy

Although there has been a dramatic increase in the use of computers in the workplace and a demand for home broadband Internet connectivity, this does not mean all health care practitioners have the skills to navigate around the electronic databases or effectively utilise the World Wide Web in the pursuit of information. Without the necessary skills the very tool that should liberate could actually frustrate the health care practitioner.

Information overload

This phenomenon is captured in the idea of not being able to see the wood for the trees. With so much information available in a variety of differing media it is difficult to know how to filter good from poor information. Effective search patterns help to reduce the amount of information presented, making the whole process more manageable.

Effective searching

Being able to develop and use search patterns and transfer these from one database to another allows efficient use of search time, and means you are more likely to find the information you need. Having these skills and knowing what the different databases have to offer makes searching the literature so much easier and less time-consuming. It does takes a bit of time and effort to learn, and you are likely to make some frustrating mistakes along the way. Help is at hand though as there are plenty of resources that will lead you through the process; libraries and librarians are particularly helpful when learning how to search the literature. Most education institutions or libraries have individuals available to spend time to help you learn about and explore these valuable tools.

Sources of evidence

There is a staggering array of health care information available to practitioners. As well as local policies and procedures, information is available from books, journals, colleagues, electronic databases and indexes, the Internet, professional organisations, policies and reports and clinical guidelines. Of course, each source has its advantages and disadvantages.

Local policies and procedures

Local policies and procedures are usually readily available and sometimes take the form of clinical guidelines (see below). However, they can become out of date very quickly unless there is a conscious effort to keep them under review in the light of new and emerging evidence.

Books

Books are perhaps the most easily accessible form of information and many now contain a substantial evidence base. However, information in books can become out of date very quickly. In subject areas in which new knowledge is emerging rapidly a book, which may take around 6–9 months to reach the shelves once the manuscript has been delivered, may be almost out of date on publication. Nevertheless, not everything in books becomes out of date so quickly so the trick is to know which information within a book is likely to need updating and which is likely to remain current. The information about, for example, Piaget's theory of child development is unlikely to change from old to new editions of general introductory textbooks on psychology, although recent research evidence supporting or disputing his theory will obviously not appear in older editions. It would only be if you needed evidence about some very specific aspect of Piaget's theory that you would need to look beyond books. Some books are published in electronic as well as hard copy versions but the popularity of the physical presence of a book shows little sign of diminishing.

Journals

Journal articles have the advantage of being more current than books because the turnaround time between acceptance and publication can be much shorter. However, some journals now have so many papers of publishable quality submitted that the publication time can be even longer than it is for some books. Nevertheless, journals are the first choice place of publication for research reports because the journal is where most research gets published. However, there is a hierarchy of journals, with those that insist on peer-review of papers at the top of the pile. Nevertheless, there is a need to recognise that just being published in a peer-reviewed journal does not mean a particular article or research report is of high quality or that it necessarily represents valid evidence.

Colleagues

One thing that you can always rely on is that your colleagues will have an opinion. However, one thing you cannot rely on is the accuracy of their opinion. There is tendency for students to assume that qualified nurses have up-to-date and comprehensive knowledge on a huge range of topics and issues. The reflective nursing student asks such questions as: why is it done this way?

If your answer is on the lines of: 'because my mentor says this is how it is done' then you are in danger of following the 'sister knows best' school of justification. If however, your answer is on the lines of: 'because my mentor has shown me the current evidence from a reliable source that recommends this way of doing it as best practice' then there is a good chance you are using evidence-based practice.

Electronic databases and indexes

Electronic databases and indexes allow you to search and cross-reference journals using keywords, author details or journal title. These range from large international databases through to databases on very specific topic areas. While each database or index can be searched individually it is becoming increasingly common to make use of 'portals', such as Ovid. Portals allow you to search a number of different databases using a common interface. This means you do not have to learn how to use each different database. Some of the more commonly used (and perhaps most generally useful) electronic databases are MEDLINE, British Nursing Index, CINAHL, EMBASE, Midwifery and Infant Care, Alt HealthWatch and the Cochrane Collection. Each of these databases are designed to search in a particular way or for a particular purpose: using them in combination will normally result in the most successful search.

The Internet

A **search engine** is an automated software program that trawls the Internet collecting data from web pages and then cataloguing them. This is presented to the user as an indexed list ranked in order of the best match to your search parameters. Search engines complete this task astonishingly quickly.

The Internet has made it possible for more individuals than ever to access information and to learn in new and exciting ways. The power of the Internet to transform the educational experience is awe-inspiring, but it can also be a frustrating and time-consuming pastime, particularly if you are unfamiliar with or unaware of the tools that can make it easier. One of the most efficient ways of retrieving information from the Internet is to use a 'search engine'. Search engines trawl the Internet in different ways so it is worth trying different search engines to maximise your results. Commonly used search engines include: Google (http://www.google.co.uk); Yahoo (http://uk.yahoo.com); and Alta Vista (http://uk.altavista.com/web/default). This list is by no means comprehensive: it is merely a starting point and you are encouraged to try out other search engines.

Professional organisations

Professional organisations provide an important source of evidence and information ranging from professional guidance or legislative change through to archives of relevant journals. Useful information and differing perspectives can be gained by searching the websites of professional organisations. For example, the Nursing Midwifery Council website (http://www.nmc-uk.org) gives a nursing perspective on nurse prescribing whereas the Royal Pharmaceutical Society of Great Britain website (http://www.rpsgb.org.uk) offers a similar strategic message but with a somewhat different professional slant.

Policies and reports

There has been a myriad of reports produced on a wide range of topic areas from international, national and local perspectives. Local Intranets that search local Trust databases are a useful first step to find polices on all manner of themes specific to your locality. Reports and publications as well as health statistics are easily obtained from the Department of Health website (http://www.dh.gov.uk). A regional perspective on health care can also be found by accessing the relevant web pages for each UK region.

Clinical guidelines

The terms primary and secondary evidence are used regularly within the literature. Primary evidence is original and you are reading the authors' report directly as it was written. **Secondary sources** of evidence may be gathered when reading a report or document where this author refers to another author's research. Unless you then refer to the primary source you are unable to determine whether context and meaning have been altered when applied to the secondary source. As such, primary evidence is considered more reliable than secondary evidence.

Clinical guidelines are a useful source of information for the busy practitioner and may be of local, regional or national origin. They represent **secondary sources** of evidence in which a critical appraisal of the primary evidence is linked to other aspects of evidence-based practice (patient preference, professional expertise and available resources) in order to make recommendations for practice.

Clinical guidelines generated by respected national bodies tend to carry greater authority, for example those from the National Institute of Health and Clinical Excellence (NICE) are held in particularly high esteem, but as a nurse you still need to be convinced that such guidelines are appropriate for your client group.

With so much easily available information and so much new information being published it would be unreasonable to think that a nurse can keep up to date with all the evidence relevant to their area of specialty. As such the practitioner is faced with the challenge of attempting to discriminate between good and poor evidence. Reviewing the literature is both a time-consuming and a skilled activity and most practitioners have neither the time nor the inclination to undertake a comprehensive appraisal of the literature. Nevertheless, there is a need to understand why appraisal is necessary and to have an idea of the process if nursing practice is to be based on the current best evidence available. This level of engagement with evidence has been described as being 'research aware' or 'research literate' (Hek and Moule 2006) and it is to appraisal that we now turn in Part 3 of this chapter.

Part 3: Exploring evidence-based practice

Appraising the evidence

Hewitt-Taylor (2006) reminds us that many nursing actions appear to be based upon tradition, habit or on the unsubstantiated preferences of influential health care professionals. It is possible that in some instances traditional practice is perfectly safe and may even be best practice, but it is difficult for a nurse to justify such practice without evidence supporting its effectiveness. Some nursing practices have changed little in 20 or more years, others have changed in light of evidence demonstrating beneficial patient outcomes, but one of the expectations of evidence-based practice is that nurses should continue to review practice in order to introduce change to practice where the evidence suggests this is necessary.

Whatever form the evidence takes it is necessary to make a judgement about its value or worth. This is to say that there is a need to find out whether or not a particular piece of evidence can or should be used to inform practice. In other words it is necessary to appraise the evidence.

The appraisal process starts with an identification of the category in which a piece of evidence belongs. Merely determining whether it is research evidence or non-research evidence is already to make a judgement about its value. Research evidence is generally considered to be more reliable than non-research evidence. Thus in any hierarchy of evidence **randomised controlled trials** (RCT) will be placed higher than clinical expertise or professional opinion (see Figure 6.2). For those seeking the kind of hard evidence that offers 'beyond reasonable doubt'-type conclusions the RCT sets the standard to which other forms of evidence aspire. Some consider studies that do not meet the RCT standard to have little part to play in evidence-based practice.

Evidence that stems from experimental designs such as **randomised controlled trials** provides an effective way of determining the cause–effect relationship between intervention and outcome (Morrow 2008). If well designed, RCTs can form the scientific basis of high-quality change. If flawed or poorly designed incorrect inferences may result in inappropriate care being delivered.

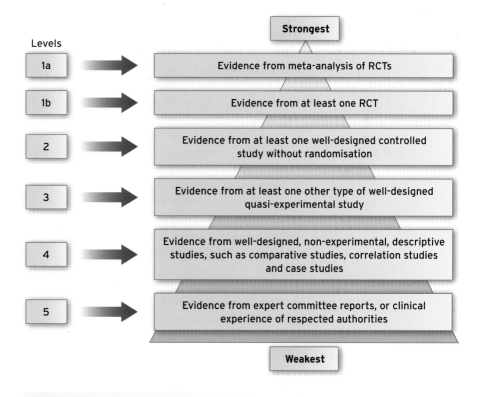

Figure 6.2 Hierarchy of evidence.
Source: Flemming and Fenton (2002, p. 114).

Hierarchies of evidence

Hierarchies of evidence take different forms. The hierarchy of evidence reproduced in Figure 6.2 is used by Flemming and Fenton (2002) and takes a familiar form. In this hierarchy the strongest form of evidence is at the top in the form of meta-analyses (level 1a in the diagram) closely followed by what they call 'Evidence from at least one RCT' (Flemming and Fenton 2002 p. 114). This would include single RCT studies as well as **systematic reviews**.

In this hierarchy it is evidence from levels 1a and 1b that meets the 'beyond reasonable doubt' standard. All the other levels from 2 down to 5 provide evidence that might meet the 'balance of probability' standard. Flemming and Fenton note that 'As you move down the hierarchy the chances of reaching reliable, accurate and unbiased answers decrease' (p. 113) but reject the idea that only the evidence of RCTs should be used in clinical decision-making. While RCTs, systematic reviews and **meta-analyses** provide the strongest evidence, this type of research can only answer those types of questions where direct comparisons between interventions and outcomes can be made.

Thus if you want to know the most effective way of transferring an immobile patient from bed to chair level 1a and 1b studies can provide the answer, but only within a set of detailed parameters. For example, well-designed level 1-type studies can tell you the quickest or the most efficient method because these things can be measured, counted and quantified (hence they are **quantitative research**) but such studies will struggle to provide meaningful data on patient comfort or preference, or information about which equipment staff find easier to use.

Just as the most fuel-efficient car is unsuitable if you cannot reach the pedals, so the equipment needed for the most efficient method of transferring immobile patients from bed to chair will be unsuitable if patients cannot tolerate the level of discomfort experienced when that equipment is used.

Thus RCTs, systematic reviews and meta-analyses cannot provide answers to all practical nursing questions. For many nursing activities the best that might be said is that evidence from these types of studies will provide a firm foundation from which to add other evidence and information when making decisions about practice. Thus evidence-based practice is not the same thing as research-based practice. For Hek and Moule (2006 p. 7) evidence-based practice involves taking three things into account:

1. Best available current evidence
2. Preferences of individual clients and patients
3. Expertise and experience of the professional.

For Flemming and Fenton (2002 p. 114) it requires a combination of the following:

- Clinical experience.
- Research evidence.
- Patient preference.
- Available resources.

A **systematic review** will critically summarise the literature using a process of quality assessment and appraisal of material. Studies that are unsound are rejected leaving the reader with a concise, reliable account to work from (Glasziou *et al.* 2001).

Meta-analysis is a technique for quantitatively combining the results from multiple studies. A meta-analysis of RCTs would produce evidence which would be considered even more valid and reliable than that from a single RCT.

Porter and Carter (2000) define **quantitative research** as 'a formal, objective, systematic process of obtaining quantifiable information about the world, presented in numerical form and analysed through the use of statistics' (p. 19).

This last point is an often-neglected item on the list of requirements for evidence-based practice. Even if the equipment recommended from level 1 studies is both the most effective and the most comfortable, it may not be available but this does not necessarily represent a failure of evidence-based practice.

The Scottish Intercollegiate Guidelines Network

Being able to rank or categorise evidence assists the health care practitioner in the pursuit of reliable evidence for guiding practice. Since the 1970s, a growing number of organisations have been involved in classifying and reviewing evidence for the benefit of health care practitioners. If nurses are to have confidence in the recommendations of systematic reviews and clinical guidelines then there must be a systematic and robust approach (Grade Working Group 2004). The system used in the development of guidance for many clinical and public health intervention involves the hierarchy used by the Scottish Intercollegiate Guidelines Network (SIGN) and reproduced by the National Institute for Health and Clinical Excellence (NICE) to explore the review and grading of evidence (see Figure 6.3).

As noted earlier, a hierarchy of evidence provides an indication of the relative confidence you can place in a particular piece of evidence. In the SIGN hierarchy evidence at levels 1^{++} and 2^{++} is deemed to be research of the highest quality and it is papers meeting the criteria of such studies that are used in generating a systematic review. This provides the best chance of producing reliable evidence of effectiveness.

1^{++}	High-quality meta-analyses, systematic reviews of RCTs, or RCTs with a very low risk of bias
1^{+}	Well-conducted meta-analyses, systematic reviews of RCTs, or RCTs with a low risk of bias
1^{-}	Meta-analyses, systematic reviews of RCTs, or RCTs with a high risk of bias
2^{++}	High-quality systematic reviews of case–control or cohort studies High-quality case–control or cohort studies with a very low risk of confounding, bias or chance and a high probability that the relationship is causal
2^{+}	Well-conducted case–control or cohort studies with a low risk of confounding, bias or chance and a moderate probability that the relationship is causal
2^{-}	Case–control or cohort studies with a high risk of confounding, bias or chance and a significant risk that the relationship is not causal
3	Non-analytic studies (for example, case reports, case series)
4	Expert opinion, formal consensus

Figure 6.3 The Scottish Intercollegiate Guidelines Network hierarchy.
Source: SIGN (2004).

Evidence at both levels 1^- and 2^- and levels 3 and 4 involves the use of research approaches that are variations of the scientific experiment or studies that do not use an experimental approach. Such approaches have additional limitations and, as a result, findings from these studies are placed lower down the hierarchy. Thus the chance of producing reliable results of effectiveness is lower than that obtained using higher-level studies.

Qualitative research may be any type of research that produces findings not arrived at by statistical procedures or any means of quantification (Strauss and Corbin 1998. p. 10). This is an all-embracing term that attempts to understand human behaviour and a rationale for that behaviour.

Qualitative research findings are not included in this hierarchy. This is not to say that qualitative research has no value or that it is unreliable; it is merely to recognise that it does not offer evidence of effectiveness in the way that quantitative research evidence does. Qualitative research does have a contribution to make to evidence-based practice, although not everyone agrees on the value of that contribution. Qualitative research methods are used to study events or experiences in their natural setting, attempting to make sense of poorly understood areas of care. In some cases a better understanding of a situation that emerges from a qualitative study may identify a particular phenomenon amenable to research using quantitative approaches.

Research focus 6.2

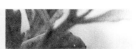

What counts as evidence?

Paley (2005) takes to task those he calls 'inclusionists' for trying to include all sorts of things that should not count as evidence under the rubric of evidence-based practice. In Paley's account the inclusionists are guilty both of confusing belief with evidence and of undermining the science project.

Paley describes the purpose of science as an attempt to distinguish between knowledge (that is, things about which we have some objective grounds to believing as true) on the one hand and belief (that is, things about which we have no objective grounds to believe as true) on the other. To help make this distinction he offers what he calls the 'error criterion' as a minimal test to be applied to claims of knowledge.

The error criterion is, he claims, neutral insofar as it does not presuppose any particular form of enquiry as satisfying the criterion, although he is quick to note that it does preference quantitative research precisely because the scientific experiment is designed to meet the sort of criterion he describes. The error criterion is purely a way of asking about the test by which the possibility of error has been minimised or reduced. So any study should be able to meet this criterion if it can be shown how we can be confident that what is claimed as knowledge is not merely the collective fantasy of a group of like-minded individuals.

Perhaps unsurprisingly, Paley comes to the conclusion that anything other than research evidence fails to meet the error criterion and therefore should not count as evidence.

Paley's is a strong and persuasive argument and it is not possible to do it justice here. What he does particularly well is to throw down the gauntlet to the inclusionists to put their claims of what counts as knowledge and therefore what counts as evidence to the test against his well-argued and clear account of the nature of evidence. Whether or not one agrees with Paley, anyone who is serious about their claims for 'other forms of knowledge' cannot afford to ignore his arguments.

A	At least one meta-analysis, systematic review, or RCT rated as 1^{++}, and directly applicable to the target population; or a systematic review or RCTs or a body of evidence consisting principally of studies rated as 1^+, directly applicable to the target population, and demonstrating overall consistency of results
B	A body of evidence including studies rated as 2^{++}, directly applicable to the target population, and demonstrating overall consistency of results; or extrapolated evidence rated as 1^{++} or 1^+
C	A body of evidence including studies rated as 2^+, directly applicable to the target population, and demonstrating overall consistency of results; or extrapolated evidence rated as 2^{++}
D	Evidence levels 3 or 4; or extrapolated evidence rated as 2^+

Figure 6.4 Level of evidence table.
Source: SIGN (2004).

It is now accepted in some circles that both quantitative and qualitative research has a part to play in evidence-based nursing practice. For example, a RCT is a frequently utilised approach when exploring the efficacy of drugs, while qualitative approaches will help us understand the experiences of clients undergoing particular treatments. Throughout your professional career you are likely to read reports that have utilised both quantitative and qualitative research approaches.

In the SIGN hierarchy, expert committee reports, professional opinion and clinical expertise represent the least reliable forms of evidence in terms of effectiveness. However, sometimes this is the only type of evidence available in which case it cannot be dismissed out of hand, but it still needs to be viewed with a critical eye. The message here is that whatever form of evidence is being used, there is a need to appraise its value in terms of its application to any particular nursing action.

The recommendation table that accompanies the SIGN hierarchy (Figure 6.4) provides an indication about the level of evidence you are using to provide care in any particular situation.

Deciding how the literature you are examining compares to the level of evidence in Figure 6.4 will give a reasonable idea of the strength and rigour of the design and of the evidence base for your practice. However, you need to remember that evidence in any category will not necessarily meet the standards of reliability set for that form of evidence: hence the need for critical appraisal.

Critical appraisal

Journals provide an excellent source of recent research papers, although as we pointed out earlier, not everything that gets published is of high quality. Using the skills of critical appraisal will help you to make a judgement about the value of a particular piece of evidence. Regardless of the form of evidence under review the process of critical appraisal is broadly similar. Undertaking a critical appraisal is a bit like being an effective detective. The purpose of both is to sift the weak from the strong evidence.

Just like effective prosecution and defence lawyers in a trial, effective critical appraisal relies on asking the right sort of probing questions. There are a number of critiquing frameworks designed just for this purpose: that is, to ask specific and probing questions of evidence to help you make a judgement about its quality. For example, LoBiondo-Wood and Haber (2002) provide a framework for evaluating qualitative research and a separate one for evaluating quantitative research. Similarly, there are frameworks specifically designed to appraise systematic reviews and clinical guidelines. While the questions in one framework will be different from the questions in another, and will be different again for appraising, for example, clinical guidelines and RCTs, the basic premise in each will be the same. In all instances a framework will seek answers to questions designed to assess whether the accepted standards of the particular type of evidence have been met. If those standards have been met then there is a greater chance that the evidence is reliable.

> . . . whatever the evidence we need to decide three things:
>
> - whether we can *trust the results*
> - what the results *mean*
> - whether they are *relevant* to our practice.
>
> (CASP and HCLU 1999 Unit 3, p. 5)

Effective critical appraisal is something that you can learn. Just as you have learned not to trust your eyes when faced with railway tracks, and just as you have learned not to be deceived by the appearance of a partly submerged stick, so you can learn what to look out for when reviewing evidence.

The chances are that at some point during your pre-registration nurse education programme you will be asked to make an appraisal of some evidence. It is likely that you will be expected to appraise evidence using a critiquing framework and you may wonder why you are being asked to do this. Well, the answer is that in order to be an autonomous and accountable practitioner you need to be able to make an independent judgement about the evidence you use to guide your practice. It is no more acceptable to use clinical guidelines (or any other form of evidence) uncritically than it is to practise on the basis of the discredited 'sister knows best' model that evidence-based practice is trying to replace. Being able to do a bit of critical appraisal means you may be able to avoid basing your actions on unreliable evidence which can be worse than not using evidence at all (CASP and HCLU 1999). The more critical appraisals you do, the easier it becomes, and the more likely it is that it will become a normal part of your reading technique.

Case 6.1 (continued)

If we return to the situation on Charterhouse Ward you will remember that Kathy acquired a copy of a local guideline on manual handling: because this document makes recommendations for practice it can be classed as a clinical guideline. Maurice remembers that one of the lecturers mentioned something about an appraisal tool for clinical guidelines and he eventually tracks it down. It comes as part of the CASP package and he and Kathy make a stab at using it to appraise the clinical guidelines on manual handling.

Naturalistic research
or inquiry sets about
understanding how individuals
construct reality within their
own natural setting (Polit and
Beck 2004).

The CASP package is an open learning source (CASP and HCLU 1999) specifically designed for health care professionals. It contains a framework for appraising
RCTs, one for appraising **naturalistic research**, one for appraising systematic
reviews and one for appraising clinical guidelines. The framework for appraising clinical guidelines was developed by Cluzeau *et al.* (1997) and contains
4 dimensions with a total of 37 questions to which a simple, 'yes', 'no', or 'not
sure' answer is sought. The first 20 questions relate to 'rigour of development'
and as with the other appraisal frameworks in the CASP package, answers to the
early questions can help you to decide how far to subject the evidence to the
full framework. For example, it may be that answers to the early questions
quickly give rise to a sense of whether or not we can trust the results.

Activity 6.3

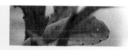

Have a look at Kathy and Maurice's answers to the first three questions of this appraisal framework (Figure 6.5). Do you think Kathy and Maurice are going to be able to trust the results of
this piece of evidence?

In this example (Figure 6.5) the author of the guideline is clearly stated. Although
she is unknown to Kathy, the author had been employed by the hospital some
years ago in the role of nurse development manager but had since left. So while
the author was identified, there is no statement about who was responsible for
the development. If the answer to two later questions (questions 18 and 19)
about who has responsibility for reviewing and updating the guideline and
when this should be done are equally unclear then the signs are that this guideline may be out of date, especially if no date of publication is given.

Responsibility for guideline development	Yes	No	Not sure
O1 Is the agency responsible for the development of the guidelines clearly identified?			✓
O2 Was external funding or other support received for developing the guideline?	✓		
O3 If external funding or support was received, is there evidence that the potential biases of the funding body(ies) were taken into account?		✓	

Figure 6.5 Example of answers to questions in the CASP framework for appraising
clinical guidelines.

Source: After Cluzeau *et al.* (1997).

Similarly, the support of a company that manufactures lifting and handling equipment is acknowledged, but there is no mention of any steps taken to make sure that support did not influence or bias the results.

So merely by answering the first three questions (with a quick look at questions 18 and 19) Kathy and Maurice are already beginning to think they may not be able to trust the results of this evidence. In this case both Kathy and Maurice are surprised (even a little shocked) to find that it looks as though this guideline will turn out to be unreliable evidence. They have no way of knowing how recent (or old) it is; they have no way of knowing if it has been recently reviewed and updated; and they have no way of knowing if the equipment recommended was influenced by the financial support given by the manufacturer.

As Polit and Beck (2006 p. 430) suggest, regardless of the framework used, a critiquing tool should take into consideration the following aspects of the evidence (whatever form that evidence takes):

- The credibility and accuracy of the results.
- The meaning of the results.
- The importance of the results.
- The extent to which the results can be generalised or have the potential for use in other contexts.
- The implications for practice, theory or research.

To even think about making a change in practice on the basis of evidence that has not been subject to some form of appraisal is to fail to understand your own professional accountability. It may be tempting to encourage change on the basis of one piece of research evidence but the only professional approach is to have some idea of the validity of that piece of evidence: thus some form of critical appraisal is a necessary skill for effective nursing practice.

Boring as it may be to read the sections on research method, sample selection and data collection, in addition to the best bits (the introduction, discussion and conclusion), this really is the only way that a critical appraisal can be undertaken. Questions on the lines of the following are common in critiquing frameworks and provide information for making a judgement about the value of a piece of research evidence.

1. Is the chosen methodology the most effective for the topic area?
2. Is there sufficient sample for the chosen method?
3. Is the data collection tool available for scrutiny and does the author give sufficient information to judge issues of reliability and validity?
4. Is sufficient data published to allow scrutiny of the figures for accuracy?
5. Does the researcher answer their research statement, question or hypothesis?
6. Does the author's discussion and conclusions stem from the data collected?

By looking for answers to these sorts of questions you will be analysing and reviewing the literature rather than merely reading uncritically. Critical appraisal is about coming to a balanced review of a research paper (or other form of evidence) while looking for both positive and negative aspects. It should not be just an account of all that is wrong with the paper. As Hibbard (2004) states: 'Critiquing research is a very high order cognitive skill. It requires knowledge of the conceptual, methodological and ethical components of research' (p. 37).

The more often you try appraising evidence using a critiquing framework the more analytical and natural the critiquing process will become. As a result of this process you will become a more informed practitioner whose care is based on evidence. Think back to your first clinical experience, sitting in the Charge Nurse's office and receiving a handover report. Remember how complex and bewildering it all seemed then, yet now you know what is going on (most of the time) and you may even be involved in giving handover. Understanding the research process and becoming comfortable with critical appraisal is a very similar learning experience.

Changing practice

In purely practical terms, making a change to existing or established practice is perhaps the most difficult phase of evidence-based practice. A willingness to change is a fundamental requirement; if you are not prepared to change the way you do things there is little point in either reviewing practice, or finding and appraising the evidence. The whole point of engaging with these activities is to try to find out whether or not existing practice is supported by current best evidence. If you are unwilling to make changes to your practice in the light of evidence suggesting that change is needed then the purpose of evidence-based practice is undermined.

Case 6.1 (continued)

Both Maurice and Kathy have already demonstrated they are willing to make changes to practice. As ward manager Kathy has tried to implement other changes with varying degrees of success. In this respect she has, at least, some experience; enough to know that there is nothing easy about making and sustaining changes to practice. Maurice, on the other hand, finds it difficult to understand why people are reluctant to change, particularly when there is so much evidence to show a need for that change.

Managing change is far from straightforward. On the face of it, it is reasonable to expect people to want to change practice when the evidence is sufficiently compelling. If only it were so simple! The reality is that people do not always behave in reasonable ways and not everyone is willing to change the way they do things. While some people embrace change, others will resist it; some people are more easily convinced of the need for change than others; some will only change once they recognise the inevitability of it and even then may resist in subtle and not so subtle ways. Yet others may be too willing to change, or seek change merely for the sake of change. In other words, change is dependent on people and managing change is a skilled and complex activity. The skilled change agent can draw from a range of different change management theories and you can find more information about these theories in Chapter 12 of this book.

Research focus 6.3

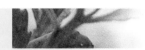

On being willing to change

Sellman (2003) claims open-mindedness as a prerequisite for evidence-based practice on the grounds that the two failures of open-mindedness (closed-mindedness and credulousness) help explain the tendency of nurses (and other health and social care practitioners) to adopt the comfort of ritual and routine. For Sellman being open-minded requires a capacity to recognise the possibility that one's current beliefs and/or practices might be incorrect, together with a willingness to change those beliefs and/or practices in the light of compelling evidence.

On this account closed-mindedness (an unwillingness to acknowledge the possibility that one might hold an erroneous belief) and credulousness (a tendency to adopt a belief in the absence of supporting evidence) are both person-located barriers to evidence-based practice.

As Sellman notes, the person who is closed-minded is unlikely to engage with evidence that contradicts their beliefs – so a nurse who believes there to be nothing wrong with using the underarm lift and thinks on the lines of: 'well, I've been using it for 35 years and it hasn't done me any harm' is not going to be convinced easily of the need to change their practice.

Similarly, Sellman notes that the credulous person is someone who might, for example, accept uncritically and act on a call from an eminent professional who merely expresses an opinion that nurses should no longer be involved in the manual handling of patients.

Sellman also notes that being open-minded requires being open-minded about what counts as evidence. This is seemingly in direct contrast to Paley's position (see Research focus 6.2).

There are, of course, different levels of change, each requiring a different level of engagement with other people in a range of positions in the hierarchy of the organisation. Campbell *et al.* (2006 p. 507) identify four levels of change:

1. A significant change that needs to be addressed immediately, such as a new treatment algorithm for resuscitation following a cardiac arrest.
2. A change so slight and obvious it can be immediately implemented, such as turning off unnecessary lights at night to improve patients' sleep and maintain normal night and day sleep–awake patterns.
3. A change that needs to be addressed by the local team, such as a new practice protocol to be developed from the latest evidence.
4. A change that needs addressing by the organisation as a whole, such as care delivery throughout the patient journey in the organisation, using national standards or guidelines.

It should be apparent that you would need to use a different approach for each level of change. Changes that involve only yourself should be easy to implement while those that affect whole organisations will require engaging with different individuals and negotiating through a raft of bureaucratic processes. One of the implications of the four different levels of change that Campbell *et al.* (2006) identify is that as the number of people involved in or affected by the change increases so does the complexity of managing that change. It is, after all, likely to be easier to effect change in a small team of nurses than to introduce change to practice across a large organisation. Nevertheless, even attempts to implement change among, for example, a small team working in a single hospital ward can easily flounder, especially if planning for the change is hasty or ill-conceived, or if change is being fostered on an unwilling staff.

It is relatively easy to change your own practice. For example, Maurice might decide never again to take part in underarm lifting but this will have only limited effect on patient care if other members of the ward team continue the poor practice. In fact, in this situation Maurice may find himself becoming unpopular and possibly isolated; and if he begins to worry this might have a negative effect on his placement assessment, then his resolve might start to slip. Such pressures are not entirely fanciful and point to the difficulty of expecting students to act as agents of change in practice areas.

However, if Kathy decides to lead by example, she will make sure everybody understands the need for change and she will work with each individual in order to demonstrate there is a different way of achieving the same or better outcomes. Of course, to do this she will need to become knowledgeable about safer techniques and proficient in using specialist equipment. If she does this there is a chance that the other staff will begin to change their behaviour, at least while Kathy is present. If it happens that some others begin to adopt the better practice that Kathy is trying to introduce there is a chance that the change in practice will continue to spread among the team until those who continue to use the underarm lift are in the minority. At this point the pressure to conform will come to bear on those resisting change rather than on those implementing it. If this happens then a lasting change may have occurred but even then you will need to recognise that, if the weight of new evidence points to it, further change may be necessary. As a result it may be best to think of change as a continuous process: as evolution rather than revolution.

This is not a theory of change, neither is it offered as a recipe for change management. For this you should turn to Chapter 12. Rather it is merely an illustration of the need to plan carefully when trying to implement change, and of the need to recognise change as inevitable.

Activity 6.4

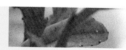

Make a list of the reasons you think the staff on Charterhouse Ward would give you if you asked them why they continue to use the underarm lift.

A time delay between the reporting of research findings and a more general recognition of the significance of those findings is common; in some cases it can be many years. It is sometimes suggested that because of this time lag, evidence for change only gradually filters into the general awareness of nurses, providing a sort of knowledge creep. When enough nurses recognise their practice is out of step with current evidence a suitable environment for change may have been created and change is then more likely to happen as those affected are, in theory at least, more likely to be receptive to it. Even then, resistance may occur, especially if individuals think the changes will affect them in negative ways. While a nurse may be convinced of the need to stop using the underarm lift they will not be motivated to change if the alternatives are too complicated, time-consuming or demanding. Resistance to change is often very powerful and should never be underestimated.

Activity 6.5

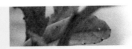

Having considered the rationale for using the underarm lift presented in Activity 6.4, why do you feel staff may be reluctant to embrace the research literature?

Polit and Beck (2006) provide a helpful breakdown of what they consider the four most important factors that get in the way of applying research findings to practice. Recognising these barriers can be half the battle in making it possible to look at the best ways to eliminate or minimise them. The four barriers highlighted by Polit and Beck are:

Research-related barriers

In many instances research that directly addresses the practice issues faced by nurses is in its infancy, which means there may be few reports of sufficient quality on which to base practice decisions. This is one reason why it is so important to be able to understand the critical appraisal process. It is not necessarily that the pressing questions of nursing cannot be answered by high-quality and trustworthy research, but it does mean that the evidence base is just too small to make it sufficiently reliable as a guide to practice. Thus while it is still developing, nurses can make decisions on the basis of whatever evidence is available at a particular point in time. This is one reason why you need to keep up to date with evidence as it becomes available.

Nurse-related barriers

Although an improving picture overall, the research awareness of health care professionals remains inadequate. Research modules are available in most courses studied at higher education institutions but it takes more than the ability to critique to implement research findings. It is also well documented that there is a lack of motivation and a resistance to change.

Organisational-related barriers

The 'culture' of an organisation can make a huge difference in the way colleagues respond to research. Some organisations actively encourage innovation and improvement. In others, the effect of established priorities and procedures can stifle innovation. With the implementation of the national Research Governance Strategy (DH 2006) research awareness is beginning to gain a higher profile throughout the NHS and Trusts are expected to identify their research strategies. As a result a more coherent research strategy to deliver evidence for practice is beginning to emerge. This has been reinforced as nurse education has become more integrated in the higher education system in the UK, with an associated focus on the application of research to practice.

Barriers related to the nursing profession (and barriers between professions)

It is useful to think about two categories of professional barriers:

1. *Barriers between health care professionals and researchers.* Researchers and health care professionals do not always see things in the same way and the priorities of each can sometimes conflict. In addition researchers and practitioners do not always trust each other. Research by its very nature attempts to control or focus in on predefined problems. This is seen as alien to many practitioners who view the care of their clients from a holistic perspective.
2. *Barriers between different health care professions.* It is not uncommon for a single piece of research to have implications for members of different health care professions. Again, the track record here is not always a good one, although progress is certainly being made.

Activity 6.6

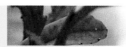

Have another look at the lists you compiled for Activity 6.4 and Activity 6.5.

- Do the reasons you think the staff might give for not abandoning the underarm lift fit neatly into Polit and Beck's four categories?
- If not, do you think there is another category?
- If you think there is a missing category, how would you describe it?

Other authors categorise the barriers to the implementation of evidence in different ways, but the characteristics Polit and Beck outline have been identified consistently over time and similar barriers are evident in many professional groups. Although a little old now, an interesting and comparatively brief literature review on the topic of getting research into practice (Tordoff 1998) highlights barriers under four similar headings of:

1. Problems with the research itself.
2. Individual resistance to implementation.
3. Organisational factors.
4. Cultural issues.

If you identified a missing category of barriers, you may find it is covered in the Tordoff model.

Reviewing practice in relation to current evidence takes place in an environment where many other factors influence the decisions we make. Muir Gray (2001) suggests there are three factors that influence the assimilation or otherwise of evidence into everyday health care and these factors are represented by interlinking circles in Figure 6.6. Muir Gray argues that the quality or otherwise of the evidence is only one factor in the complex activity of decision-making. Values and resources have a significant influence on the decisions that are made regardless of the weight or quality of evidence supporting change. Proposals for changes that have significant resource implications are likely to be modified in an effort to keep costs down to that which the organisation can afford, while those proposed changes that appear inconsistent with the strongly held values

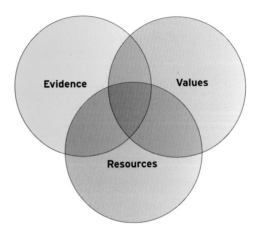

Figure 6.6 The influence of values, resources and evidence on actual decisions.

Source: Adapted from Muir Gray (2001).

of nurses are likely to be resisted, subverted or even ignored altogether. Muir Gray claims that the influence of values and resources on actual decisions made is greater than the influence of evidence, regardless of the quality of that evidence.

Campbell *et al.* (2006) provide a number of case studies of change and these are recommended reading for anyone thinking about making changes to practice. In their examples they link the evidence to planning for and implementing and evaluating the change. Implicit in these examples is the influence of both values and resources.

In *Managing Change and Making it Stick*, Plant (1987 pp. 33–34) suggests six key activities for maximising commitment to change, designed to help others to accept and come to terms with the change, to maximise their commitment to it and to lower their resistance to it.

1   Help individuals or groups face up to change

This involves helping people to accept the need for change. In particular, you need to work with those who are positive so that you harness the power of the supporters. You also need to decide what you can do that will let the more hesitant people come round in their own time.

2   Communicate like you have never communicated before

Make sure that everyone knows everything that is relevant to them, and do not assume they will find out through the grapevine. Rumour and misinformation flourish where real information is missing, and trust can be weakened as a result.

3   Gain energetic commitment to the change

This means identifying 'what's in it for them', and showing that it is better, and less painful, than standing still. You can stress both the positive sides, such as the benefits to patients or clients, and the potential for avoiding something negative, such as unnecessary costs, wasted time and effort and so on.

4 Ensure early involvement

One unit of energy spent early on avoids having to spend many units later, when you may have the active opposition of people who otherwise might have been with you, had they shared the level of insight you have.

5 Turn perceptions of threat into opportunities

Stress the benefits to patients and clients and also sell the benefits to the practitioners themselves. There is a tendency to assume that innovations necessarily bring additional work with them. This is not always true. If you have a good case for arguing that the result will be both a better job *and* an easier job, be prepared to make this case loud and clear.

6 Avoid over-organising

Planning is not a one-off process. Protocols and guidance may need to be revised in the light of experience; if you are asking other people to be flexible, you need to show flexibility yourself when it is needed.

Conclusion

The whole point of evidence-based nursing practice is to ensure practice is based on best available evidence and that any changes made have benefit to those in receipt of nursing care. Making a decision to change, or wanting changes to be implemented, is only one part of this. There always needs to be some way of finding out if a change has produced a beneficial outcome. This is the essence of evaluation. Just as there are significant barriers to overcome in implementing changes in practice so there are some really difficult aspects of trying to measure the benefit of changes made. In a way, evaluation is part and parcel of reviewing practice in a reflective way. Merely asking the sorts of questions reflective practitioners routinely ask (e.g., Why do it this way? Is there a better way to do it?) is to be engaged in evaluation of practice, and if this leads to another round of finding the evidence and subjecting it to critical appraisal with a willingness to change if the evidence is sufficiently compelling then one can say that evaluation is taking place. In this way evidence-based practice is one way to guard against a slide towards poor practice.

By reading this chapter we hope that you have begun to understand the importance and relevance of evidence-based practice for nursing. We also hope that the information contained in these pages will help you to think about and review practice so that you can play your part in influencing nursing practice in positive and beneficial ways.

Suggested further reading

DH (2005) *Research Governance Framework for Health and Social Care* (2nd ed.), London: DH.

Gerrish, K. and Lacey, A. (2006) *The Research Process in Nursing* (5th ed.), Oxford: Blackwell.

Sackett, D. L., Straus, S. E., Richardson, W. S., Rosenburg, W. and Haynes, R. B. (2001) *Evidence-based Medicine: How to practice and teach EBM*, London: Churchill Livingstone.

Internet pages

Department of Health: http://www.dh.gov.uk

Welsh Assembly Government (Health): http://new.wales.gov.uk/topics/health/

Scottish Executive: http://www.scotland.gov.uk/Topics/Health

Northern Ireland Assembly: http://www.niassembly.gov.uk/health/healthhome.htm

National Institute of Health & Clinical Excellence: http://www.nice.org.uk

Healthcare Commission: http://www.healthcarecommission.org.uk/homepage.cfm

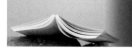

References

Campbell, S. Hancock, H. and Lloyd, H. (2006) Implementing evidence-based practice. In *The Research Process in Nursing* (5th ed.), Gerrish, K. and Lacey, A. (eds). Oxford: Blackwell, pp. 506–520.

CASP (Critical Appraisal Skills Programme) and HCLU (Health Care Libraries Unit) (1999) *Evidence-based Health Care: An open learning resource for health care practitioners*. Oxford: Update Software.

Cluzeau, F., Littlejohns, P., Grimshaw, J. and Feder, G. (1997) *Appraisal Instrument for Clinical Guidelines*. London: St George's Hospital Medical School.

DH (2006) *Best Research for Best Health: A new national health research strategy*. (http://www.dh.gov.uk).

Flemming, K. and Fenton, M. (2002) Making sense of research evidence to inform decision making. In *Clinical Decision Making and Judgement in Nursing*, Thompson, C. and Dowding, D. (eds). Edinburgh: Churchill Livingstone, pp. 109–129.

Glasziou, P., Irwig, L. and Colditz, C. B. G. (2001) *Systematic Reviews in Health Care: A practical guide*. Cambridge: Cambridge University Press.

Grade Working Group (2004) Grading quality of evidence and strength of recommendations. *British Medical Journal* **328** (7454), 1490–1498.

Hek, G. and Moule, P. (2006) *Making Sense of Research: An introduction for health and social care practitioners* (3rd ed.). London: Sage.

Hewitt-Taylor, J. (2006) *Clinical Guidelines and Care Protocols*. Chichester: Wiley.

Hibbard, C. (2004) Accessing sources of knowledge. In *Research into Practice: Essential skills for reading and applying research in nursing and health care* (2nd ed.), Crookes, P. A. and Davies, S. (eds). Edinburgh: Bailliere Tindall, pp. 23–28.

LoBiondo-Wood, G. and Haber, J. (2002) *Nursing Research: Methods, critical appraisal, and utilization*. St Louis: Mosby.

Morrow B. M. (2008) Randomized controlled trials: fundamental concepts. *International Journal of Therapy and Rehabilitation* **15** (7), 290–297.

Muir Gray, J. A. (2001) *Evidence-based Health care: How to make health policy and management decisions.* Edinburgh: Churchill Livingstone.

NMC (Nursing and Midwifery Council) (2004) *Standards of Proficiency for Pre-registration Nursing Education.* London: NMC.

Paley, J. (2005) Evidence and expertise. *Nursing Inquiry* **13** (2), 82–93.
Plant, R. (1987) *Managing Change and Making it Stick.* London: Fontana.
Polit, D. F. and Beck, C. T. (2004) *Nursing Research: Principles and methods* (7th edn). Philadelphia: Lippincott, Williams & Wilkins.
Polit, D. F. and Beck, C. T. (2006) *Essentials of Nursing Research: Methods, appraisal and utilization* (6th ed.). Philadelphia: Lippincott, Williams & Wilkins.
Porter, S. and Carter, D. E. (2000) Common terms and concepts in research. In Cormack, D. (ed.) *The Research Process in Nursing* (4th edn). London: Blackwell, 17–28.

SIGN (Scottish Intercollegiate Guidelines Network) (2004) *SIGN 50. A guideline developer's handbook.* Edinburgh: SIGN.
Sellman, D. (2003) Open-mindedness: a virtue for professional practice. *Nursing Philosophy* **4** (1), 17–24.
Strauss, A. and Corbin, J. (1998) *Basics of Qualitative Research: Techniques and procedures for developing grounded theory* (2nd ed.). California: Sage Publications.
Tordoff, C. (1998) From research to practice: a review of the literature. *Nursing Standard,* **12** (25), 34–37.

Walsh, M. and Ford, P. (eds) (1989) *Nursing Rituals: Research and rational actions.* Oxford: Butterworth Heinemann.

Chapter 7

Assessment

Derek Sellman, Stephen Evans and
Jackie Younker

Learning outcomes

After reading and reflecting on this chapter, you should be able to:

- Explain the importance of assessment for nursing practice;
- Describe the skills needed for effective assessment;
- Consider the usefulness of assessment tools;
- Discuss the relationship between systematic assessment and safe care.

Related NMC Standards of Proficiency for Pre-registration Nursing Education (NMC 2004)

- Select valid and reliable assessment tools for the required purpose.

- Systematically collect data regarding the health and functional status of individuals, clients and communities through appropriate interaction, observation and measurement.

- Analyse and interpret data accurately to inform nursing care and take appropriate action.

- Establish priorities for care based on individual or group needs.

- Develop and document a care plan to achieve optimal health, habilitation, and rehabilitation based on assessment and current nursing knowledge.

- Identify and respond to patients and clients' continuing learning and care needs.

- Identify, collect and evaluate information to justify the effective utilisation of resources to achieve planned outcomes of nursing care.

- Collaborate with patients and clients and, when appropriate, additional carers to review and monitor the progress of individuals or groups towards planned outcomes.

- Analyse and revise expected outcomes, nursing interventions and priorities in accordance with changes in the individual's condition, needs or circumstances.

- Review and evaluate care with members of the health and social care team and others.

Introduction

As Barrett *et al.* (2009) note 'Assessment . . . is as much about finding out what the patient can do as it is about what they cannot do' (p. 22). In this chapter we emphasise this 'finding out' aspect of assessment as the foundation for nursing care. Without finding out appropriate information about patients and clients it is difficult to know what nursing care might be suitable. Being systematic about assessment seems to be the only way to be sure of gathering all the information necessary to deliver safe and effective care. As such, assessment is an integral part of becoming a nurse in any of the four branches of nursing in the UK.

The chapter is divided into three parts.

In Part 1, we offer some information about assessment in general and emphasise the importance of effective patient assessment in particular.

In Part 2, we explain some general aspects of the skills of observing, measuring and interviewing which are all necessary for effective assessment. We also offer some examples using specific assessment tools, the general principles of which are transferable to other assessment tools.

In Part 3, we detail some aspects of the head-to-toe physical assessment and begin to outline the nature of assessment beyond the physical realm.

Part 1: Outlining assessment

Case 7.1

Maureen is a first-year student nurse. Today is the end of her first week on her second placement: a busy ward at the local hospital. She is having difficulty making sense of much of what she sees going on around her and she is beginning to worry that she will never manage to prioritise her workload in the way that her mentor (Alia) seems to do so effortlessly. Maureen is struggling to understand how Alia seems to know intuitively when to do what to whom and is starting to think she may never get the hang of managing her own workload effectively. By way of an example, when they enter a bay of patients together, Alia seems to notice all sorts of things that Maureen does not, and Maureen is beginning to understand that unless she can find a way of seeing the types of things that appear obvious to Alia, she is in danger of missing important aspects of patient care.

Activity 7.1

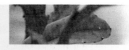

Imagine you are a friend of Maureen (see Case 7.1) and she has asked you for advice. Write down a few suggestions that might help Maureen to find a way of seeing those things that appear obvious to Alia.

The importance of patient assessment cannot be overstated. As a student or registered nurse, every time you approach a patient you will be making some kind of assessment. At one extreme this may be as simple as noticing that a patient looks better than they did yesterday; or thinking that they look uncomfortable, or worried, or happy and so on; at the other extreme this may involve the purposeful, deliberate and systematic collection of information, some of which will be objectively measurable. Using only the former approach you may notice some things but not others and so may or may not obtain accurate information, particularly if you do not check out your suspicions or assumptions against an external source. For example, if you decide to change the position of a patient you think looks uncomfortable without checking with that patient about whether or not they *are* uncomfortable, then you may inadvertently cause rather than relieve discomfort, as well as adding to your workload. Using a systematic approach, you will be less likely to miss information important to making decisions about patient care.

What Maureen has yet to work out for herself is that she needs to start making her observations count: that is, she needs to learn to become attentive to the environment in which nursing takes place so as to be able to discriminate between relevant and irrelevant information about patients and their treatments and care. This process of becoming appropriately selective is one that Alia has learned from her experiences working as a nurse. In fact, much of what Alia does is so 'second nature' to her now that she sometimes finds it difficult to understand why things that are obvious to her are not obvious to others. Indeed, there was a time when Alia was as inexperienced as Maureen. At that point Alia would have been a novice, just as Maureen is now. Benner (1984) eloquently describes how nurses develop from novice to expert (although not all nurses become experts in the sense Benner understands this). In our vignette Maureen is clearly a novice whereas Alia is not.

Benner recognises being a novice as an essential starting point for developing expertise in nursing: the novice will tend to rely on some kind of checklist approach and the need for checklists diminishes as the nurse moves through stages towards becoming an expert. Medicine may offer a relevant example insofar as doctors are trained to undertake a systematic approach to the assessment of patients. In the physical domain this is reflected in the 'head-to-toe' assessment of body systems which once learned and ingrained informs doctors' subsequent systematic approach to decision-making. We will say more about the 'head-to-toe' approach to assessment in Part 3 of this chapter (and information about decision-making can be found in Chapter 8). At present we shall concentrate on an overview of assessment.

Human beings make assessments all the time. In our everyday activities we make rapid and complex assessments, yet we usually fail to recognise these as assessments as such, nor do we acknowledge that the relative success of these assessments is dependent on how well we learned the skills to enable us to make those assessments. Many of the assessments we make are related to seemingly minor aspects of our lives, but all of them reflect our ability to adapt to our environment and some are necessary for our continued survival as individuals and as a species.

One important fact about assessment is that it precedes action. At the mundane level we assess how much toothpaste we need *before* we brush our teeth, we assess how much shampoo is left in the bottle *before* we wash our hair and we assess how much cheese we need *before* we make ourselves cheese on toast. If our assessments are not very good before we engage with these sorts of tasks it does not matter all that much: the effects of too little or too much toothpaste, shampoo or cheese will only affect us as individuals. Too much toothpaste may leave us with overly minty breath, too little shampoo may leave us with hair not quite as clean or shiny as we intended and too little cheese might mean a slightly lower intake of fat; none of these things affect others (or at least, if they do, they do so in relatively minor ways).

A second important fact about assessment is that it is something we learn to do, and if it is something we learn then we may learn it well or poorly. We learn to assess the speed of an oncoming vehicle *before* we cross the road (and it is worth remembering that there was a time when we were either unable to do this or when we were not very good at doing it – we each needed to learn this at the side of older and more experienced pedestrians); we assess the amount of time it will take us to get to the airport *before* we leave the house to catch a plane (we may have learned to allow extra time to account for un-expected delays en route, particularly if we have previously missed an important flight); and we assess how much debt we can afford *before* we take out a mortgage to buy a house (we may have learned to balance our income with our proposed expenditure). If we get our assessments wrong for these types of tasks then the consequences can be more harmful both to ourselves and to others. If we get hit by a car when we step into the road because our assessment of its speed was inaccurate, the effects may be felt by a number of different individuals including the driver and any passengers of the car, and has the potential to involve the police and/or rescue services as well as emergency and hospital services. If we miss the plane it may ruin a holiday for our friends or may mean we miss an important meeting, and if we failed to account for the total costs of home ownership we may end up causing considerable hardship to our families.

A third important fact about assessment is that in professional life ineffective assessment has the potential to result in serious harm to patients. The nurse who undertakes an ineffective assessment of routine observations (temperature, pulse, respirations and blood pressure) of a postoperative patient may fail to notice a significant change in that patient's condition resulting in, for example, a delay in recognition of and action about a serious postoperative complication.

A fourth important fact about assessment in relation to nursing in particular is that it stretches beyond the mere physical. This is to recognise that patients and clients have psychological, social and spiritual as well as physical needs and that the claim that nurses provide holistic care rings hollow if patient assessment is restricted to the physical only. We recognise that this chapter will appear to concentrate on physical aspects of assessment, although we will attempt to incorporate other aspects in some places. In some ways the chapter reflects the realities of practice (at least for adult nurses) because the tools for physical assessment are well established and largely uncontroversial in comparison with tools of assessment for these other, non-physical domains. Indeed, while most nurses will acknowledge the interdependence of the physical, psychological, social and spiritual in terms of health, it is neither clear that nurses are sufficiently skilled to undertake assessment in all four domains nor that the role of the nurse is to provide holistic care.

Thus we have identified four important aspects of assessment:

1. Assessment precedes action.
2. Effective assessment skills need to be learned.

3. Ineffective assessment can have harmful consequences.
4. Comprehensive assessment necessarily involves the assessment of a patient's psychological, social, spiritual and physical needs.

To act without undertaking an assessment (to act without thinking, as it were), not to learn the skills of effective assessment and to be ineffective at the assessment of patients and their care needs is to fail to recognise one essential aspect of becoming a safe and competent registered nurse. Like Maureen, all first-year student nurses are novices and like novices in other walks of life, the student nurse as novice will need to spend time and expend effort in moving on from being a mere novice to being a safe and competent practitioner (the minimum level for registration as a nurse). In learning to become effective in patient assessment it is helpful for a novice to adopt a checklist approach in order to be both thorough and systematic. For, as illustrated above, the importance of effective assessment in professional practice is reflected in the potential for harm to patients of ineffective assessment.

In this chapter you will find information about the observing, measuring and interviewing skills you will need to develop if you are to become effective at assessment, together with details of some specific aspects of assessment to illustrate and highlight the importance of developing a systematic and thorough approach to the assessment of patients and their nursing care needs.

Part 2: Explaining assessment

Case 7.1 (continued)

Despite her concern that she does not notice all the things that Alia (her mentor) notices, Maureen does have some basic skills in observation, measurement and interviewing. Some of these skills she brought with her as part of her everyday skills of assessment; others she is beginning to learn as she continues on her pre-registration nursing course. The fact that Maureen knows that she needs to develop these skills is a sign that she is beginning to recognise some of the things she will need to learn if she is to become a safe and effective practitioner.

Effective assessment requires a systematic approach to the collection of data using a variety of sources as appropriate to the particular focus of assessment in any given situation. In our everyday lives our assessments are based on familiarity and assumptions that usually serve us well enough. However, in our professional lives the need to be systematic in the assessment of patients is crucial in order to ensure nursing actions are based on accurate information. This need to be systematic in the gathering of information, together with the recognition that patients' health status is likely to change over time (and thus require continuous and ongoing assessment) is the only way that nurses can be sure they are delivering care that relates to, and meets, a client's needs at any point in time. Thus the skills required for effective assessment are essential features of what it means to be a safe and effective practitioner.

Assessment and the nursing process

The nursing process is a systematic problem-solving cycle that includes assessment, planning, implementation and evaluation.

Subjective data is information told to you by the patient or others (relatives, friends and so on). It might include, for example, information about a person's feelings of anxiety, or their experience of pain or stress. It is difficult to measure subjective information against external criteria.

Objective data is information that can be measured against external criteria. It is information gained from, for example, undertaking a physical assessment including the measurement of blood pressure, and from the results of laboratory and diagnostic tests.

Assessment is the first step in the **nursing process**. Amongst other things the nursing process enables nurses to recognise that each patient is an individual whose situation is unique, despite having presenting signs and symptoms common among particular patient populations. Without an effective assessment not only are the experiences of individual patients likely to be subsumed within a category (surgical, cardiac, dementia and so on) but also the care provided is likely to meet collective rather than individual needs.

Assessment requires gathering information and this information can be either **subjective data** or **objective data**. A nursing assessment will aim to gather information about a client's health status, which includes biographical data, a health history, health patterns, cultural, social and other norms, as well as the findings of a physical examination (Weber and Kelley 2007).

The skills of effective assessment

Observing, measuring and interviewing are the essential skills required for effective patient assessment. Learning to becoming appropriately observant requires learning to pay attention to the information presented to the senses as well as learning to discriminate between relevant and irrelevant information. Learning to measure is learning to be accurate and consistent; and learning to interview is learning to make effective use of a particular set of communication skills.

Observation

Our senses are bombarded with information all the time; as human beings we learn to screen out much of this information and allow it to fade into the background while we get on with our lives. It is only when we enter unfamiliar environments that we become aware of information that makes up this sensory background. During a first night away from home we notice the noises a building makes, the general odour of a room, the texture of the bed sheets, the way the shadows move across the room and so on. Yet by the second or third night what we thought was a slightly scary creaking becomes part of the reassuringly normal background noise of the building and after a week or so we only notice these particular sounds if there is some sudden or unexpected change to their tone, pitch or intensity. It is not that the noises have gone away; rather it is that we have stopped paying attention to them. The same phenomenon occurs with other senses.

This phenomenon goes some way to explain why our first-year student nurse (Maureen) finds it difficult to know what needs doing to whom when she enters a bay of patients. For Maureen, the hospital ward is still a relatively unfamiliar environment that bombards her with all sorts of sensory information (sights, sounds, smells etc.), much of which will eventually become part of the unnoticed background of her professional working life. Unlike Maureen, Alia (Maureen's mentor) only notices if there is something significant lurking within this background of sensory information. Alia may detect subtleties in the sounds, sights and smells that confront her as she enters a bay; things that Maureen has not yet learned to distinguish as significant from the cacophony of sensory information coming her way. Alia may hear sounds in one patient's breathing that give her cause for concern where Maureen hears only normal breathing; may see early indications of pallor in another patient where Maureen does not; or may recognise the beginnings of an odour of infection masked to Maureen by the stronger smells of disinfectant and other standard hospital smells.

Measurement

We are constantly engaged in measuring, whether this is measuring the time before our working shift ends; the distance between our ward and the canteen; or the number of potatoes we need to peel to feed four people. Generally speaking, measurement of this kind can be 'rough and ready' for we might estimate around 3 hours to the end of our shift, about 300 metres to the canteen; or a large pan full of potatoes. We have the equipment to be more precise in these measurements but normally we would not bother: we could use a clock to establish that we have 2 hours 51 minutes and 30 seconds to go before we finish work; we could use a tape measure to find the canteen is precisely 322 metres from the ward; and we could use scales to weigh out 200-gram portions of potatoes per person. We do not do this, and we would find it odd for someone to do this unless there were good reasons to do so, yet we know that in other circumstances more accuracy is required. A space shuttle launch requires precise timing, an Olympic running track must have a specific length, and precise quantities of carbohydrates, proteins and fats are required in the preparation of enteral feeding solutions.

Interviewing

Similarly, we make use of the basic skills of interviewing in our everyday lives. To interview is merely to inquire about something, usually by asking questions. Asking a friend about their favourite colour or asking directions to a cinema is to seek information, although we would not normally describe this as interviewing as such. Yet the skills we would use in these examples are the same skills we need if we are to find things out about patients and their nursing care requirements. Effective interviewing skills rely on and are closely related to communication and interpersonal skills (more detail about communication and interpersonal skills can be found in Chapter 9).

A comprehensive assessment of a patient requires using the skills of observation, measurement and interview to gather data in relation to their physical, psychological, social and spiritual well-being. In the UK there are four branches of nursing: adult, children's, learning disabilities and mental health nursing. Because it is issues of physical well-being that brings patients into contact with the majority of adult and children's nurses, it is the physical assessment that tends to be the priority for these two groups of nurses. In contrast, the majority of learning disabilities and mental health nurses are less concerned with this type of assessment, although there are good reasons for all nurses to be familiar with physical assessment in order to ensure that the physical problems of all patients and clients are not neglected. Similarly, patients under the care of nurses in all branches will have psychological, social and spiritual needs. To neglect psychological, social and/or spiritual assessment is to fail to recognise that people are more than mere physical beings. However, in the current climate of target-driven health care provision and given the time pressures under which most nurses in the UK are working, it is unsurprising that many nurses find the time restrictions of their practice causes them to focus predominately on physical aspects of care. Thus we begin with the physical assessment.

Activity 7.2 Doing the observations

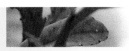

Think back to the most recent occasion when you did some patient observations. Imagine that you are a senior student charged with teaching Maureen (Case 7.1) all about doing patient observations. Do you think you know enough about the measurement, purpose and recording of patient observations to ensure that Maureen becomes safe and effective at doing the observations? Write some brief notes about the things you definitely know about doing the observations, and try to identify any gaps in your knowledge.

Starting the physical assessment

While most nurses will become adept at 'doing the observations' not all will develop their observational skills beyond efficient task performance. Yet there is more to doing observations than mere technical proficiency. Those who progress from novice to expert will have learned to pay attention to a range of sensory information from patients and their environments. A systematic physical assessment begins with a general observational survey of the patient along with the measurement of their temperature, pulse, respirations and blood pressure. The general observational survey begins at the start of the encounter between nurse and patient, and continues for the duration of the physical examination (Seidel *et al.* 2006). It includes paying attention to such things as the patient's height and weight, posture, mood and alertness, skin colour, signs of distress, grooming and personal hygiene, facial expression, as well as body and breath odours. On first encounter, Maureen may have noticed nothing more than an older woman sitting in bed, asking for a nurse. Because of her limited experience Maureen may not have realised that during the few moments it took her to generate this first impression, Alia had already begun a general survey of the patient. In those first few seconds Alia had processed a range of sensory information as part of her initial assessment of the patient's general state of health. While Alia might not have systematically asked herself a set of specific questions, her observations were guided by such questions as:

Maureen's initial impression	Alia's initial impressions
Maureen perceives an older woman sitting up in bed asking for a nurse, and rambling on a bit.	Alia perceives an older woman sitting forward in bed looking anxious and short of breath. She is asking for a nurse but also calling out for her sister who is not present. On seeing Maureen and Alia she immediately asks: 'where am I and why am I here?'
	The patient looks flushed and sweaty. She has removed one sleeve of her hospital gown and it looks as though she has been trying to get rid of the bed covers. The bedside locker door is open and the contents appear to have been rummaged, some have fallen on the floor along with the call bell.
	To Alia this indicates that the patient is restless, possibly confused and may have a raised temperature.

Figure 7.1 Maureen's and Alia's initial impressions.

- How does the patient look?
- Is she anxious, distressed, acutely ill, frail?
- Is she awake, alert, and responsive to other people in the environment?
- Did she hear/notice the nurses entering the room?
- What items are on the bedside table? (get-well cards, flowers, religious reading material, an empty water jug, an emesis basin).
- Is she interacting with visitors?
- Is she short or tall, thin or stocky?
- Are there any unusual odours?

Each of these observations helps Alia to build up a picture of the patient's general health and offers initial clues not only about how she might begin to shape a plan of care but also how best to proceed with the assessment.

Figure 7.1 illustrates the things that Maureen and Alia might notice from the same sensory information available to both as they enter the room of patient.

Alia's experience has allowed her to sift out relevant information from the background and leads her to an initial impression of a patient who is acutely unwell and in need of urgent attention. Her experience has enabled her to pay attention to significant information from among the clutter of sensory data that confronted both Maureen and Alia as they entered the room. In her general survey, Alia had noticed important clues including the patient's colour and appearance, the apparent confusion that had not been present the previous day, the call bell on the floor that may have added to the patient's distress by making it difficult for her to summon assistance, her position in the bed (sitting forward in the bed is a position often adopted by patients experiencing shortness of breath) and the absence of relatives or visitors. Alia captures this information in the brief moment it takes to reach the patient. For Alia, doing the observations will help to confirm her suspicions about the unwellness of the patient, whereas for Maureen, it merely represents the starting point for more comprehensive assessment of the patient.

Observations. Temperature, pulse, respirations, and blood pressure (commonly referred to as 'vital signs', 'the observations' or simply 'the obs') are a set of physiological measurements that provide the basis for the physical examination.

The general survey continues while doing the **observations**. The observations (temperature, pulse, respirations, and blood pressure – commonly referred to as 'vital signs', 'the observations' or simply 'the obs') are a set of physiological measurements that provide the basis for the physical examination. Whatever underlying disease processes may be going on, a patient's vital signs offer important objective data about their level of wellness or illness. Thus there is a real need for nurses to be effective in both doing the observations and noticing other indicators of patients' wellness and illness. Effective observation of patients' vital signs requires the use of effective communication skills in explaining what you plan to do and why the procedure is necessary. This is particularly important for patients or clients who are confused, anxious, agitated or fearful of medical procedures.

Temperature

A patient's temperature is measured against an objective scale but even before using a thermometer, Alia suspects the patient will have a raised temperature because she appears flushed and sweaty. This is confirmed by the use of touch (the patient's skin feels hot and clammy) as, using calm and measured language, Alia acknowledges the patient with a '*Hello Mrs Swinbourne*' followed by a simple explanation of the need to '*take some routine observations*'. Alia knows there is a chance that in her distressed and possibly confused state the patient may not cooperate and so does her best to explain carefully every action she plans to take, together with some polite conversation designed to help orientate Mrs Swinbourne.

Body temperature can be measured at different sites (e.g., mouth, rectum, axillae, and tympanic membrane) but it should be noted that these are all peripheral sites so each reflects a slight variation from the core body temperature. Thus an apparent change in temperature over time may not be a change if the measurements were made at different sites. Tympanic membrane (ear) measurement is the least invasive and most widely used. Tympanic thermometers are simple to use but can be challenging for patients who are confused, agitated or fearful of medical technology. Fortunately in this instance, Mrs Swinbourne was familiar with their use and remained cooperative. The reading was 38.5° centigrade. This is a high temperature and suggestive of the presence of infection. It will need further investigation.

Alia pointed out to Maureen that if a patient is uncooperative or becoming distressed it may be useful to consider if other clinical signs make the need for a temperature measurement essential. For example, if there is no reason to suspect a raised temperature, if all the other observations are within the normal range, if the patient does not feel hot to the touch, or does not appear flushed then it may be appropriate to leave temperature measurement temporarily. However, if the patient is recently admitted, apparently confused and appears unwell then this may be indicative of an infection and an accurate measurement of temperature is essential.

Pulse

Another routine observation involves assessing the pulse. Sensory information from a patient's pulse contributes primarily to the assessment of cardiovascular function, although other useful information can be obtained at the same time. The standard recording is of the pulse rate, which is a measurement of the number of heartbeats (or cardiac cycles) per minute. Typically the pulse is palpated at the radial artery while counting the number of pulsations in one minute. For patients with a strong, steady and regular pulse, it is accepted practice to count the number of beats for only 15 or 30 seconds and then multiply whatever number is reached by four or two respectively. However, if there is any indication that the pulse is weak or irregular, then the rate should be counted for a full minute. So while 'taking' a pulse involves measurement, assessment requires interpretation of a wider range of sensory information.

Variation of the pulse rate is normal and relates to the physiological need to get blood to those tissues that need it. So an individual will have a faster pulse rate when engaged in strenuous activity than they do at rest. Maureen records Mrs Swinbourne's pulse as 100 beats per minute. This is a faster rate than her normal at rest rate as recorded on her chart and may be a reflection of physiological deterioration or of her restlessness and apparent anxiety.

Tachycardia (fast heart rate) can occur with activity or movement, exercise, anxiety and stress, pain or high temperature. Bradycardia (slow heart rate) is usually a sign of heart problems and needs to be reported immediately. However, some drugs can lower the heart rate so it is necessary to consider a patient's history as well as information from the drug chart to assist in the assessment of the significance of a slow heart rate.

Normally a pulse will have a steady, regular rhythm. Some irregularities in the electrical conduction of the heart can cause the rhythm of the pulse to be irregular. A rapid, irregular heartbeat is usually a sign that the patient is unwell and needs urgent attention. The other observations (blood pressure and respirations) will provide useful additional assessment information. Some patients with known heart disease may have an irregular heartbeat being treated with medication so being aware of (or finding out about) a patient's medical history, medications and other findings from the general survey will assist in the overall assessment. A patient's pulse is usually easy to palpate. Difficulties arise for patients with cardiovascular collapse and decreased peripheral circulation. This is also likely to be reflected in a low blood pressure (see below) and indicates the patient is critically ill.

Information that will assist in the overall assessment when a patient has either a fast or slow pulse rate will come from the answers to questions such as:

* Is this normal for this patient?
* Is the patient engaged in any activity that increases heart rate?
* Are there other important clinical signs such as a change in blood pressure or an elevated temperature?
* Is the patient known to have heart disease?
* Is the patient taking any drugs that affect the heart?

These and other similar questions can help in the overall assessment of the patient and will contribute to decision-making in relation to a plan of care. Of course, other sensory information is available when 'taking' a pulse. A pulse rate taken manually allows the nurse to feel the patient's skin and this can provide sensory information about skin temperature, tone, general condition and so on, all of which provides further data to add to the patient assessment.

Respirations

Changes in respirations can be an early indication of deterioration in patients' health status. Often regarded as something of a poor relation in the observations, the value of accurate measurement of respiratory rate and effort can be underestimated. Respirations are counted by observing the rise and fall (one respiratory cycle) of the chest over one minute. The normal respiratory rate is about 10–20 breaths per minute. While counting the number of respiratory cycles is important, significant information can be obtained by paying attention to the pattern of a patient's breathing, as well as the nature of their respiratory effort. A patient who is struggling for breath may still have a normal respiratory rate, so this measurement is only part of the assessment of respirations. For example, a patient may have a respiratory rate of 12 breaths per minute yet have shallow chest movements and may be unable to complete a sentence when talking without gasping for breath. Clearly the care needs of this patient cannot be determined merely on the basis of their respiratory rate. Factors that affect the respiratory rate include pain, a raised temperature, respiratory disease, airway problems, central nervous system problems, drugs, muscle weakness and anxiety, so it is important to consider all of these possible causes when making an assessment of a patient's respirations.

A single measurement of respiratory rate can offer some information towards an assessment of respirations, but the trend of respiratory rate over time is of more use. For example, it would not be unusual to find a respiratory rate of 24 breaths per minute returning to, say, 12 breaths per minute in a patient once that patient has been reassured about impending surgery. Whereas a steady increase in respiratory rate over an 8-hour period from 12 breaths per minute to a consistent 24 breaths per minute would indicate a respiratory problem in need of urgent attention. This last point reinforces the importance of understanding assessment as a continuous ongoing process where measurement takes place against a background of knowledge of normal and abnormal physiological function in relation to what is normal for any given patient at any particular time.

Blood pressure

Blood pressure is the peripheral measurement of cardiovascular function. 'Taking' a patient's blood pressure has become routine but accurate assessment requires paying attention to detail and taking account of factors that might give false or inaccurate readings.

An accurate measurement of blood pressure requires the use of a **blood pressure cuff** of the correct size: one that is too narrow or too short may give a falsely high reading. The cuff needs to be positioned correctly on a patient's arm (about 2.5 cm above the antecubital crease over the brachial artery). The patient's arm should be free of clothing, supported, relaxed and positioned at about heart level. If these conditions are not met there is a danger of getting a

Whether using a manual or automated system, the **blood pressure cuff** must be the correct size for the patient. The blood pressure cuff houses an inflatable bladder. The width of the bladder should be approximately 40 per cent of the upper arm circumference (about 12–15 cm for the average adult). The length of the bladder should be around 80 per cent of the upper arm circumference (almost long enough to encircle the arm).

false reading, and if the conditions vary (e.g., on a general hospital ward over a 24-hour period a patient's blood pressure may be measured by several different nurses each of whom may approximate these ideal conditions to a different extent) then there is the possibility that the pattern of readings recorded may reflect these variations rather than changes in health status of the patient. Of course, such ideal conditions are not always possible as some patients may be unable or unwilling to cooperate.

A 'high' blood pressure may be 'normal' for some patients. A high reading may occur if a patient has been active, if their arm was unsupported or not relaxed, and can accompany anxiety or distress. Thus accurate assessment of blood pressure is not merely taking and recording a reading on a chart: it requires making sense of that reading in relation to other aspects of the patient's condition and environment.

Activity 7.3

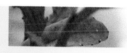

Have another look at your responses to Activity 7.2 and make notes about what you have learned from reading the section about the routine observations of temperature, pulse, respirations and blood pressure. Can you identify any further gaps in your knowledge base in relation to doing the observations?

Case 7.1 (continued)

Alia and Maureen perform Mrs Swinbourne's observations together. Their findings are as follows:

- Temperature: 38.5°C
- Pulse: 100 beats per minute
- Respirations: 32 breaths per minute
- Blood pressure: 110/50 mmHg

Alia knows from reading Mrs Swinbourne's notes and from the information given during handover that the patient is not on any cardiac medications and her blood pressure is normally about 140/90 mmHg. She also knows that 12 hours ago Mrs Swinbourne was sitting up in bed comfortably with a temperature of 37.5°C. Together, Maureen and Alia review the information on the patient's observations chart and note that since her admission Mrs Swinbourne's observations have been as follows:

- *Temperature.* Previously recorded within the range of 37.2°C to 37.7°C. The present reading of 38.5°C represents a change in her health status and indicates the presence of infection and a need for further investigation.
- *Pulse.* Previously recorded within the range of 72 and 80 beats per minute. The new reading of 100 beats per minute is also a change from normal and may be a reflection of a physiological deterioration or of her apparent anxiety and restlessness.

- *Respirations*. Previously recorded within the range of 15 to 18 breaths per minute. This new measurement of 32 breaths per minute is a significant increase in respiratory rate and together with the position she has adopted in bed indicates a breathing problem.
- *Blood Pressure*. Previously recorded within the range of 135/85 to 150/90 mmHg. While this new measurement of 110/50 is within what is considered a 'normal' range, it is not normal for this particular patient and therefore represents a significant change in health status.

The information gathered thus far has required skills of measurement (illustrated by, for example, the use of a thermometer); the skills of interview (in asking specific questions); and the skills of observation (by, for example, using the senses to notice the texture of the patient's skin). Having completed the general survey together with the measurement of a standard set of observations, Maureen and Alia now have considerable information to contribute to their initial assessment of Mrs Swinbourne. The findings of the initial assessment indicate that the patient is having problems of a respiratory nature and that a more in-depth assessment of her respiratory system will be necessary. In Part 3 of this chapter we will return to Alia's physical assessment of Mrs Swinbourne.

The assessment of pain

Case 7.1 (continued)

Maureen and the drug round

While assisting on drug rounds during her first placement, Maureen noticed that closed questions such as *'do you want any pain killers?'* were routinely used by the nurses for patients prescribed 'as required' pain medication. Closed questions of this type invite brief responses such as 'yes', 'no' or 'don't know'. While closed questions have their place, their usefulness in the assessment of pain is limited. Rather than asking, *'do you want any pain killers?'* the nurses on Maureen's second placement tend to ask, *'do you have any pain or discomfort?'* and for patients who say 'yes' they follow this up with other more probing questions such as *'can you show me where it hurts?'*, *'is the pain in the same place as yesterday?'* or *'is it less or more painful than it was yesterday?'* Consequently, the drug round takes longer here but patients' pain does seem to be better managed with a reduced incidence of complications arising from unrelieved pain (Brennan *et al.* 2007; Cousins *et al.* 2004; Lynch 2001; RCA and PS 2003).

Nurses make a significant contribution to the management of pain, particularly through the use of effective assessment. The amelioration of patients' pain is notoriously poor (Coulling 2005, Layman Young *et al.* 2006). There are many reasons for this, including suggestions that nurses tend:

- to underestimate how much pain patients have (in relation to how much pain patients report);
- to overestimate the danger of morphine addiction and respiratory depression;
- to make correlations between conditions and analgesia requirements rather than assess individual need for pain control.

On this last point, it is not unusual to hear nurses say things such as: *'he shouldn't need morphine now because he had his appendicetomy three days ago'*. In fact the patient might indeed need morphine, although reports of severe pain from a patient under these circumstances should alert the nurse to the possibility of serious postoperative complications. Similarly, it is not unknown for nurses to continue to administer doses of morphine to cancer patients on the assumption that their pain is associated with their cancer, when in fact their pain is the pain of constipation: one of the familiar side effects of morphine. In both these examples it is the failure to assess the patient's pain that has led the nurse to respond inappropriately.

Activity 7.4

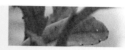

List the pain assessment tools you have seen used in assessing patients' pain. Write some notes about the advantages and disadvantages of each tool you have listed.

There are a number of different tools available for the assessment of pain, but unlike the tools used for collecting information about temperature, pulse and blood pressure (e.g., different types of thermometer and sphygmomanometer) the tools used for the assessment of pain typically rely on more subjective measures. It is important to address potential communication barriers when conducting pain assessment in order to achieve an objective outcome (McDonald *et al.* 2000). There are some observable behavioural and physiological indicators that can be suggestive of pain, but these indicators (Lynch 2001) may be present under other circumstances and for other reasons so cannot be relied on as sole indicators when assessing a patient's pain. For example, rubbing an area of the body, a general restlessness, facial grimacing, mood changes, flushing and sweating, a rise in blood pressure and/or pulse rate may all suggest the presence of pain, but are not definitive of it. It may be that for individuals unable to verbalise such observable phenomena may be the only indicators of a patient's pain (RCP, BGS and BPS 2007; Zwakhelan *et al.* 2004).

A self-reporting scale is probably the most commonly used type of pain assessment tool (Kim *et al.* 2005). The essential feature of a pain scale is that it provides a patient with an opportunity to indicate how much pain they are experiencing in terms of a continuum that ranges from no pain at all at one end to unbearable pain at the other; with choices along the continuum reflecting increasing levels of severity between the two extremes. There are different forms of pain scales (verbal, numeric and pictorial) and each has its advantages and disadvantages. While some clinical areas may adopt a particular type of scale, there will always be situations in which an alternative scale will be more appropriate for a specific individual. The essential point is that if a scale is to have any chance of providing an effective assessment of a patient's pain then the patient must be able to understand it. Hence, a pictorial scale might be most appropriate for someone who has limited verbal skills or whose cognitive function is compromised. In addition, differences in both attitudes to pain and to its meaning at the individual level make it difficult to generalise. Nevertheless, it is reported that older people may need a more proactive approach to pain assessment as they tend to have a set of 'attitudes and beliefs . . . [that] may generate barriers to good pain control' (José Closs 2007 p. 12). There may be all sorts of reasons for this, or it may be a combination of expectations and language. Older people may use words such as 'ache' or 'soreness' to describe their pain and thus may say no to the question 'Do you have any pain?' Responsibility for such failures of communication and thus failures of effective pain assessment lies with the nurse rather than the patient.

The subjective nature of pain scales can be illustrated by a comparison with the scale for measuring blood pressure. Blood pressure is measured using a standardised and objective scale and (assuming a threshold competence in measuring blood pressure among different individuals performing the observation) variations in readings obtained will reflect actual and verifiable changes in a patient's blood pressure. There is no guesswork involved here; anyone who has the necessary skill can make an accurate measurement of a patient's blood pressure (it is therefore objective data) and it can be compared directly with the blood pressure measurements of other people. This is one reason why it is possible to make meaningful statements about the normal range for blood pressure in healthy individuals; or to know that a diastolic blood pressure of less than 80 mmHg will compromise kidney function. In contrast, pain can only be measured from the perspective of the person experiencing it; there can be no objective standardised numerical scale comparable to that for measuring blood pressure. This is partly because individuals have different tolerances to pain and partly because such numerical scales as exist for pain assessment rely on patients choosing a number that has no meaningful external reference point. The number chosen by a patient bears no necessary relationship either to other numbers on the scale or to numbers as chosen by other patients: on a scale of 0–10, a score of 8 for one patient bears no necessary relation to a score of 8 listed by any other patient. So it is not possible to generalise from self-reported (or even nurse-estimated) pain scores.

Pain scales are simple to use and provide a way of capturing information about how much pain a patient has (pain intensity) and therefore are especially useful for evaluating whether or not a patient's pain is better, worse or unchanged following analgesia. However, intensity is only one aspect of pain and thus pain scales offer only limited information towards a comprehensive assessment of an individual's pain.

One way to add to the assessment of a patient's pain is to ask them to indicate its location and to describe the pain. Location can be determined by asking a patient to mark the site of their pain on a body diagram, and the simple question *'is your pain in the same place as you indicated on this diagram?'* is an easy way to ensure changes in the location of a patient's pain are quickly identified. Similarly, asking a patient to choose a word that best describes their pain can both add to the overall pain assessment and provide a common language between health care professional and patient. Mrs Swinbourne tends to describe her pain using the words 'ache' and 'soreness' so it would be appropriate to use these words when asking her about her pain. For example: *'can you point to where your ache is today?'*; or *'is your soreness better or worse than it was yesterday?'*

One further issue that makes the assessment of pain more difficult than, for example, measuring blood pressure, is the complicated relationship between pain and mood. There is a recognised association between depression and the experience of pain although it is not clear which has the greater effect on the other: there is a suggestion that pain, particularly constant pain, can lead to depression which in turn can worsen the experience of pain. This can add a further layer of complexity because in addition to physiological aspects, there may be psychological, social and/or spiritual factors involved in the pain experienced by any one person, which means that a comprehensive pain assessment requires assessment in all four domains. The McGill Pain Questionnaire (Melzack 2005, first published in 1971), which attempts to provide this level of assessment of pain, is considered the most reliable and sophisticated pain assessment tool. However, its comprehensiveness is such that it is extremely time-consuming and therefore unsuitable in the busy and pressurised clinical environment, although there is a short-form McGill Pain Questionnaire (Melzack 1987).

However, it may be useful to extract some features from the McGill pain assessment tool, especially in relation to asking the patient questions about the frequency of their pain, if it is worse at particular times of the day, and whether it is related to specific activities or moods. Of course, these types of questions begin to take on aspects of the psychological, social and perhaps spiritual assessment and while there may be appropriate assessment tools for each, it is not clear that nurses are sufficiently qualified or trained in their use.

Assessing a patient's pain is a complex activity requiring skills of interview, observation and measurement. In the busy practice environment the use of a pain-intensity scale together with a location chart will provide sufficient information to enable appropriate measures to be taken to reduce or eliminate a patient's pain in the short term. However, for some patients (those with chronic pain and those whose cognitive capacities are compromised) there is a need for a more comprehensive (e.g., for those with chronic or long-term pain) or more imaginative (e.g., for those with compromised cognitive capacities) pain assessment.

Part 3: Exploring assessment

We know from experience that first impressions can be misleading. Nevertheless, our initial impressions of a patient at each and any encounter can offer clues about their health status at a given time. In Part 2 of the chapter we highlighted the apparent ease with which Alia was able to recognise the potential significance of some aspects of the sensory information available when approaching a patient. Some of the things she notices may turn out to have little or no significance, but in remaining responsive to potential clues among the background of sensory information Alia is retaining the capacity to pay attention to information that may be of importance in relation to the care of patients. Thus first or initial impressions can offer a starting point for assessment but it is just a starting point, and the assessment still needs to progress in a systematic and thorough manner if it is to be effective. Just as we suggested in Part 1 that a nurse should check with the patient to see if they are as uncomfortable as they appear before making any attempt to change their position, so it is important not to be misled by the apparent significance of some tantalising clue about a particular problem being experienced by a patient. The danger of focusing assessment predominately on one aspect of a patient's health status suggested by a first impression is that it may be at the expense of other areas of the assessment. In other words, if you prejudge your assessment of a patient you may stop looking for (or stop noticing) things that do not fit with that prejudgement and in so doing miss what might turn out to be important information to contribute to an assessment. This is one reason why being systematic and thorough is so important.

We have also made the point that while the systematic collection of data is an essential feature, an effective assessment requires the information so gathered to be interpreted in the light of the specific circumstances of a given patient at a particular point in time. To illustrate the point, not every patient with a blood pressure of 110/80 mmHg and a pulse rate of 110 will be critically ill: some will but this will depend on, amongst other things, what the usual blood pressure and pulse rate is for a particular patient. It may also depend on the patient's previous level of health. A fit, healthy 32-year-old male may be able to cope physically with a change in heart rate and blood pressure following a routine operation; while an 80-year-old female with multiple health problems may become very unwell with small physiological changes in the heart rate and blood pressure after a simple procedure.

Completing the physical assessment

In Part 2 of this chapter we explored some aspects of the general survey together with observation of vital signs and noted that this initial assessment provides clues about how a more thorough assessment of a patient might proceed. A complete physical assessment requires a full head-to-toe examination but this may not be necessary if the initial assessment indicates the need for an in-depth assessment of a particular area of the body. For example, the focus of assessment for a patient identified as having shortness of breath and rapid breathing will be a detailed respiratory assessment. In this section we will outline the head-to-toe approach of physical assessment.

In the UK head-to-toe physical examination has traditionally been the preserve of doctors. Recently nurses have begun to expand their roles in line with government policy aimed at developing new ways of working in order to deliver improvements in care (DH 2001). Some nurses have begun to develop the skills necessary for a variety of roles including prescribing, case management and advanced practice, and for this last, the skills of physical examination have become increasingly important. While it may not be necessary for all nurses to undertake head-to-toe examination, a working knowledge of it will add to the knowledge base from which effective assessment takes place.

The head-to-toe examination

Advance preparation of an environment conducive to physical examination together with having all necessary equipment ready for use allows the examination to be conducted without interruption. The examination may take place in different locations (e.g., GP surgery, hospital ward, patient's home) but wherever it occurs consideration needs to be given to patient privacy, noise levels, temperature, adequate lighting, a bed or examination table for the patient, and a table or tray to hold equipment. Effective hand washing and having gloves readily available is a further part of preparation for the examination (Bickley and Szilagyi 2007).

It is helpful to begin the examination with familiar and less intrusive procedures such as blood pressure, pulse and respirations. This will help the patient to feel less anxious about the full examination. Throughout the examination, it is important to explain what you are doing and why you are doing it. It may also be a good time to integrate health promotion and teaching (e.g., while examining the skin it may be appropriate under some circumstances to help the patient learn to look for changes to the colour, size or shape of moles). The physical examination is generally done from the patient's right side because most examination techniques are done with the examiner's right hand. If it is necessary to change the patient's position during the examination it is important to explain to the patient what you want them to do in clear, simple terms.

There are four basic techniques that are used during head-to-toe examinations: inspection; palpation; percussion: and auscultation with each is adapted as appropriate for the body system being examined (Bickley and Szilagyi 2007).

Inspection

Inspection begins from the moment that you meet the patient and continues throughout the examination. It involves using the senses of vision, smell and hearing to observe and detect normal and abnormal findings. The following guidelines should be considered to help with inspection:

- A comfortable room temperature – a room that is too cold or too hot may alter the patient's behaviour and skin appearance.
- Fluorescent lights may alter the skin's appearance – it is best to use natural lighting where possible.
- Completely expose the body part you are inspecting and keep the rest of the patient covered as much as possible.
- Note colour, patterns, size, location, consistency, odours, movement and sounds during the inspection.
- Compare the symmetry of body parts on both sides of the body (e.g., eyes, ears, hands, legs).

Most inspection only involves the use of your senses; however a few body systems require equipment for thorough inspection (e.g., ophthalmoscope for the eyes and otoscope for the ears).

Palpation

Palpation involves using the hands to touch the patient. Characteristics noted by palpation include:

- Texture (rough, smooth).
- Moisture (dry, wet).
- Temperature.
- Consistency (soft, hard, fluid-filled).
- Mobility (movable, fixed, vibrating).
- Strength of pulse.
- Size.
- Shape.
- Degree of tenderness.

Palpation may be done with three areas of the hand, depending on the nature of the examination. The fingerpads are most often used to feel pulses and check size, texture, consistency and shape. The ulnar or palmar surface of the hand may be used to feel for vibrations. The dorsal surface of the hand is best for checking temperature. Palpation may be light, moderate or deep depending on the depth of the structure being palpated and the thickness of the tissue overlying the structure. For example, it is good practice to use light palpation to assess the abdomen and this is followed by deeper palpation to check for location of internal organs such as the liver.

Percussion

Percussion is tapping over a body part to produce a sound wave. The sound produced helps the examiner to determine the underlying structures. Percussion has a few different assessment uses that include:

- Determining density – percussion helps determine whether an underlying structure is filled with air or fluid or is a solid mass: for example, the lungs are generally filled with air and percussion should produce a resonant sound – if there is a pleural effusion, the sound will change to dull, indicating a fluid-filled area.
- Determining location, size and shape: percussion may be used to note changes between borders of an organ.
- Eliciting pain: percussion is used to help identify inflamed underlying structures – when an inflamed area is percussed, the patient may say it feels tender, painful or sore.

Percussion is most commonly used as part of the respiratory and abdominal examination.

Auscultation

Auscultation involves using a stethoscope to listen to body sounds that are not otherwise audible to the human ear. Sounds heard with the stethoscope include heart sounds, movement of blood through the cardiovascular system, bowel sounds and movement of air through the lung fields. The sounds are described by their intensity, pitch, duration and quality. The following points should be considered to help with auscultation:

- Eliminate noises in the environment that are distracting or competing.
- Auscultate over the patient's bare skin – listening through the clothing may obscure the body sound.
- The diaphragm (flat part) of the stethoscope can be used for high-pitched sounds such as normal heart sounds, lung sounds and bowel sounds.
- The bell of the stethoscope is used for low-pitched sounds such as abnormal heart sounds and bruits (loud sounds heard over major blood vessels such as the carotid artery or aorta).

Case 7.1 (continued)

We last encountered Maureen and Alia in Part 2 of this chapter as they had completed their initial assessment of Mrs Swinbourne. Based on their findings of the general survey and on the significance of the temperature, pulse and respirations, Alia's hypothesis is that the patient may have a chest infection. This prompts her to undertake a more comprehensive assessment of Mrs Swinbourne's respiratory system.

Examination of the respiratory system

Here we will outline in some detail the way in which the four basic techniques of inspection, palpation, percussion and auscultation help to examine and assess a patient's respiratory system.

Inspection

- Look at the patient's overall pattern of breathing and note their respiratory rate. Inspect the chest movement as they breathe to look for symmetry and ease of breathing.
- Assess the colour of the face, lips and chest. Cyanosis is a late sign of hypoxia and will make white skin appear blue-tinged. Hypoxia may also cause the lips or nails to look pale.
- Inspect the front and back of the chest noting size, shape and symmetry. Patients with chronic emphysema may have a characteristic barrel chest appearance.
- Look at the client's position. Normally breathing is relaxed with arms at the side or on the lap. Often patients with chronic obstructive pulmonary disease (COPD) will lean forward and use their arms to support their weight and lift the chest to increase breathing capacity (tripod position).
- Inspect for use of accessory muscles. Normally breathing uses the diaphragm and abdominal muscles. Patients with breathing problems may use the trapezius or shoulder muscles to help with inspiration.

Palpation

- Palpate the anterior and posterior thorax to assess for symmetry and general condition.
- Assess thoracic expansion. Place the hands around the chest and ask the patient to take a deep breath. Note whether both sides of the chest move symmetrically.

Percussion

- Percuss over the anterior and posterior lung fields. The sound should be resonant over all areas of the lungs and dull over major organs (heart, liver, spleen).

Auscultation

- Ask the patient to breathe deeply through the mouth. With the diaphragm of the stethoscope, listen to the anterior and posterior lung fields, starting at the apex and moving to the base. It is important to listen from side to side to make comparisons while listening through a full inspiration and expiration cycle at each point. Normal breath sounds are described as:
  (a) Vesicular – heard over most of the lung fields; soft and clear; low pitch; expiration sound is short;
  (b) Bronchovesicular – heard over main bronchus and upper right posterior lung field area; medium pitch; expiration equals inspiration;
  (c) Bronchial – heard over the trachea; high pitch; expiration sound is loud and longer than other areas.

- Breath sounds may be difficult to hear or absent. Fluid or secretions in the lungs or airway will change the sound (e.g., crackles or rhonchi). Narrowing of the airway will also affect lung sounds (wheeze).

Case 7.1 (continued)

Alia's findings:

- Mrs Swinbourne appears short of breath; she is not using accessory muscles; she is sitting forward in bed (which may indicate anxiety or a breathing problem); she also has a non-productive cough that is worse when she lies supine.
- There is symmetry between the anterior and posterior thorax. Both sides of the chest move when the patient takes a deep breath, however the breaths are shallow and it is difficult for her to breathe deeply.
- Percussion reveals dullness over both bases.
- Crackles heard at both bases of the lungs that do not clear with coughing. The breath sounds are also diminished in both bases.

Alia now has information that has been collected by using a systematic approach. This information allows Alia to make an informed assessment of Mrs Swinbourne's well-being and to begin to shape an appropriate plan of care. The assessment includes findings from the history, basic observations, the general survey and a more thorough assessment of the respiratory system. All these findings support Alia's initial impression of an acutely ill woman in need of urgent care, but now Alia has a clear set of data drawn from her systematic assessment of the patient to communicate to other professionals (such as other nurses, doctors and physiotherapists) involved in the patient's care. This thorough assessment led to a well-planned package of care and Mrs Swinbourne's speedy recovery led to a focus on arrangements for transfer home.

Assessment for transfer

Arrangements for the transfer of a patient from hospital to home or to a different care facility (often referred to as 'discharge planning') requires a comprehensive assessment of a patient's capacities for self-care. Ideally, the assessment for transfer begins on admission and continues during a patient's hospital stay. All patient assessment relies on the same set of core skills; the skills of observing, measuring and interviewing. In assessment for transfer the focus shifts from assessment of a client's nursing needs towards assessment of the client's capacities for self-care. In many instances this will necessitate the involvement of professionals from different disciplines.

Case 7.1 (continued)

Prior to Mrs Swinbourne's transfer home Maureen has been working with several other professionals in an attempt to ensure that the discharge arrangements are suitable. Maureen and Alia had met with Mrs Swinbourne and the Intermediate Care Team (a community-based team comprising a nurse, a care manager, a physiotherapist and an occupational therapist who work alongside Mrs Swinbourne's GP). The team advised Mrs Swinbourne that they would continue to provide medical care and rehabilitation once the hospital-based team determined that she was well enough to return home. During the meeting Mrs Swinbourne told everyone that prior to this hospital admission she had managed very well at home. She needs no assistance with personal care, she can cook a hot meal every day at lunchtime, and that she shops for her own groceries from the small local supermarket across the road who then deliver to her door. The care manager reported that Mrs Swinbourne received home help once a week for two hours to do the heavy housework, such as vacuuming and laundry. Mrs Swinbourne stated that she thought that the home help was unnecessary and complained that they 'always put things back in the wrong place'.

The care manager advised the meeting that before her admission to hospital, Mrs Swinbourne had been living alone in a second-floor, local authority-owned flat. Despite her 82 years, she had until recently been working as a volunteer in the hospital's gift shop. Prior to this admission she had had very little contact with the health services. A neighbour had called an ambulance when she found Mrs Swinbourne sitting at the bottom of the stairs inside their block of flats, unable to respond and looking very pale. The neighbour had reportedly advised the paramedics that she had been very concerned about Mrs Swinbourne for quite some time. In the meeting it was decided that Maureen would accompany Mrs Swinbourne on a pre-discharge home visit, to be met there by Melissa (the Intermediate Care Team nurse) and Raina (the occupational therapist).

The Intermediate Care Team service is based on government policy intended to ease the transition from hospital to home for older people, as well as to reduce the likelihood of re-admission and to allow timely discharge (DH 2008). Of course, nursing and other care and rehabilitation processes continue once a patient is deemed suitable for transfer home (or to another care setting). This continuity of care will be essential to ensure the problems that Mrs Swinbourne was facing prior to her hospital admission, both in terms of her health and other aspects of her home life, do not reach such an acute level that she needs to be re-admitted to hospital. Partnership-based Intermediate Care Teams have been developed in most localities across the United Kingdom in recent years to bridge the gap between hospital care and other established community-based health and social care services.

The focus on the physical aspect of the nursing assessment in the earlier parts of this chapter reflects the patient journey in as much as the priority for most hospital patients is to improve their physical health so that they are well enough to return home. Generally speaking, the acute hospital environment, with its emphasis on minimising the duration of patient stay, is not particularly conducive to systematic evaluation of a person's psychological, social and spiritual well-being. This is in part because in being removed from their familiar surroundings an individual may feel socially and spiritually detached. Clearly, the acute health reason for the initial hospital admission must take priority and once this had been addressed, other non-physical or less urgent physical health and environmental factors can be assessed. As we noted in Part 2 of this chapter, to entirely neglect these matters from the nursing assessment is to fail to realise that people are more than mere physical beings. To continue to do so up to the point of transfer is likely to endanger the patient and substantially increase the risk of rapid re-admission to hospital. While they may have been acknowledged earlier during her hospital stay, it is the meeting with the Intermediate Care Team that begins to systematically take account of these other types of issues that can help Maureen to assess how safe and independent Mrs Swinbourne will be when she goes home; as well as what further nursing input and other supports will be required to ensure that she can remain at home.

The things that Maureen has observed

The first thing that Maureen may have observed from the meeting with the Intermediate Care Team is that Mrs Swinbourne is a very independently minded lady. She is of the opinion that she can manage personal activities of daily living, such as self-care and feeding, for herself, and also suggests that she does not require the services she previously received to help with domestic activities of daily living. This may contradict Maureen's own observations of how Mrs Swinbourne has been coping with her self-care while in hospital, as well as the data provided by the care manager on the home help provided for Mrs Swinbourne prior to her admission. It may also indicate to Maureen that Mrs Swinbourne may be lacking some insight into her current physical health problems and their impact on how much she can do for herself. This may be indicative of more than simply an independent spirit: it could be an early sign of other undiagnosed health problems, such as dementia. This shows that Maureen needs to continue to assess Mrs Swinbourne's ability to self-care while she is on the ward, and perhaps refer her to a hospital occupational therapist who can work with Mrs Swinbourne on some other activities of daily living (e.g., cooking simple meals) until her discharge.

The reader will note that as the emphasis of care moves away gradually from physical health and well-being towards non-health factors that could be obstacles to a successful and sustainable discharge home for Mrs Swinbourne, so the assessment methods rely less on the interpretation of objective, measured data, such as vital signs, and more on subjective data from the nurse's personal observation of the patient's behaviours, from the reports of others members of the multidisciplinary team, as well as those of the patient, carers and other people within their social circle.

Maureen will have noted that Mrs Swinbourne's neighbour had been concerned about her before the event that led to her admission. This may lead Maureen to obtain more information from the neighbour if she sees her visiting Mrs Swinbourne on the ward. Thus the process of assessment (gathering information, interpreting it and acting upon it) is a cycle which continues throughout each patient episode. All the information gathered by Maureen can be used to feed into Melissa's assessment for an individualised community care plan for Mrs Swinbourne.

Case 7.1 (continued)

On the day of the visit, Maureen accompanies Mrs Swinbourne to her home by hospital transport to meet Melissa (the nurse) and Raina (the occupational therapist) from the Intermediate Care Team. When they arrive, they find that Mrs Swinbourne's flat is in a very dishevelled state, with her clothing lying all around the floor, as well as dozens of chocolate wrappers. In her kitchen there are several opened bags of frozen food that have been spilt and left to go mouldy, with the freezer door left open. Mrs Swinbourne offers her visitors a cup of tea, but is unable to find the switch on her kettle. When she eventually does, she finds two cups in a cupboard which Maureen notices are not clean. Also, Mrs Swinbourne misses the cups and spills hot water from the kettle onto the worktop. On the worktop there are several bottles of pills, which are open, and Maureen notices that most of them have passed their expiry date.

Maureen's earlier concerns regarding Mrs Swinbourne's ability to cope at home seem to have been confirmed by her observations during this visit. Assessment through observation of how a person behaves, or appears to be behaving in their own home environment is crucial for successful and sustainable community living for people with complex health problems. Maureen's interpretation of what she has observed during her visit to Mrs Swinbourne's flat could include the following:

- Mrs Swinbourne may have been unable to keep her home tidy prior to admission.
- Mrs Swinbourne's diet and nutritional intake may have been poor prior to admission.
- Mrs Swinbourne may have a visual impairment causing her not to see the kettle switch or the dirty cups (although the kettle should be familiar to her).
- Mrs Swinbourne may have a cognitive impairment causing her not to see the switch on the kettle or the dirty cups.
- Mrs Swinbourne may have a visual-perceptual deficit causing her to spill the hot water when attempting to pour hot water into the cup.
- Mrs Swinbourne may have impaired upper limb strength and/or mobility causing her to spill the hot water when attempting to pour hot water into the cup.
- Mrs Swinbourne may not have been able to manage her own medication prior to her admission.

This list is not exhaustive and the only way that all possibilities to explain the patient's behaviour can be explored and the reasons for her behaviour identified, in order to determine whether discharge home is feasible, is through a systematic assessment from individuals from the appropriate professional groups.

On return to the hospital and after talking things through with Raina, Maureen begins to realise that the priorities she has as a nurse (with emphasis on the physical) are not shared by occupational therapists. This became clear as Raina explained that the distinctions that Maureen (and other nurses) tend to make between physical, social, psychological and spiritual assessment (while understandable in the acute stages of a patient's illness) are less important for other professional groups such as occupational therapists who tend not to compartmentalise medical and health issues as separate from other factors that contribute to (or inhibit) a person's well-being.

Case 7.1 (continued)

On the day before transfer home, Maureen notices Mrs Swinbourne leaving the ward bathroom and walking with her wheeled walking frame, as she usually does, back towards her bed. However, on this occasion Mrs Swinbourne passes by her bed and makes her way out of the ward. Maureen follows and asks if she is looking for something, to which Mrs Swinbourne replies that she is trying to find her spectacles because one of the doctors had taken them from her. Maureen suggests that she may have left them by her bedside or in the bathroom and that she will help look for them. Maureen accompanies Mrs Swinbourne back to the bed, but they cannot find her spectacles there; Maureen helps Mrs Swinbourne to sit comfortably by her bed and then proceeds to the ward bathroom where she finds the spectacles on the floor. She notices the washbasin taps have been left running and water is spilling over into large puddles on the floor.

Later that day, Mrs Swinbourne is visited by Charlotte, one of the hospital social workers. Charlotte chats to Mrs Swinbourne for about half an hour, after which she writes something in the medical notes and promptly leaves the ward without speaking to anyone else. Maureen looks at the medical notes and sees that Charlotte has written that no services are required to be put in place for Mrs Swinbourne's discharge tomorrow, other than reinstating the existing home help.

Maureen is distressed by this cursory assessment of Mrs Swinbourne by the social worker and with her new-found understanding about the complexities involved in comprehensive assessment recognises how important it is for all professionals involved in the care of a patient such as Mrs Swinbourne to communicate with each other and work together constructively. In effect, Maureen now realises the importance not only of developing effective skills of assessment but also of interprofessional working (see Chapter 5).

Conclusion

It is not possible in a chapter of this length to cover all aspects of patient assessment: as a result we have tried to focus on the skills needed for effective assessment regardless of what aspect of a patient is under assessment. While the physical domain predominates we are at pains to point out that this is meant to be illustrative: that is, we take it that the skills of observation, measurement and interviewing detailed in this chapter can be put to use in the assessment of any domain of patient experience. Thus these skills are (in modern parlance) transferable.

We would just like to make three final points before leaving the reader to find the best way to make use of the learning that will have occurred as a result of reading this chapter.

1. Effective assessment lies at the heart of safe and effective nursing practice, wherever and whenever that practice takes places.
2. There are many different assessment tools available that can assist in the pursuit of effective assessment but these tools should not be mistaken as replacements for the need for careful observation, measurement and interviewing. Even with the most valid and reliable assessment tools there remains a need for professional judgement and discretion in interpreting the information gathered from using such tools.
3. A focus on assessment in the physical domain is a necessary component of all the assessments that nurses undertake, and the need for effectiveness in physical assessment will remain

whatever other domain is being assessed. According to the NMC (2004) nurses are expected to perform assessment in all domains of patients' experiences including the physical, the psychological, the social and the spiritual. As we intimated in Part 1 of this chapter, it is not clear that pre-registration education prepares individual nurses to undertake assessment in all these domains. Indeed, in the case of spirituality, it is not even clear that nurses have a common understanding of what a spiritual need is (see Paley 2008).

Despite this last reservation, we hope that by reading this chapter you will have gained a deeper understanding of the importance of effective assessment and of the relationship between systematic assessment on the one hand and safe and effective care on the other.

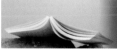

Suggested further reading

Baid, H. (2006) The process of conducting a physical assessment: a nursing perspective. *British Journal of Nursing* **15** (13), 710–714.

Barker, P. J. (1997) *Assessment in Psychiatric and Mental Health Nursing: In search of the whole person*. Cheltenham: Stanley Thomas.

West, S. L. (2006) Physical assessment: whose role is it anyway?' *Nursing in Critical Care* **11** (4), 161–167

Wheeldon, A. (2005) Exploring nursing roles: using physical assessment in the respiratory unit. *British Journal of Nursing* **14** (10), 571–574.

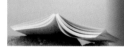

References

Barrett, D., Wilson, B. and Woollands, A. (2009) *Care Planning: A guide for nurses*. Harlow: Pearson Education.

Benner, P. (1984) *From Novice to Expert: Excellence and power in clinical nursing practice*. Menlo Park, CA: Addison-Wesley.

Bickley, L. S. and Szilagyi, P. G. (2007) *Bates' Guide to Physical Examination and History Taking* (9th ed.). Philadelphia: Lippincott, Williams & Wilkins.

Brennan, F., Carr, D. B. and Cousins, M. (2007) Pain management: a fundamental right. *International Anesthesia Research Society* **105** (1), 205–221.

Coulling, S. (2005) Nurses' and doctors' knowledge of pain after surgery. *Nursing Standard* **19** (34), 41–49.

Cousins, M. J., Brennan, F. and Carr, D. B. (2004) Pain relief: A universal human right. *Pain* **112** (1–2), 1–4.

DH (Department of Health) (2001) *The NHS Plan*. London: DH.

DH (Department of Health) (2008) *Older People's NSF Standards* (http://www.dh.gov.uk).

José Closs, S. (2007) Assessment of pain, mood, and quality of life. In *Pain in Older People*, Crome, P., Main, C. J. and Lally, F. (eds). Oxford: Oxford University Press, pp. 11–19.

Kim, H. S., Shwartz-Barcott, D., Tracy, S. M., Fortin, J. D. and Sjostrom, B. (2005) Strategies of pain assessment used by nurses on surgical units. *Pain Management Nursing* **6** (1), 3–9.

Layman Young, J., Horton, F. M. and Davidhizar, R. (2006) Nursing attitudes and beliefs in pain assessment and management. *Journal of Advanced Nursing* **53** (4), 412–421.

Lynch, M. (2001) Pain as the fifth vital sign. *Journal of Intravenous Nursing* **24** (2), 85–94.

McDonald, D. D., McNulty, J., Erickson, K. and Weiskopf, C. (2000) Communicating pain and pain management needs after surgery. *Applied Nursing Research* **13** (2), 70–75.

Melzack, R. (1987) The short-form McGill Pain Questionnaire. *Pain* **30** (2), 191–197.

Melzack, R. (2005) The McGill Pain Questionnaire: from description to measurement. *Anesthesiology* **103** (1), 199–202 (first published in *Anesthesiology* in 1971).

NMC (Nursing and Midwifery Council) (2004) *Standards of Proficiency for Pre-registration Nursing Education*. London: NMC.

Paley, J. (2008) Spirituality and nursing: a reductionist approach. *Nursing Philosophy* **9** (1), 3–18.

RCA and PS (The Royal College of Anaesthetists and The Pain Society) (2003) *Pain Management Services: Good practice*. London: RCA and PS.

RCP, BGS and BPS (Royal College of Physicians, British Geriatrics Society and British Pain Society) (2007) *The Assessment of Pain in Older People: National guidelines. Concise guidance to good practice series, No 8*. London: RCP.

Seidel, H. M., Ball, J. W., Dains, J. E. and Benedict, G. W. (2006) *Mosby's Guide to Physical Examination* (6th ed.). London: Mosby.

Weber, J. and Kelley, J. (2007) *Health Assessment in Nursing* (3rd ed.). Philadelphia: Lippincott, Williams & Wilkins.

Zwakhelan, S. M. G., Katinka, K. A., Hamers, J. P. H. and Huijer Abu-Saad, H. (2004) Pain assessment in intellectually disabled people: Non-verbal indicators. *Journal of Advanced Nursing* **45** (3), 236–245.

Chapter 8

Judgement and decision-making

P. Anne Scott, Pádraig MacNeela,
Gerard Clinton and David Pontin

Learning outcomes

After reading and reflecting on this chapter, you should be able to:

- Describe the field of judgement and decision-making research;
- Identify and discuss the kinds of clinical judgements and decisions that arise in nursing practice;
- Identify contextual influences on judgement and decision-making;
- Discuss the main approaches, trends and findings of judgement and decision-making research in nursing.

Related NMC Standard of Proficiency for Pre-registration Nursing Education (NMC 2004)

● Problem-solving – demonstrate sound clinical decision-making which can be justified even when made on the basis of limited imformation.

Introduction

Nurses make judgements and decisions every day in relation to all sorts of situations ranging from the mundane to the complex. Much of this judgement and decision-making activity remains unnoticed because it operates in relation to the routines and procedures that dominate nursing work. In many instances this level of judgement and decision-making is sufficient for getting things done under increasingly time constrained pressures of work. However, sufficiency in judgement and decision-making may not result in actions that are in the best interests of patients and their families; and it may be efficiency rather than sufficiency that is required. This chapter offers an introduction to some aspects of judgement and decision-making theory that have a bearing on the everyday work of nurses.

The chapter is divided into three parts.

In Part 1, we make a distinction between judgement on the one hand and decision-making on the other and note how both relate to safe and effective nursing practice.

In Part 2, we offer some explanation of normative, descriptive and prescriptive models of judgment and decision-making together with some initial comments on the influence of individual and organisational factors on the way nurses approach decision-making.

In Part 3, we explore some of the differences between intuitive and analytical approaches and suggest that because nursing practice takes place in the pressured environment of time constraints intuition plays a significant role in the judgements and decisions that nurses make every day.

Part 1: Outlining judgement and decision-making

Case 8.1

Natasha is a first-year student nurse. She is surprised when her mentor (Valerie) refuses to sanction the transfer home of Mr Chin (an 84-year-old man) who has no further medical needs from an acute medical unit on the grounds that the family are insufficiently prepared for caring for him at home. Natasha has always assumed that once medical staff say a patient is ready for discharge it is the nurse's job to make this happen; it is certainly what she has seen happen before. When asked about this by Natasha, Valerie says that in her view there is more to be lost than gained by sending this patient home. His family are clearly unprepared for the heavy nursing care demands he will require. If sent home without the necessary support services in place it is likely that Mr Chin will be re-admitted within a matter of days and the family will then doubt their ability to cope. This in turn may mean that in the longer term they may be reluctant to take on the burden of caring for him at home. Valerie explains that she plans to influence the doctor's decision about discharge by convincing him of the need to wait a couple of days in the hope of avoiding further complications.

Nurses make hundreds of judgements and decisions every day. Many of these go unnoticed, many are made with only minimal information and most are made rapidly. For many nurses the processes involved in making judgements and decisions remain unconscious, unexamined and unarticulated. Indeed, it is not uncommon to hear judgement and decision-making (JDM) spoken of as if it were a natural ability that some but not all nurses possess. The problem with this view is that it assumes that a nurse cannot improve their JDM. In reality, JDM is a skill and just like any other skill, it can be studied, broken down into its component parts (analysed) and learned. Few judgements and decisions are made under perfect conditions and, as with so many other aspects of nursing, nurses generally try to do the best they can under difficult circumstances: very often with incomplete information, under pressure of work and within time contraints imposed by rapidly changing conditions. Not ideal circumstances for effective decision-making.

In Case 8.1 it can be seen that Valerie is *making a judgement* about the family's ability to cope with the care the patient needs and also *making a decision* about what she is going to do. Valerie is thus demonstrating JDM. However, she would also have demonstrated JDM had she gone along with the original discharge plan, it is just that this JDM would have gone unnoticed.

Although it may not be obvious to you now, the judgements and decisions you make as a student nurse and later as a registered nurse will be a feature of your professional practice. Whatever your current stage on a pre-registration nursing programme you will already be making judgements and decisions. What you may not be aware of is whether or not you are effective at making judgements and decisions. The importance of effective JDM cannot be overstated. The judgements and decisions you make will have an effect not only on the quality of the care for which you are responsible but also for how you manage your time as a registered practitioner.

In the process of becoming a nurse, you are expected to gain experience in making judgments and decisions as you progress through your programme. It may be acceptable and appropriate during your first year to rely on more experienced and more qualified staff, but as you approach qualification and increased accountability it is important not only to make but also to justify your independent judgements and decisions. Effective JDM is something that can be learned, but it does require knowing something about decision-making theories and being able to put (at least) some of those ideas into use in the practice environment.

The literature on judgement and decision-making can be confusing. A variety of different terms are used (e.g., clinical judgement, clinical inference, clinical reasoning, diagnostic reasoning) and not all authors differentiate between judgements and decisions (e.g., Bucknall 2003, Connolly *et al.* 2000). In this chapter we take the view that **judgement** is different from (but related to) **decision**-making.

A judgement is a conclusion reached in relation to a set of information, whereas a decision involves choosing between alternatives. The International Council of Nursing define judgement as:

> *a clinical opinion, an estimate, or determination of professional nursing practice regarding the state of a nursing phenomenon, including the relative quality of the intensity or degree of the manifestation of the nursing phenomenon.*
> (ICN 2002 p. 75)

A **judgement** is a conclusion reached in relation to a set of information.

A **decision** involves choosing between alternatives.

Judgements may relate to a patient state (e.g., distress, anxiety, happiness, hypotension, being in pain or discomfort) but may also relate to wider contextual issues (e.g., the ability of a family to manage the care of a relative at home or the appropriateness of a treatment of intervention being offered to a patient). Whereas Wickens *et al.* (2004) suggest a decision requires choosing between different possible actions where that choice is related to known available options (although the best alternative may not be obvious), requires some thought (i.e., is not instantaneous) and involves some risk.

Activity 8.1

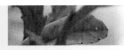

Think about your most recent shift on placement. Take 5 minutes to jot down the sorts of judgements and decisions you made throughout the shift.

You should not be surprised if you found it difficult to identify the judgements and decisions you made during your most recent working shift. This is because JDM is all-pervasive within everyday nursing and it is sometimes difficult to get a clear picture of the JDM process. Some of your judgements and decisions may have been made when, for example:

- Assessing patients or clients; monitoring patient condition or progress against nursing interventions.
- Evaluating treatment efficacy.
- Choosing different interventions and working with patients and families to co-ordinate their care.

Of course there are differences in the types of judgements and decisions made in different parts of nursing, for example, mental health services, acute and community-based physical health care, children's services and services for people living with learning disabilities.

Nursing work involves uncertainty, and nowhere is this more apparent than in the realm of JDM. Making judgements and decisions means sometimes getting it wrong: this is after all a feature of working in the busy environment of constant demands and interruptions (Hedberg and Larsson 2004) as well as the stresses of time pressures, performance indicators and targets that all serve to increase the risk of human error (Patel and Currie 2005). There are two more important and related points to mention here:

1. *That there is no necessary relationship between experience and effective JDM.* It is tempting to think that more experienced nurses will be better at JDM. However, as an example, Solomon (2001) found that not only do nurses underestimate the pain patients experience compared with patients' self-rated pain scores but also that it is the most experienced nurses who underestimate patients' pain the most.
2. *That effective JDM is not merely a function of individual capacity.* It is all too easy to blame individual nurses for ineffective JDM, but this fails to account for the shaping influence that organisations have on our ability to make effective judgements or decisions at a given time and in a given place.

Part 2: Explaining judgement and decision-making

Case 8.1 (continued)

Clearly Valerie has already made a judgement (about the lack of suitable arrangements in place for Mr Chin to be transferred home) and she has also made a decision (to influence the doctor's decision on the timing of Mr Chin's discharge). Valerie is experienced enough to understand that merely putting together a logical argument about the high risk of rapid re-admission will not be sufficient to convince the doctor of the need to keep Mr Chin in hopsital for extra time, so she now needs to make a decision about which course of action will best achieve what she perceives to be in the best long-term interests of the patient in this situation. In order to make the best decision possible in this instance, it wil be helpful for Valerie to have some knowledge about different models of judgement and decision-making.

Activity 8.2

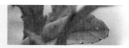

Make some notes on how Valerie might go about making a decision on how to ensure that suitable home care arrangements can be put in place before Mr Chin's discharge home.

Models of judgement and decision-making

Chapman and Sonnenberg (2000) identify three main models of JDM processes:

1. Normative (how a decision can best be made).
2. Descriptive (how decisions are actually made).
3. Prescriptive (how decision theory can be used to improve decision-making).

The normative model

Normative refers to norms and values and is used to suggest what ought to happen.

The **normative** model of decision-making is based on ideas of what people ought to do in order to be rational decision makers. The key word here is *rational*, and there is an assumption in the model that we wish to be rational both in our decision-making and in our subsequent actions. Central to the model is the Expected Utility theory of human behaviour. This theory assumes two things:

1. That people make decisions fully aware of all the information they need to make the decision.
2. That people are aware of all the possible alternatives of potential outcomes.

Utility is the usefulness of some thing, some event or some outcome for a person.

In other words, by following the rationally determined best course of action, the **utility** of people's decision-making will be maximised; that is, they will achieve the optimum outcome (Baron 1994).

Operating on the basis of expected utility here refers to favouring a decision option with the highest expected utility. However, it is recognised that people's JDM is influenced by other factors, in particular how we respond to the way that nearly all of the task environments we encounter involve some limitation on our knowledge or level of certainty. So it is important to know how people make choices in the face of uncertainty, that is, where the outcome of the decision cannot be easily predicted. In this type of situation the risks involved in decision-making become writ large. The classic mode of research inquiry in the normative model is to ask people to evaluate trade-offs (Goldstein and Hogarth 1997). For example, to ask a client to choose between alternative interventions on the basis of the likelihood of side effects (such as choosing between psycho-surgery or cognitive behaviour therapy to reduce socially unacceptable behaviour and avoid compulsory detention in a forensic mental health unit).

The descriptive model

Information processing. Human cognition is based on processing information. An analogy can be made with a computer (i.e., input-throughput or processing-output). JDM is viewed as a technical exercise using intuitive, heuristic and/or analytical processes. Information processing provides insight into underlying thinking structures and processes but is less helpful in understanding interpersonal or organisational factors.

Heuristic is a rule of thumb strategy that circumvents the need to analyse a problem through logic (Kahneman and Tversky 1973). As a form of cognitive bias it cannot provide the most reliable form of decision-making but it is relatively effortless and therefore valuable in adapting to limited information or time.

In contrast to the normative model, the descriptive model of JDM aims to illustrate how people actually make decisions (rather than how they ought to). Underpinning the descriptive model is the idea that in reality people are not particularly effective decision makers. According to this model, we can never really hope to achieve rational decision-making because of our limited **information processing** capacity or bounded rationality. Proponents of the descriptive model acknowledge that modes of thinking that serve us well for our everyday decisions can lead to ineffective decision-making in complex situations (Payne *et al.* 1993) such as those encountered in nursing practice. Our everyday JDM is based on the notion that we adapt to the environment in which the decision is to be made and we use cues we have found helpful previously to inform our understanding of the situation. The descriptive model emphasises that people base their decisions on what they understand, believe or feel rather than objective evidence and logical analysis. An important issue arising from this is the accuracy of judgements. In health contexts, this tends to focus on intuitive or clinical judgement being less accurate than a simple statistical combination (Daly 2005). Health care practitioners tend to make judgements about patients and clients on the basis of inferences drawn from incomplete and fallible cues (Goldstein and Hogarth 1997).

Although we may not be rational decision makers, proponents of the descriptive model point out that we are able to make intelligent use of our limited cognitive resources to make decisions by the use of **heuristics**. Heuristics are rules of thumb we use in the attempt to overcome our bounded rationality. According to the model, people will stop searching for a decision once they find an option that meets their minimal acceptable criteria (Goldstein and Hogarth 1997). In other words, they may not select the best decision because they foreclose on alternatives before they know the extent of available options. It should not come as a surprise that nurses often adopt a descriptive model of decision-making because of the enormous pressure to make rapid decisions with only partial information, but this can lead to falling into a routine of choosing the familiar when a little more thought might offer a better decision in a given situation. In other words, an over-reliance on heuristics can lead to routine and ritual (I always do it this way) that in turn can hinder the development of novel solutions to individual patient problems.

The prescriptive model

The prescriptive model also acknowledges that we are poor decision makers but recognises that there are techniques and aids that can be used to improve the quality of our JDM. In particular, proponents of the model set out to describe the underlying cognitive processes that support and influence JDM (e.g., attitudes, biases or **schemas**) in order to offer effective ways of making decisions (Connor and Norman 1996). The focus thus becomes the different strategies that people use for addressing different problems, the level of mental effort involved in making the decision, and the importance of accuracy to the quality of decision-making.

The prescriptive model recognises factors that impinge on the quality of decision-making. According to Maule (1997) these factors include:

- The time pressures under which decisions are made.
- The stress and associated emotional states (e.g., fear, anger) experienced by the decision maker.
- The level of engagement the decision maker has with the problem to be addressed.

In acknowledging these factors the prescriptive model allows for the requirement of different types of decisions for different types of prescriptive action (Klein 1997). According to Olson (1996) there are three main ways that decision-making can be developed to support people's decision-making:

1. Structured sequencing of activities using decision analysis techniques and decision trees.
2. Scenario planning where strategic decisions for medium- to long-term outcomes may be developed. These are not ascribed to probabilities of events happening but rather are positive or negative scenarios which describe how the future may unfold, and allow people to choose the best action regardless of which sequence of events occurs.
3. The development of training packages or materials allowing people to follow rule-based or formal models of decision-making which are constructed from statistics or logic and probability theory.

Schemas are cognitive structures that represent general and specialised knowledge about objects, people or situations and the relationships between them (Fiske and Morling 1996). Intuitive or experiential nursing knowledge can be seen as a set of clinical schemas. Another form of knowledge structure is an exemplar. While a schema may suggest a general, average case, exemplars represent specific cases or instances. Nursing knowledge includes abstract knowledge, schemas and case exemplars.

Judgement and decision-making in nursing practice

Judgements are generally carried out for a purpose. The nature of the judgement made often varies according to the purpose or the task to which it is related. For example:

- *Initial assessment*: nurses carry out initial assessments of patients and clients for the purpose of achieving an overall sense of the person's functioning, health state or abilities or a specific assessment of a presenting problem.
- *Monitoring*: ongoing assessment of people is different from initial assessment. Having established some basic patient parameters, nurses update these judgements and form evaluative judgements that detect stability and change.
- *Discharge assessment*: here a judgement is made about whether someone's condition has improved or stabilised enough to recommend discharge home or to a step-down facility, or to recommend transfer to a specialist service if the condition has worsened.
- *Knowing the patient*: this requires nurses to form a view on several different aspects of patient functioning, looking at the 'whole person'.
- *Risk assessment*: here the judgement is framed to identify a particular vulnerability or threat to the patient (e.g., risk of infection, risk of violent behaviour, risk of being abused).
- *Compliance with treatments*: assessing the degree to which patients and/or their families or carers have adhered to treatment plans or nursing care plans (e.g., activity or diet recommendations) or complied with medication prescriptions.

Intervention choice	Choices related to choosing between different care interventions. Special attention may be given to targeting particular people. So while several patients may require skin care, the person with the highest priority for this intervention is targeted first and the best time is chosen to give the care
Communication	Choices related to the ways and means of gathering and sharing information. This may involve patients and clients, their families or carers, other members of the multidisciplinary team and other agencies. An example here would be safeguarding vulnerable adults
Service organisation, delivery and management	Choices related to the delivery of specific services at designated times and places (e.g., deciding which staff are required to work a particular shift because of the anticipated needs of the patients/clients)

Figure 8.1 Three major types of decisions taken by nurses.

Source: Adapted from Thompson *et al.* (2000).

The taxonomy of decision types offered by Thompson *et al.* (Figure 8.1) illustrates the point that the student or the registered nurse is likely to be exposed to different levels of decision-making. Some decisions focus on activities directly related to patient care (e.g., patient positioning in acute hospital nursing or anxiety reduction in mental health nursing) while others relate to indirect interventions carried out for the benefit of patients (e.g., trying to get a patient with acute health needs admitted to a ward or place of safety). Because nurses usually work in a complex health care environment, many judgements and decisions relate to the system of health care delivery as much as to direct patient care. It has been noted that nurses have a tendency to deny their individual decision-making activities and tend to talk about (at least by implication) collective decision-making (McGovern 2001). We argue that effective JDM is part and parcel of what it means to be a competent nurse (Scott *et al.* 2006).

The influence of the organisation on JDM

Like other health care practices, nursing takes place within (or under the jurisdiction of) organsations, and the influence of organisational arrangements tends to be underestimated. In other words, JDM is not solely related to the cognitive abilities of individual nurses because there may be a whole range of organisational constraints that facilitate or get in the way of effective decision-making. For example:

- The reality of working within organisational arrangements may be quite different from the formal vision of organisational structure.
- Organisational status is a way of giving more or less autonomy in JDM according to seniority.
- Care settings present different kinds of JDM problems and different resources for their resolution.
- Formal aids to JDM may vary from organisation to organisation, and within organisations.
- Different professional groups will exhibit different cultural norms and beliefs about medical and biopsychosocial models of illness, drug-based and psychosocial treatments, the involvement of patients in decision-making, and openness to organisational change.
- Professional working relationships between different occupational groups may encourage or discourage effective JDM at the level of the individual.

Critical social theory sometimes positions nurses as belonging to an oppressed professional group. Manias and Street (2001) argue that:

> *the status and development of nurses' knowledge has been largely influenced by the dominance of medical power . . . this dominance has supported the view that medicine operates from a foundation of 'superior', legitimated knowledge (p. 129).*

Which is one reason why doctors are often considered to have more legitimacy than nurses in relation to JDM. However, the 'doctor–nurse game' (Porter 1991) is one strategy that allows nurses to covertly steer medical decision-making in particular ways and this may be the only way that Valerie can influence arrangements for Mr Chin's discharge (Case 8.1).

Research focus 8.1

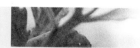

Manias and Street's (2001) study of critical care in Australia identified several ways in which nurses were formally excluded from decisions about patients yet still exerted considerable influence over decision-making. Nurses possessed knowledge that doctors needed but did not have. Nurses used their role as informants on patient status to get their views acted on, and presented information to suggest actions to doctors. It can be seen from this that it is not enough merely to possess information, combine it well and identify an appropriate decision. It is also necessary to be able to work effectively in a system where you cannot automatically, or directly, put your views into effect. Knowing how the system works can be as important as knowing the patient.

Carmel's (2006) ethnographic case study of medical and nursing work in intensive care questions the degree to which nursing and medicine are actually different in the practice environment. He concludes that 'what is perhaps more noticeable are the similarities in practice and perspective between nursing and medical staff'. Both appear to value psychosocial as well as physiological information about patients. In a similar vein, Montgomery's (2005) analysis of medical knowledge highlighted the use of heuristics and narratives in medical practice, concluding that physicians work more from 'art' than 'science', as nurses also appear to do in many cases.

Activity 8.3

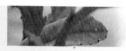

Try to identify a situation you have witnessed in which a nurse has found a way to influence the JDM of a doctor. What strategy did they use? Can you work out why the nurse felt it necessary to use a subtle approach rather than just refer to their own JDM?

Making judgements and decisions about patient care necessarily occurs within a system of limited resources; where time, expense, effectiveness and use of staff all have a bearing. This gives rise to informal and undocumented strategies for making decisions about resources (e.g., bed management in forensic psychiatry units, Grounds *et al.* 2004). In addition, the relationships between different professional groups can impact on JDM (Bucknall 2003, Bucknall and Thomas 1995, Hancock and Easen 2006). The influence of these relationships is made more complex by the autonomy and authority (or lack thereof) of nurses in decision-making (Bucknall and Thomas 1995). In both the USA and the UK, increased visibility of the nursing contribution to JDM is seen as important in improving the standing of the profession in multi-professional teams (Buckingham and Adams 2000, Havens and Vasey 2005).

Crow and colleagues (1995) argue that the JDM process differs between medicine and nursing. Other researchers see little intrinsic difference (Buckingham and Adams 2000, Rashotte and Carnavale 2004) as both use evidence to categorise patients accurately (at risk/not at risk; suitable/unsuitable for discharge, etc.). In practice, doctors are often seen as privileging biomedical knowledge and exercising decision-making in a hierarchical manner (Coombs and Ersser 2004). In this environment, nurses' experiential knowledge base may be seen as inferior, perhaps because of the medical interest in diagnosis supported by empirical knowledge (di Giulio and Crow 1997). Experiential

Attention. We do not and cannot attend to all environmental information, so we select information for processing through attention. Attention is used for different tasks – to orient us to important environmental events (e.g., a cry for help), to filter out information (e.g., routine monitoring sounds), to conduct a goal-directed search (e.g., to monitor patients' level of eye contact) and to direct our senses in line with our expectations (e.g., detecting smells from body fluids) (Coren *et al.* 1994). Focused attention has a single target while divided attention involves monitoring of several targets (e.g., multitasking).

knowledge links to JDM through **attention** and memory. Henneman *et al.* (1995) identify the need for experiential knowledge to be recognised and used in teamwork in order to promote successful interdisciplinary collaboration. It is claimed that the richest source of knowledge informing clinical JDM for nurses is gained through continuous involvement in patient care (Coombs and Ersser 2004). Nurses generally spend more time with patients than do doctors, and of course each carries out different tasks. Knowledge derived from caring for patients is largely experiential, and has the potential to complement an approach that emphasises formal empirical scientific knowledge (Kikuchi and Simmons 1999, Rashotte and Carnavale 2004). Coombs and Ersser (2004) argue that nurses are not empowered to make clinical JDM to the same extent as doctors, although greater levels of decision-making responsibility are seen among nurses at a higher organisational status (Bucknall 2003).

Part 3: Exploring judgement and decision-making

Intuition is a form of knowing or understanding about something that cannot be explained by reference to facts, previous experience or the experience of others. This might be expressed in a sentence such as 'I have a gut feeling about this but I cannot tell you why'.

One of the claims implied in this chapter is that within JDM nursing tends towards **intuition** and heuristics rather than analysis because (at least in part) of the constraints of environment and time. Here we will begin to explore the role of intuition in JDM for nursing.

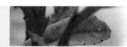

Activity 8.4

Spend some time thinking about the way you approach judgement and decision-making. Do you think others would describe you as intuitive or analytical in your judgements and decisions?

Intuitive judgements and decisions

Intuitive JDM rests on the outcome of a process of perceiving or apprehending something that triggers previous knowledge, experience or skill in such a way that it is knowable to the decision maker. This pattern recognition is a relatively automatic judgement response to a set of cues (e.g., facial grimacing and muscular tension trigger prior knowledge and can lead us to make a judgement about a patient's pain). However, it takes practice, expertise and familiarity to exercise selective perception or 'see' things in this way, rather than having to think

Descriptive judgement	Using a label to describe a relevant state (e.g., anxious, uncomfortable, pyrexial)
Evaluative judgement	Making a comparison in relation to time, situation or other people (e.g., better/worse than yesterday, it was different last time, she is responding better than him)
Inferential judgement	Making a prediction about what may happen (e.g., I don't think she will be ready for discharge tomorrow)
Causal judgement	Stating a cause of a state (e.g., anaemia due to poor diet, erratic behaviour due to drug misuse)

Figure 8.2 Four types of judgements characteristic of nursing.
Source: Adapted from Lamond et al. (1996).

consciously. Judging that someone is anxious is of a different order to judging that they are more anxious today than they were yesterday ('descriptive judgement' and 'evaluative judgement' respectively, see Figure 8.2). Both descriptive and evaluative judgements can be reached through an intuitive process using sensory evidence to prime existing knowledge, although each requires different kinds of information. The intuitive descriptive judgement is based on an automatic recognition of cue patterns associated with anxiety; whereas the intuitive evaluative judgement requires two descriptive judgements at different times and an unconscious comparison of the two.

These judgements could serve several purposes: in knowing the patient and thinking about the causes of a problem (making a causal judgement); assessing people's post-intervention state (a broad descriptive judgement); or making a prediction about likely rate of improvement (an inferential judgement). Making a judgement of anxiety is also closely linked to decision-making as recognising someone's anxiety may prompt a decision about what to do next. Natasha's mentor made a prediction that the patient would have to be re-admitted within days, having mentally simulated what would happen in the absence of adequate family support.

A consideration of intuitive judgements triggers three important issues.

1. We have a limited capacity to process information but with practice we can learn to recognise particular patterns. With limited capacity for attention and reasoning, it may be more time-efficient to trigger judgements using patterns and categories than to think deliberately about each one.
2. Fluency and flexibility in categorising environmental information is an acquired skill. Experts are able to make quick and accurate judgements based on experience and/or knowledge acquired over a long period of time and/or specific to a specialist area of practice.
3. Some tasks require rapid intuitive judgements – time pressure, stress, limited information and varied tasks may demand a quick response (Hammond 1996). Our attention is impaired by information overload, fatigue and stress from difficult or unfamiliar situations (O'Neill et al. 2005).

There is inevitably a trade-off between speed and error: the more rapid the JDM the higher the risk of error. This is perhaps a particular issue for the novice nurse (student or qualified) who may have little experience of making intuitive judgements on which to draw and so is more likely to be faced with unfamiliar situations. As a result the novice will need to consciously engage with the features of unfamiliar situations in order to make judgements that will be in the intuitive realm for the expert nurse (some elements of such intuition can be seen in the different approaches to patient assessment of the student and mentor in Chapter 7).

Research focus 8.2

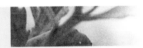

Novice to expert

Some nurses move from novice through intermediate levels of performance to expert with experience (Benner *et al*. 1999). This parallels Rasmussen's (1993) levels of task performance. At the highest level, task performance is skill-based (i.e., intuitive) at the intermediate and low level it is rule-based (e.g., protocol or procedure driven). Performance is knowledge-based among novices (i.e., the novice needs to think through the different options on how to approach a task). In contrast the expert nurse demonstrates skilled performance in a particular domain and it is suggested that this takes approximately ten years to attain (Ericsson 2005). However, experience alone does not lead to expert performance; it is the learning and development that arises from and with experience that offers a route to expert practice (and this provides one of the basic justifications for the need for nurses to engage with reflective practice – see Chapter 13). Thus higher levels of practice combined with appropriate feedback can lead to a high level of skill (deGroot 1965). Expert performance involves knowing what to do when things go wrong, as well as knowing how to make sure things go right.

Heuristic thinking

In the previous section we presented a case for regarding intuitive JDM as a range of separate strategies. With practice it is possible to develop skill in noticing clusters and patterns of symptoms experienced by patients and clients. This is an impressive skill as health care problems rarely present themselves in textbook fashion. According to Bargh (1994) a truly automatic judgement is one that is:

- efficient (requires few resources);
- lacks intentionality (you cannot help but see the pattern);
- outside conscious control (it happens and you are aware of the result);
- outside awareness (you are unable to say what information was used to reach the judgement).

Very few judgements fulfil all these criteria. Yet many judgements come close, although the accuracy of those judgements is a different matter. This still leaves us needing to account for a number of thinking strategies and judgements that are more conscious than unconscious. We describe this mode of thought as heuristic thinking, based on 'rules of thumb' and simplified forms of analytical thinking.

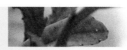

Activity 8.5

Think about a client or patient who was leaving your placement area to return home, go to a step-down facility or transfer to a more intensive environment. Write some brief notes identifying the sequence of events and the key players involved in making judgements and decisions in relation to this patient's transfer.

Wigton (1996) found that health workers normally use only a small number (generally between two and four) of information cues in making a judgement or decision. Despite the low number, there is no guarantee that each practitioner is paying attention to the same cues. In the case of a discharge decision these information cues might include family support, the patient's wishes and their mobility status. Seeking out information on particular information cues and forming a judgement is likely to involve some conscious thinking, especially if the information cues are contradictory and hard to reconcile. While some work is involved, a heuristic of targeting a small number of cues cuts down on mental workload. Various 'stopping rules' (Gigerenzer 2002) may also be employed. For example, if there is a very low level on any one information cue, then a default recommendation may be that discharge does not take place, or if the person is under 50 years of age and wishes to go home, then a default recommendation may be to recommend discharge. Are there any stopping rules you identified in your scenario developed from Activity 8.5?

A basic set of heuristics is applicable to most situations (Cioffi and Markham 1997, Kahneman and Tversky 1973, Thompson 2003). These deal with judgements based on:

- *Similarity* (representativeness heuristic).
- *Ease of recall* (availability heuristic).
- *Ease of projection* (simulation heuristic).
- *An initial starting point* as a guiding reference (anchoring and adjustment heuristic).

The representativeness and availability heuristics rely on prior knowledge and are more automatic than conscious. The simulation, and the anchoring and adjustment heuristics are likely to involve some conscious mediation. At some level, experiential knowledge is required for each of these heuristics.

Human judgement and decision-making is characterised by heuristics researchers as being prone to errors and biases. This view presumes we tend towards inaccuracy and misjudgement because we are cognitive misers; that is, we are unwilling or unable to think analytically so as to conserve our processing power (Fiske and Taylor 1984). This view has been challenged recently with an increased emphasis on considering human judgement as good enough to satisfy most task requirements. Gigerenzer (2002) argues that heuristic methods based on experience are generally sufficient for us to adapt to our environment. Klein (1999) points out that experts' use of simulation to think about future possibilities and consequences and the ability to think ahead is a source of strength, rather than a weakness.

In a study of specialist practice nurses, Fonteyn (1998) proposed a set of thinking strategies or heuristic types and identified several specific heuristics

Planning	Thinking how to proceed with a task (e.g., I think this client will respond well to active listening, how can I best accomplish this intervention today?)
Predicting	Thinking that is designed to anticipate outcomes (e.g., I've noticed that this patient tends to be more anxious in the mornings, it's probably better to engage him later in the day)
Guessing	Thinking to form hunches or hypotheses prior to determining the solution to a problem (e.g., my assessment is that active listening is an effective means of reducing this person's sense of isolation)
Monitoring	Thinking designed to assess progress toward problem resolution (e.g., the client seemed rather concerned about some of his problems, maybe I should try using distraction first and then move on to active listening related to his problems)

Figure 8.3 Heuristic types.
Source: Fonteyn (1998).

within each broad category (see Figure 8.3). There are many other heuristic 'rules of thumb' that remain to be identified or analysed from a JDM perspective. Discussion of a case with peers can be used heuristically, for instance. If several colleagues think you are incorrect in your assessment of a patient, you may reconsider your judgement (due to informational/normative social influence). Structure can be given to assessments and decisions through other more formal means. Judgement aids range from the conceptual (e.g., a nursing model as an aid to making judgements) to the formal and specific (e.g., rating scales as a means to categorise a patient). A decision aid differs from a judgement aid in that the former guides action whereas the latter helps in the assessment of a patient. Some decision aids (e.g., a decision tree) are derived from decision-making research. Other aids to decision-making provide a general framework for care (e.g., a care pathway) or specific guidance (e.g., a protocol for choosing an intervention).

Analytical judgements and decisions

Intuitive JDM is in stark contrast to an analytic JDM, which is characterised by conscious thinking and use of formal reasoning methods (e.g., Hastie and Dawes 2001). Normative models of JDM suggest how logic, utility analysis and propositional thinking should be used to yield the correct judgement or decision. This is a useful perspective, but in any given situation we are likely to lack the ability, time and information levels required to support the normative approach. Heuristic thinking strategies borrow from both analytical and perceptual methods. A heuristic is partly a conscious form of JDM, but individuals tend to make use of informal strategies, for example peer discussion, rule of thumb or simplified analytical strategies such as using a practice guideline or a decision tree. An analytical judgement is reached through a relatively slow, sequential consideration of information cues, as opposed to the fast and simultaneous processing happening in intuitive judgement (Hammond 1996).

Cue acquisition	Collecting information cues seen as relevant
Hypothesis generation	Coming up with one or more explanation that explains the patient's condition
Cue interpretation	Considering the information cues you have in light of the explanations you have generated
Hypothesis evaluation	Working out which explanation or hypothesis is correct

Figure 8.4 Four analytical stages in JDM.
Source: Elstein and Bordage (1988).

Short-term memory has a capacity of 7 items +/–2 (Miller 1956) and a duration of approximately 30 seconds. This limits our capacity to remember information from the environment. Working memory (Baddeley 2004) is a dynamic reading of short-term memory; the cognitive thinking and planning centre guides your strategy in a situation, aided by attention and the faculty for visualisation and language-based thought. In contrast, long-term memory is limitless. Declarative long-term memory is the store of verbal knowledge. Procedural long-term memory is the store of skilled knowledge. Once sufficiently well practised, task performance becomes proceduralised and increasingly automatic (Solso *et al.* 2004). Perceptual skills (such as pattern recognition) and skilled performance (in relation to a technical skill) are based on procedural memory. Episodic memory is the store for memories of specific events.

Probabilistic terms refers to levels of certainty such as probability, maybe or sometimes, but without a specific numerical indicator.

Hypothetico-deductive reasoning is seeking information or fact to confirm or disprove a statement about the world that has yet to be proved.

Montgomery and colleagues (2005) assume that the majority of our JDM is intuitive and heuristic and that this is to be expected given our limited **short-term memory** and difficulty with logical and propositional reasoning (Wason 1966). While we often employ **probabilistic terms** they tend to be used fairly loosely. In addition, the ambiguity or time pressure associated with nursing work makes it difficult to adopt an analytic approach. As a result, our bounded rationality tends to discourage us from thinking in genuinely analytical ways precisely because of environmental and personally imposed constraints (Simon 1956).

We would argue that nursing practice has the built-in conditions for making it easier to rely on experiential knowledge. Nursing often requires multi-tasking in a busy environment where the slowness and resource-intensiveness of analytical thinking is a disadvantage. Nursing work also requires high levels of certainty and accuracy, underscored by adverse potential consequences for patients if the JDM is wrong. We often try to adapt to this tension by engineering the environment: if you are not proficient in mental calculations, you can use a calculator; if errors in medication administration or dosage calculation are likely, you need a system that is as error-proof as possible through checks and balances (Sharpe 2004).

One of the main trends of analytical thinking in the JDM literature is **hypothetico-deductive reasoning**. Elstein and Bordage (1988) outline four analytical stages when making a judgement or decision about patients and clients (see Figure 8.4).

Most formal clinical judgements can be viewed in terms of generating hypotheses and working deductively to analyse which one is most likely to be correct. If you wish to judge whether a patient or client is under the influence of street drugs you would begin by collecting information. This might come from your observations, from patient notes, or from family members and colleagues. From this you can generate one or more hypotheses, for example: that the patient is using heroin, that she is not using any street drugs, that she is using some other drug, that she is using some combination of drugs and so on. In the cue interpretation stage, you consider the meaning and relevance of the information you have collected (e.g., your observation of the client's pupils). In the hypothesis evaluation stage you come to a conclusion as to which hypothesis is best supported, with different weight placed on different information cues (e.g., the presence of constricted pupils would constitute a high weight) and attempt to reconcile any contradictions or inconsistencies among the information cues (e.g., the person's insistence that they have not been using street drugs as opposed to your opinion based on observation).

Nurses certainly seek out relevant information as characterised by the hypothetico-deductive model. This is a skilled activity and in this instance would involve knowing what information to obtain from the family. While you might not think in terms of 'hypotheses', you may often have identified more than one explanation or possible cause for a set of symptoms or presenting features. Most information cues need to be interpreted in terms of quality and relevance to a particular situation at hand. Sometimes individuals will think through the cause of a problem, comparing and considering the best fit with the evidence.

This four-stage model also helps us to understand how groups make judgements. A multidisciplinary team working on a clinical problem in a formal way will find the stages in the model useful as a guide for how to resolve the problem. However, the conditions required for a thoroughly analytical approach to JDM are seldom met. A heuristic rather than prescriptive approach is likely to be used in many cases, leading to a decision such as requesting a physiological test to confirm or refute a hypothesis. In most cases it is presumed that we use intuition and, to a lesser extent, analysis. Klein's (1997) recognition-primed decision model is typical of this view. It is an example of a naturalistic decision-making theory developed to account for situations that are continually changing, which is often the case in nursing where time is of the essence in patient assessment, and where information changes rapidly requiring immediate attention and rapid updating of judgements.

Nursing researchers have tended to focus on the hypothetico-deductive model, although it may not be the best way to describe all of what nurses do in practice. We suggest that naturalistic decision-making research is needed because it focuses on complex environments where highly skilled responses are needed within short time frames in situations such as, for example, air traffic control, fire fighting and military command. It has been used less often in the nursing literature and there is a smaller pool of work from which to draw than the hypothetico-deductive research tradition. Klein argues that people make use of experiential knowledge first to judge whether a situation is typical or not. A conscious, analytical approach is considered appropriate only if the situation or patient condition is perceived as atypical or unusual. If not, the person proceeds to consider a set of situation-specific expectations. For instance, for a person who is two hours post-surgery the typical problems that may be expected are bleeding, oliguria and shock. The most telling pieces of information may be seen as pulse rate, blood pressure, urinary output and skin tone. The JDM heuristic model proposes that one conclusion is drawn quickly, making the link between judgement and decision seamless. Making relevant judgements about patients' conditions speeds up the identification of actions typically used in these situations. Experienced individuals find it effective to base many decisions on prior knowledge, applied through intuitive and heuristic means. This seems to be the default position, with further analysis carried out as appropriate when and if it is possible to do so. Klein's model presumes that making a judgement or decision may well involve pattern recognition, use of varied heuristic strategies and formal analysis if required.

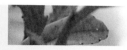

Activity 8.6

Think about your most recent time in placement and try to identify a situation in which you witnessed or took part in a formal analytical JDM process.

So far we have explored the range of models within JDM and acknowledged that nursing tends towards intuition and heuristics rather than analysis because of the constraints of environment and time. Another criterion for exploring analytical/intuitive thinking in nursing is the quality of the decision made. Hypothetico-deductive reasoning seems better than intuitive thinking because several hypotheses will have been consciously compared against the available evidence. Developing only one explanation of an event suggests confirmation bias and lack of motivation. Intuition also seems at odds with the demands of evidence-based care, which requires statements on how a judgement was reached and the form of supporting research evidence. In medical decision-making doctors often select a hypothesis early on in a patient consultation and this can be interpreted in various ways. It suggests that doctors may be closed to revising their judgement; that is, that they are not open-minded (Sellman 2003). It might also be interpreted as meaning that doctors use their knowledge and experience to explain patients' conditions in an efficient manner (i.e., it is a good thing). However, a judgement need not be arrived at through logical analysis to be accurate (Hammond 2000), and using logic does not guarantee accuracy. Lack of evidence on JDM quality means it is difficult to make pre-scriptive recommendations as to the best approach. Certainly, as people acquire experience they tend to become more intuitive in their approach, but experience should not always be taken as a proxy for effectiveness.

Establishing the quality of JDM in nursing

Cognitive task analysis (CTA) uses techniques designed to uncover and analyse task-related knowledge and skills (Hoffman *et al.* 1998a, Militello and Hutton 1998) and is one way to establish the quality of JDM. Four types of CTA have been identified (Wei and Salvendy 2004), and observation and interview methods are one useful approach. Interviewing is useful when studying task performance if direct observation is not possible and the skill is based on expert knowledge (Rasmussen 1993). Given our aim of articulating the judgement and decision-making process in nursing the use of interview methods to shed light on the process would seem highly appropriate.

CTA interviews are associated with the naturalistic decision-making perspective (Zsambok and Klein 1997). One method, critical decision method (CDM), is frequently used for retrospective analysis of difficult cases (Klein *et al.* 1989).

CTA interviews have been used in health care for work-based training, identifying task performance criteria, implementing information systems and classifying clinical practice (Christensen *et al.* 2005, Crandall and Getchell-Reiter 1993). However, because interviews are based on subjective recall, information may be omitted, misremembered or reinterpreted. Nevertheless, CTA interviews are valid and reliable when supported by rigorous development and training (Hoffman *et al.* 1998b).

The Knowledge Audit (Klein and Militello 2005) is another example of a cognitive task analysis interview used to articulate judgements and decisions to determine quality. It is based on eight probe questions, each of which has further explanation and follow-up questions. Probe questions are used to gather information on key events and examples related to performing a particular task. For example:

- *Big picture*. Follow-up question: can you give me an example of what is important about the big picture for this task; what are the major elements you have to know and keep track of?
- *Self-monitoring*. Follow-up question: can you think of a time when you realised that you would need to change the way you were performing to get the job done?
- *Anomalies*. Follow-up question: can you describe an instance when you spotted a deviation from the norm or knew something was amiss?

Research focus 8.3

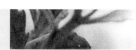

Themes in nursing research on clinical judgement and decision-making

- *Knowledge informing the process*: Specialist, domain-specific knowledge is integral to JDM in health care. O'Neill *et al.* (2005) describe nurses' knowledge as pre-encounter data. Clinical and general knowledge are used to anticipate and control risk. Armed with this resource, information is taken from the environment.
- *The nature and use of cues*: Nurses use information cues from observation, verbal and written information and prior knowledge (Lamond *et al.* 1996). Having access to diverse information cues leads to more accurate JDM (Evans 2005, Moore 1996). However, the number and type of cues available contributes to the task complexity (Hammond 1988). Novices find it time-consuming to make sense of the cues and identifying what patterns the cues suggest. Also the presentation of information affects the interpretation and use (Hammond 1988). Using cues for JDM in real clinical settings has been studied by a number of researchers in nursing (Hedberg and Larsson 2003, King and Macleod Clark 2002, Manias *et al.* 2004). Hedberg and Larsson (2003) and King and Macleod Clark (2002) conclude that nurses focus on biomedical information cues. Manias *et al.* (2004) found that medically specialised work settings increase the use of biomedical cues such as blood pressure measurements, radiating chest pain and electrolyte levels.
- *Autonomy*: Nurses perceive themselves to be lesser partners in care provision alongside other health care professionals (Cassidy 2002). However, specialist and autonomous nurse practitioner roles, nurse prescribing and other movements toward autonomy are becoming prevalent (An Bord Altranais 2000, DH 2005). One rationale for this is the supposed link with positive patient outcomes (Curley 2002). There is no agreement on nursing autonomy (Keenan 1998), but there seems to be a link between autonomy and JDM in nursing (Buckingham and Adams 2000, Havens and Vasey 2005). Autonomous spaces can be found in acute settings (Bucknall 2003), but autonomy is most associated with community-based practice (McCarthy 2003). Community practice tends to bring a relatively high level of accountability and responsibility. Working autonomously often changes the way in which JDM is reached.

Conclusion

In this chapter we set out to link JDM concepts and research to everyday nursing practice. We argue that being able to analyse one's JDM is valuable in providing good-quality nursing care and in furthering the professional development of the individual nurse. We identify and highlight the basic structures and processes involved in JDM and highlight the links between JDM and nursing practice. Nurses support the JDM of other health professionals and they make independent JDM. In nursing practice this may be for purposes of assessment, monitoring, discharge planning, risk assessment, assessing adherence to treatment and so on. Lamond *et al.* (1996) identify four types of nursing judgements and provide a useful framework for investigating nursing JDM: descriptive, evaluative, inferential and causal. Thompson *et al.* (2000) identify three major types of decisions taken by nurses: intervention choices, communication, service organisation, delivery and management.

Two of the key approaches to JDM in the literature are intuition and analysis. In most instances it is assumed that we use elements of both. However, in practice we tend towards relying on intuition rather than analysis because of environmental and time limitations. This has implications for nursing practice, education and research as we move to embrace concepts such as evidence-based practice and try to ensure such concepts are incorporated in the care provided to individual patients by practising nurses.

In this chapter we also touch on the influence of organisations and groups on JDM, as well as highlighting issues regarding JDM within the ethical domain of practice. This is to encourage nurses to consider and explore not just the cognitive processes involved in JDM, but the wider range of influences on JDM in daily practice. These influences range from nursing peers, formal guidelines and resource constraints to medical power, multidisciplinary team working and the organisation of care. Ultimately, we argue that the cognitive, social and pragmatic factors that affect nursing work need to be articulated so that we can identify the nursing contribution to care and continue to make further improvements in care delivery.

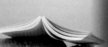

Suggested further reading

Adair, J. (1999) *Decision Making and Problem Solving*. London: Institute of Personnel and Development.

Thompson, C. and Dowding, D. (2002) *Clinical Decision Making and Judgement in Nursing*. Edinburgh: Churchill Livingstone.

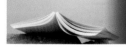

References

An Bord Altranais (2000) *Review of Scope of Practice for Nursing and Midwifery – Final Report*. Dublin: An Bord Altranais.

Baddeley, A. (2004) *Your Memory: A user's guide*. London: Carlton Books.

Bargh, J. A. (1994) The four horsemen on automaticity: awareness, intention, efficiency, and control in social cognition. In *Handbook of Social Cognition, Volume 2:*

Application, Wyer, R. S. and Srull, T. K. (eds). Hillsdale, NJ: Lawrence Erlbaum, pp. 1–40.

Baron, J. (1994) *Thinking and Deciding* (2nd ed.). New York: Cambridge University Press.

Benner, P., Hooper-Kyriakidis, P. and Stannard, D. (1999) *Clinical Wisdom and Interventions in Critical Care*. Philadelphia: W.B. Saunders.

Buckingham, C. D. and Adams, A. (2000) Classifying clinical decision-making: a unifying approach. *Journal of Advanced Nursing* **32** (4), 981–989.

Bucknall, T. (2003) The clinical landscape of critical care: nurses' decision-making. *Journal of Advanced Nursing* **43** (3), 310–319.

Bucknall, T. and Thomas, S. (1995) Clinical decision-making in critical care. *Australian Journal of Advanced Nursing* **13** (2), 10–17.

Carmel, S. (2006) Health care practices, professions and perspectives: a case study in intensive care. *Social Science and Medicine* **62** (8), 2079–2090.

Cassidy, M. (2002) Health strategy–from theory to practice. *World of Irish Nursing* **10** (4) (http://www.ino.ie).

Chapman, G. B. and Sonnenberg, F. A. (2000) Introduction. In *Decision Making in Health Care. Theory, Psychology and Applications*, Chapman, G. B. and Sonnenberg, F. A. (eds). Cambridge: Cambridge University Press, pp. 3–19.

Christensen, R. L., Fetters, M. D. and Green, L. A. (2005) Opening the black box: cognitive strategies in family practice. *Annals of Family Medicine* **3** (2), 144–150.

Cioffi, J. and Markham, R. (1997) Clinical decision-making by midwives: managing case complexity. *Journal of Advanced Nursing* **25** (3), 265–272.

Connolly, T., Arkes, H. R. and Hammond, K. R. (2000) General introduction. In *Judgement and Decision Making. An interdisciplinary reader* (2nd ed.), Connolly, T., Arkes, H. R. and Hammond, K. R. (eds). Cambridge: Cambridge University Press, pp. 1–11.

Connor, M. and Norman, P. (eds) (1996) *Predicting Health Behaviours: Research and practice with social cognition models*. Milton Keynes: Open University Press.

Coombs, M. and Ersser, S. J. (2004) Medical hegemony in decision-making – a barrier to interdisciplinary working in intensive care? *Journal of Advanced Nursing* **46** (3), 245–252.

Coren, S., Ward, L. M. and Enns, J. T. (1994) *Sensation and Perception*. Fort Worth: Harcourt Brace.

Crandall, B. and Getchell-Reiter, K. (1993) Critical decision method: a technique for eliciting concrete assessment indicators from the intuition of NICU nurses. *Advances in Nursing Science* **16** (1), 42–51.

Crow, R., Chase, J. and Lamond, D. (1995) The cognitive component of nursing assessment: an analysis. *Journal of Advanced Nursing* **22** (2), 206–212.

Curley, M. A. (2002) Experienced nurses + autonomy = better patient outcomes. *Pediatric Critical Care Medicine* **3** (4), 385–386.

Daly, J. (2005) *Professional Nursing: Concepts, issues and challenges*. New York: Springer.

deGroot, A. D. (1965) *Thought and Choice in Chess*. The Hague: Mouton.

DH (Department of Health) (2005) *Medicine Matters*. London: DH.

di Giulio, P. and Crow, R. (1997) Cognitive processes nurses and doctors use in the administration of PRN (as needed) analgesic drugs. *Scandinavian Journal of Caring Sciences* **11** (1), 12–19.

Elstein, A. S. and Bordage, G. (1988) Psychology of clinical reasoning. In *Professional Judgement: A reader in clinical decision making*, Dowie, J. and Elstein, A. (eds). Cambridge: Cambridge University Press, pp. 109–129.

Ericsson, K. A. (2005) Recent advances in expertise research: a commentary on the contributions to the special issue. *Applied Cognitive Psychology* **19** (2), 233–241.

Evans, C. (2005) Clinical decision-making theories: patient assessment in A&E. *Emergency Nurse* **13** (5), 16–19.

Fiske, S. and Morling, B. A. (1996) Schemas. In *The Blackwell Encyclopaedia of Social Psychology*, Manstead, A. and Hewstone, M. (eds). Oxford: Blackwell, pp. 489–494.

Fiske, S. T. and Taylor, S. E. (1984) *Social Cognition*. Reading, MA: Addison-Wesley.

Fonteyn, M. (1998) *Thinking Strategies for Nursing Practice*. Philadelphia: Lippincott.

Gigerenzer, G. (2002) The adaptive toolbox. In *Bounded Rationality: The adaptive toolbox*, Gigerenzer, G. and Selten, R. (eds). Cambridge, MA: The MIT Press, pp. 37–50.

Goldstein, N. M. and Hogarth, R. M. (eds) (1997) *Research on Judgement and Decision Making. Currents, connections and controversies*. Cambridge: Cambridge University Press.

Grounds, A., Glesthorpe, L., Howes, M., *et al.* (2004) Access to medium secure psychiatric care in England and Wales. 2: A qualitative study of admission decision-making. *The Journal of Forensic Psychiatry and Psychology* **15** (1), 32–49.

Hammond, K. R. (1988) Judgement and decision-making in dynamic tasks. *Information and Decision Technologies* **14** (1), 3–14.

Hammond, K. R. (1996) How convergence of research paradigms can improve research on diagnostic judgment. *Medical Decision Making* **16** (3), 281–287.

Hammond, K. R. (2000) *Judgments Under Stress*. New York: Oxford University Press.

Hancock, H. C. and Easen, P. R. (2006) The decision-making processes of nurses when extubating patients following cardiac surgery: an ethnographic study. *International Journal of Nursing Studies* **46** (3), 693–706.

Hastie, R. and Dawes, R. (2001) *Rational Choice in an Uncertain World: The psychology of judgment and decision making*. Thousand Oaks: Sage.

Havens, D. S. and Vasey, J. (2005) The staff nurse decisional involvement scale: report of psychometric assessments. *Nursing Research* **54** (6), 376–383.

Hedberg, B. and Larsson, U. S. (2003) Observations, confirmations and strategies – useful tools in decision-making process for nurses in practice? *Journal of Clinical Nursing* **12** (2), 215–222.

Hedberg, B. and Larsson, U. (2004) Environmental elements affecting the decision-making process in nursing practice. *Journal of Clinical Nursing* **13** (3), 316–324.

Henneman, E., Lee, J. and Cohen, J. (1995) Collaboration: a concept analysis. *Journal of Advanced Nursing* **21** (1) 103–109.

Hoffman, R. R., Shadbolt, N. R., Burton, A. M. and Klein, G. (1998a) Eliciting knowledge from experts: a methodological analysis. *Organizational Behavior and Human Decision Processes* **62** (2), 129–158.

Hoffman, R. R., Crandall, B. W. and Shadbolt, N. R. (1998b) Use of the critical decision method to elicit expert knowledge: a case study in cognitive task analysis methodology. *Human Factors* **40** (2), 254–276.

ICN (International Council of Nurses) (2002) *International Classification for Nursing Practice: Beta 2*. Geneva: International Council of Nurses.

Kahneman, D. and Tversky, A. (1973) On the psychology of prediction. *Psychological Review* **80** (4), 237–251.

Keenan, J. (1998) A concept analysis of autonomy. *Journal of Advanced Nursing* **29** (3), 556–562.

Kikuchi, J. F. and Simmons, H. (1999) Practical nursing judgment: a moderate realist conception. *Scholarly Inquiry for Nursing Practice: An International Journal* **13** (1), 43–55.

King, L. and Macleod Clark, J. (2002) Intuition and the development of expertise in surgical ward and intensive care nurses. *Journal of Advanced Nursing* **37** (4), 322–329.

Klein, G. (1997) The recognition-primed decision (RPD) model: looking back, looking forward. In *Naturalistic Decision Making*, Zsambok, C. and Klein, G. (eds). Hillside, NJ: Lawrence Erlbaum, pp. 285–292.

Klein, G. (1999) *Sources of Power: How people make decisions*. Cambridge, MA: The MIT Press.

Klein, G. and Militello, L. (2005) The knowledge audit as a method for cognitive task analysis. In *How Professionals Make Decisions*, Montgomery, H., Lipshitz, R. and Brehmer, B. (eds). Mahwah, NJ: Lawrence Erlbaum, pp. 335–342.

Klein, G., Calderwood, R. and MacGregor, D. (1989) Critical decision method for eliciting knowledge. *IEEE Transactions on Systems, Man, and Cybernetics* **19** (3), 462–472.

Lamond, D., Crow, R., Chase, J., Doggen, K. and Swinkels, M. (1996) Information sources used in decision-making: considerations for simulation development. *International Journal of Nursing Studies* **33** (1), 47–57.

Manias, E., Aitken, R. and Dunning, T. (2004) Decision-making models used by 'graduate nurses' managing patients' medications. *Journal of Advanced Nursing* **47** (3), 270–278.

Manias, E. and Street, A. F. (2001) The interplay of knowledge and decision-making between nurses and doctors in critical care. *International Journal of Nursing Studies* **38** (2), 173–184.

Maule, J. (1997) Strategies for adapting to time pressure. In *Decision Making Under Stress: Emerging themes and applications*, Flin, R., Salas, E., Strub, M. and Martin, L. (eds). Aldershot: Ashgate, pp. 271–289.

McCarthy, M. C. (2003) Detecting acute confusion in older adults: comparing clinical reasoning of nurses working in acute, long-term, and community health care environments. *Research in Nursing and Health* **26** (3), 203–212.

McGovern, S. (2001) *The Lived Experience of Staff Nurse Decision-Making in Team Nursing and Patient Allocation Wards*. Trinity College Dublin: unpublished MSc thesis.

Militello, L. G. and Hutton, R. J. B. (1998) Applied cognitive task analysis (ACTA): a practitioner's toolkit for understanding cognitive task demands. *Ergonomics* **41** (11), 1618–1641.

Miller, G. (1956) The magical number seven, plus or minus two: some limits on our capacity for processing information. *Psychological Review* **63** (2), 81–97.

Montgomery, H., Lipshitz, R. and Brehmer, B. (2005) *How Professionals Make Decisions*. Mahwah, NJ: Lawrence Erlbaum.

Montgomery, K. (2005) *How Doctors Think: Clinical judgement and the practice of medicine*. Oxford: Oxford University Press.

Moore, P. A. (1996) Decision-making in professional practice. *British Journal of Nursing* **5** (10), 635–640.

Nisbett, R. E., Krantz, D. H., Jepson, C. and Kunda, Z. (1983) The use of statistical heuristics in everyday inductive reasoning. *Psychological Review* **90** (4), 339–363.

NMC (Nursing and Midwifery Council) (2004) *Standards of Proficiency for Pre-registration Nursing Education*. London: NMC.

Olson, D. (1996) *Decision Aids for Selection Problems*. New York: Springer.

O'Neill, E. S., Dluhy, N. M. and Chin, E. (2005) Modelling novice clinical reasoning for a computerized decision support system. *Journal of Advanced Nursing* **49** (1), 68–77.

Patel, V. L. and Currie, L. M. (2005) Clinical cognition and biomedical informatics: issues of patient safety. *International Journal of Medical Informatics* **74** (11), 869–885.

Payne, J. Bettman, J. and Johson, E. (1993) *The Adaptive Decision Maker*. Cambridge: Cambridge University Press.

Porter, S. (1991) A participant observation study of power relations between nurses and doctors in a general hospital. *Journal of Advanced Nursing* **16** (6), 728–735.

Rashotte, J. and Carnavale, F. A. (2004) Medical and nursing clinical decision-making: a comparative epistemological analysis. *Nursing Philosophy* **5** (2), 160–174.

Rasmussen, J. (1993) Deciding and doing: decision-making in natural contexts. In *Decision Making in Action: Models and methods*, Klein, G., Orasallu, J., Calderwood, R. and Zsambok, C. E. (eds). Norwood, NJ: Ablex, pp. 158–171.

Scott, P. A., Matthew, A., Duffy, S., *et al.* (2006) Documenting the activities and decision-making of registered nurses in an acute Irish health care setting: a pilot study. Presentation to RCN Research Conference May 2006, York, UK.

Sellman, D. (2003) Open-mindedness: a virtue for professional practice. *Nursing Philosophy* **4** (1), 17–24.

Sharpe, V. A. (2004) *Accountability: Patient safety and policy reform.* Washington, DC: Georgetown University Press.

Simon, H. (1956) Rational choice and the structure of environments. *Psychological Review* **63** (2), 129–138.

Solomon, P. (2001) Congruence between health professionals' and patients' pain ratings: a review of the literature. *Scandinavian Journal of Caring Sciences* **15** (2), 174–180.

Solso, R. L., MacLin, M. K. and MacLin, O. H. (2004) *Cognitive Psychology.* New Jersey: Prentice Hall.

Thompson, C. (2003) Clinical experience as evidence in evidence-based practice. *Journal of Advanced Nursing* **43** (3), 230–237.

Thompson, C., McCaughan, D., Cullum, N., *et al.* (2000) *Nurses' Use of Research Information in Clinical Decision-Making: A descriptive and analytical study.* London: NCC SDO.

Wason, P. C. (1966) Reasoning. In *New Horizons in Psychology*, Foss, B. M. (ed.). Harmondsworth: Penguin, pp. 135–151.

Wei, J. and Salvendy, G. (2004) The cognitive task analysis methods for job and task design: review and reappraisal. *Behaviour and Information Technology* **23** (4): 273–299.

Wickens, C. D., Lee, J. D., Liu, Y. and Becker, S. E. G. (2004) *An Introduction to Human Factors Engineering.* Upper Saddle River, NJ: Pearson.

Wigton, R. S. (1996) Social judgement theory and medical judgement. *Thinking and Reasoning* **2** (2), 175–190.

Zsambok, C. E. and Klein, G. (1997) *Naturalistic Decision-Making.* Mahwah, NJ: Lawrence Erlbaum.

Chapter 9

Communication and interpersonal skills

Victoria Lavender

Learning outcomes

After reading and reflecting on this chapter, you should be able to:

- Explain the basic components of communication;
- Outline a range of communication and engagement skills that can be employed within a caring relationship with a client;
- Describe the skills involved in initiating, maintaining and disengaging from the therapeutic relationship;
- Discuss the importance of the development of emotional intelligence in interpersonal skills working.

Related NMC Standards of Proficiency for Pre-registration Nursing Education (NMC 2004)

- Utilise a range of effective and appropriate communication and engagement skills.

- Maintain and, where appropriate, disengage from professional caring relationships that focus on meeting the patient's or client's needs within professional therapeutic boundaries.

Introduction

The importance of effective communication as a fundamental element of nursing activity has been acknowledged repeatedly (Booth *et al.* 1999, Egan 2002, Hargie *et al.* 1994, Wilkinson *et al.* 1998, 1999) and is regarded as integral to the provision of high-quality patient-focused care (Dunn 1991, Lubbers and Roy 1990, Macleod Clark 1988). There is evidence that effective communication prior to, and during, physical procedures results in decreased anxiety, enhanced coping ability and greater adherence to treatment (Dickson 1999, Nichols 1993). Faulkner states that 'to be able to communicate effectively with others is at the heart of all patient care' (1998 p. 1) for the foundation of all practice is, arguably, the relationship between the nurse and the client. The nurse's competence in communicating will determine whether, and to what degree, the client's nursing needs will be appropriately assessed and the goals of client care provided (Attree 2001, Gallant *et al.* 2002, Thorsteinsson 2002).

Central to the healing process is the professional caring relationship (often called the therapeutic relationship) between the nurse and the client. This chapter will explore some of the essential building blocks of communication and interpersonal skills involved in creating, sustaining and disengaging from therapeutic relationships.

The chapter is divided into three parts.

In Part 1, an outline is offered of the importance of effective communication and interpersonal skills in relation to nursing practice. This is accompanied by a brief overview of the scope of the subject area.

In Part 2, a fuller explanation of why it is important for nurses to have effective communication and interpersonal skills and to be able to engage with therapeutic relationships with patients is given. I provide a brief review of verbal and para-verbal aspects of communication before beginning to explain two aspects of building and maintaining the therapeutic relationship: (i) building and maintaining trust and (ii) demonstrating respect, empathy and genuineness.

In Part 3, a deeper exploration of communication and interpersonal skills is provided with an emphasis on some of the more advanced and complex aspects of developing and maintaining a therapeutic relationship. Some information relating to barriers to and disengaging from therapeutic relationships concludes the chapter.

Part 1: Outlining communication and interpersonal skills

Case 9.1

Almira is a third-year student nurse working on a general medical ward at a local hospital. Suzanne (Almira's mentor) is a larger than life personality who was born and brought up in the community in which the hospital is situated. Almira finds Suzanne rather loud and somewhat overbearing with her seemingly unrestrained jollity (everybody definitely knows when she is on duty), her tendency to stand a bit too close, and her (over)use of physical contact. Almira notices that Suzanne tends to call everyone (both staff and patients) 'pet' and is surprised that no one seems to mind. Almira is not sure she likes being called pet, but she does not voice her objections as she finds Suzanne a bit intimidating and the practice seems to be an accepted part of the ward culture.

The importance of developing communication skills

Stickley and Freshwater argue that 'nursing involves the formation of a meaningful relationship through the development of an effective interpersonal process' (2006 p. 13). They go on to point out that despite the emphasis placed on the importance of effective interpersonal and communication skills in nursing, there remain considerable variations in the quality of nurse–patient communication and there is a need for significant improvement.

The importance of high-quality nurse–patient communication is noted by a number of nursing scholars (e.g., Burnard 1998, Peplau 1991, Tschudin 1995). Peplau's theory of nursing, originally published in 1952, helped turn attention away from internal patient pathology towards the therapeutic process between nurse and patient. In emphasising this process Peplau recognised the therapeutic opportunity for the patient to understand the circumstances of their health and with it the potential to make beneficial health-related changes. At the heart of the interpersonal process lies a requirement for nurses to develop effective and caring communication skills.

Research focus 9.1

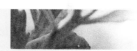

Mallett and Dougherty (2000) report in their study of patient satisfaction of care that the quality of nurse's communication was recorded as the least satisfying aspect. They go on to suggest that complacency or indifference to the goal of improving communication and interpersonal skills has no place in the preparation for becoming a registered nurse.

Activity 9.1

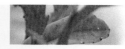

Think of someone you would describe as a good communicator.

- Make a list of what you think are the top ten skills/qualities that makes that person such an effective communicator.
- Explain why you think the top five skills/qualities on your list are the most important.

Communication and nursing

Communication can be defined as a reciprocal process of sending and receiving messages between two or more persons. Thoughts, feelings and information are sent or encoded as messages and may be conveyed verbally through speech which includes pitch, tone and inflection of voice as well as speed of delivery. Equally important are the messages conveyed through non-verbal means, such as facial expression (including eye contact), body posture, body position, movement and gestures. The receiver decodes the message or transmission in order to make sense of the sender's thoughts, feelings or information and generally returns messages in response to what they have understood. Consisting of a sender, a message and a receiver, this model of communication is described as linear (McQuail and Windahl 1981).

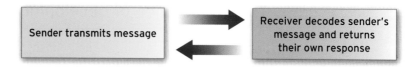

Figure 9.1 A linear model of communication.

Figure 9.1 illustrates the reciprocal nature of interpersonal communication, for both the sender and the receiver are likely to receive simultaneous transmissions from one another resulting in amendments to both the coding and the decoding process. The transmission process will also be influenced by, for example, environmental factors (such as external noise levels), the degree of privacy, or the presence of other people. Encoding and decoding messages is invariably fraught with the potential for misinterpretation or misunderstanding, and this together with additional barriers such as the specialised language of health care or differing attitudes, values or beliefs of the participants, makes the communication process both complex and highly individualistic.

Contemporary models of communication try to capture this complexity. In a circular transactional model, such as the one in Figure 9.2, communication is viewed as a circular process with communication as 'a continuous, mutually interdependent activity involving communicators who reciprocally influence each other's behaviour' (Arnold and Underman Boggs 1999 p. 16). In the circular transactional model, emphasis is placed on the contexts of communication within a relationship and, in contrast to the linear model, holds that feedback and

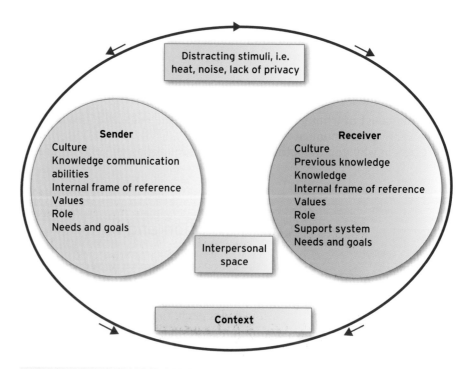

Figure 9.2 A circular transactional model of communication.
Source: After Arnold and Underman Boggs (1999).

validation are interdependent and dynamic elements. Feedback as the response from the receiver to the original message will affect all future communication. In this model feedback is conveyed even when a response is not forthcoming, and validation is understood as a form of feedback that confirms participants hold similar understandings of the message and the feedback.

Nelson-Jones (2005) categorises the basic means by which we send messages to one another as:

- Verbal messages (those sent through words and language).
- Para-verbal or vocal messages (those sent through the volume, articulation, pitch, tone and speech rate).
- Non-verbal or body messages (those sent through facial expression, eye contact and gaze, gesture, posture, physical proximity, touch, clothing and grooming).
- Action-taking messages (such as letters, reports and e-mails when sender and receiver are not face-to-face).

Because nurses spend a great deal of time in face-to-face interaction with patients, their relatives and carers as well as with other health care professionals, the focus in the remainder of this chapter is on verbal, para-verbal and non-verbal communication and interpersonal skills.

Part 2: Explaining communication and interpersonal skills

The components of communication

Given the complexity of the communication process, nurses need to pay particular attention to ensuring that they are proficient and effective in developing clarity as senders of communication messages and in the development of sensitive comprehension as receivers. By being aware of the complexities, subtleties and interdynamics of the individual components of communication the nurse can utilise a range of effective and appropriate communication skills.

Verbal communication

Language may be formal as in, for example, the choice of words used by government departments or authorities, or informal as in language used between friends or in informal situations. Nurses need to be aware of the possible distancing effect that professional language may have with clients struggling to understand and translate what is being said. Cultural differences in language affect the nurse–patient relationship and can easily get in the way of mutual understanding. For example, in Case 9.1, Almira comes from a different background to most of the staff and patients and cannot get used to being called pet. Similarly, the convention in English of saying 'please' and 'thank you' presents problems for speakers of some languages, including Urdu which has no equivalent for these words, they are instead built into the verb (Holland and Hogg 2001). So a nurse whose first language is English might think a patient whose first language is Urdu rude or ungrateful if they do not use these terms in the conventional British way. The recognition that even simple everyday conversations between nurses and patients have the potential to cause offence is an important part of understanding the need for sensitivity and respect in communication; and arguably Suzanne and her colleagues do not show sufficient sensitivity for Almira's language traditions. Thus part of developing effective interpersonal skills for nursing practice is an awareness of a need to adopt clear, precise and unambiguous words appropriate to and respectful of others (staff and clients) in professional relationships.

Para-verbal communication

Para-verbal (or vocal) communication includes vocalisations (those parts of speech that accompany words) that add to what is being said in important ways. These **vocalisations** can be interpreted as conveying information about the sender's message and include: volume, articulation, pitch, tone and speed of delivery. Each has the potential to be interpreted (or misinterpreted) by the listener regardless of the intention of the speaker.

Volume refers to loudness or softness of the words used and should be appropriate to the client's level of hearing and to the environment in which the communication is taking place. Overly loud delivery of speech may convey, or may be interpreted as conveying, anger or hostility, or may simply make others feel uncomfortable (Almira wonders if some patients find Suzanne's loudness uncomfortable); undue softness may convey uncertainty, shyness or deference.

Articulation refers to clarity of speech, whether words are clearly spoken or merely mumbled. This is related to volume in some instances; for example, a nurse who mumbles will compound communication problems with someone who has difficulty with hearing in noisy environments (and hospital wards are often noisy environments).

Pitch refers to the height or depth of the voice and tone refers to the manner of delivery. Both can be interpreted as conveying (regardless of the intention of the speaker) the underlying thoughts, feelings and attitudes of the speaker.

The rate of speech is measured not only by the number of the words spoken each minute but also by the frequency and the duration of pauses between the words. A rapid speech rate may convey the speaker's anxiety, excitement or degree of happiness. A slow speech rate may convey ponderous thinking, pomposity or condescension.

Each of these para-verbal aspects of speech has the potential to get in the way of clear and effective communication. In those instances where everyone in a particular situation understands the culturally and socially specific conventions of speech the potential for misunderstandings is minimal. So in a small, localised community with few 'outsiders', ways of communicating (including the nuances of, for example, irony, dialects and accents) between individuals will be understood by all participants. Until recently, this had been the situation on the ward where Almira is a student. However, such communities are becoming rare as society becomes increasingly multicultural and as language development diversifies across different sections of different communities. As the populations of both nurses and patients become more multicultural so the potential for misunderstandings or offence between staff and between staff and patients increases. In these types of situations the onus is on the professional (rather than on the patient) to take steps to enable rather than hinder effective communication.

Vocalisations are those parts of speech that accompany words. So volume, clarity of words, pitch, tone and rate of speech add to the meanings of spoken words and can convey messages that may or may not reflect the speaker's intent.

So here we might say that Suzanne is reliant on a form of communication that is no longer appropriate in her situation. In other words, a nurse who is serious about providing safe and effective care needs to recognise their responsibilities for developing their interpersonal skills in order to maintain methods of communication that contribute to the well-being of patients, and this includes ensuring respectful communication between health and social care individuals.

Non-verbal or bodily communication

Perhaps the main vehicle for sending non-verbal messages is through facial expressions. According to Ekman *et al.* (1972) the seven main facial expressions of emotion are:

1. Happiness
2. Interest
3. Surprise
4. Fear
5. Sadness
6. Anger
7. Disgust or contempt

The eyes, the eyebrows and the mouth shape are particularly effective in conveying expressed or unexpressed emotion. Eye contact both sends and collects information and helps to regulate turn-taking during conversations. Nelson-Jones (2005) suggests that during conversations, listeners look at speakers more often than speakers look at listeners (approximately 70–75 per cent for the former, 40 per cent for the latter). Speakers tend to look at listeners just before they intend to pause or stop speaking to collect feedback about the listener's reactions and to invite the other person to have a turn at speaking. However, conventions in the use of eye contact vary across cultures. Holland and Hogg (2001) note that the Western convention of understanding direct eye contact as a sign of honesty does not translate to some other cultures, where it may be interpreted as challenging or rude. For example, in Arabic cultures, sharing prolonged eye contact denotes respect, whereas in South Asian cultures it is regarded as aggressive or confrontational.

Gestures are physical movements that accompany speech and demonstrate, illustrate or emphasise particular aspects of verbal communication. Gestures sometimes replace words altogether when, for example, nodding or shaking the head indicates agreement or disagreement respectively. Gestures too are culturally specific, so a gesture in one part of the world may mean something altogether different in another. The classic example offered by Liberman *et al.* (1975) is the hand gesture made by the thumb and first finger meeting to form a circle in the familiar 'OK' sign in many parts of the world. For Hispanic Americans, however, the same sign is an invitation to perform a sexual act.

Posture encompasses both the relative heights of speaker and listener and the position of the body, that is, whether the body is turned toward or away from the other person. Unequal height can cause a feeling of unease; for example, a nurse standing might seem to tower over a client who is lying or sitting. Turning the body or part of the body towards the other person conveys interest. Turning the body away or crossing the arms or legs (often referred to as a closed posture) may be interpreted as lack of interest, indifference or defensiveness. An open posture, that is with arms and legs uncrossed, but in a relaxed position and held reasonably still will indicate acceptance of the other person, interest in what they are saying and a willingness to continue to communicate.

Proximity or physical closeness between communicators is an important non-verbal component. Hall (1966) suggests that for Western cultures proximity can be categorised in zones of comfort. An intimate zone (between 15 and 46 centimetres) for spouses, lovers, close friends and relatives; a personal zone (46 to 122 centimetres) for acquaintances at social gatherings; a social zone (1.22 to 3.6 metres) for people unknown to each another; and a public zone (over 3.6 metres) for impersonal public gatherings. Of course, some individuals within a culture do not observe these proximity zones and the zones may be different in different cultures: ignoring the social norms of any one group by positioning the body too closely may give rise to feelings of unease or even threat. This helps to explain why Almira feels uncomfortable in Suzanne's presence.

The inevitable intimacy of many nursing activities requires sensitivity on the part of the nurse to ensure the physical proximity that comes with such intimate physicality does not give rise to feelings of violation or distress in patients. This can be a difficult area to negotiate as touch can be a powerful conveyor of warmth, comfort and acceptance, so an awareness of the ways in which patients might show non-verbal signs of discomfort (e.g., slight facial grimacing or physical movement away from the nurse) is an important feature of effective nursing.

Activity 9.2

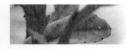

Face-to-face communication includes:

- Verbal components: words and language.
- Para-verbal components: volume, articulation, pitch, tone, rate of speech.
- Non-verbal components: facial expression, eye contact and gaze, gestures, posture, proximity and touch, clothing and grooming.

Try to identify each of these components while you are engaged in conversation with another student. The questions below might help you to think about how these components facilitate or hinder the communication process.

- Do you use all components in all conversations?
- In what ways do the different components interact with each other?
- Which (if any) components dominate?
- Which (if any) components hinder communication?
- Which (if any) components enable effective communication?

The therapeutic relationship

The **therapeutic relationship** is initiated, promoted, managed and sustained by the nurse for the express purpose of helping the client meet their treatment goals.

The recognition of the importance of a **therapeutic relationship** between nurses and clients builds on the work of humanist psychologist Carl Rogers. The therapeutic relationship is initiated, promoted, managed and sustained by a nurse for the express purpose of helping the client meet their treatment goals. The therapeutic relationship can be defined as a helping relationship and one that 'is established for the benefit of the client, whereas kinship and friendship relationships are designed to meet mutual needs' (Balzer-Riley 1996 p. 24). Arnold and Underman Boggs (1999) suggest that social relationships are distinguished from therapeutic ones that aim to:

- enhance the well-being of the patient or client;
- promote recovery;
- support the self-care functioning of the client.

In the therapeutic relationship communication is directed towards the needs of the client and is termed patient-centred communication. This has been defined as 'communication that invites and encourages the patient to participate and negotiate in decision-making regarding their own care' (Langewitz *et al.* 1998 p. 230).

Of course, the patient is not merely a passive recipient, for inherent in the therapeutic relationship is a sense of affiliation or working in partnership. Gallant and colleagues (2002) trace the emergence of the position of the client as equal partner in their own care against a background of increasing contemporary emphasis on the importance of basic human rights.

Timmins (2004) and Price (2006) suggest that partnership working acknowledges and values the patient's own knowledge and skills in managing their ill-health, particularly for long-term conditions. Essential information is likely to be omitted from the assessment, planning and evaluation of the client's care if communication between the nurse and patient is purely one-directional and where the client's experience and expertise is not sought (see Chapter 7 for more information about patient assessment). In the absence of a partnership approach, giving clients information about their care is likely to follow a pattern of 'I talk/ you listen', creating and sustaining a situation of professional dominance.

The most frequently cited benefit of partnership working is empowerment understood as enhancing the ability of a client to act in their own interest, leading to improved self-esteem and confidence (Courtney *et al.* 1996, Raeburn and Rootman 1998). Arnold and Underman Boggs (1999) describe empowerment as a method of preparing patients to cope with difficult life situations as a result of alterations in health and well-being.

Developing and maintaining therapeutic relationships

Some of the essential skills necessary for building and maintaining a nurse–patient therapeutic relationship can be summarised thus:

- Building and maintaining trust.
- Demonstrating respect, empathy and genuineness.
- Active listening.
- Listening to self and developing self-awareness.
- Setting and maintaining professional boundaries.

The first two items in this list act as building blocks for the more advanced and complex skills needed for the other three. Building and maintaining trust together with demonstrating respect, empathy and genuineness will be the focus of the remainder of this part of the chapter. Active listening, listening to self and developing self-awareness, and setting and maintaining professional boundaries will be considered in Part 3.

Building and maintaining trust

Trust can be defined as the firm belief in the honesty, integrity and reliability of another person. The importance of trust in the caring relationship cannot be overestimated: a therapeutic relationship always begins with trust (Arnold and Underman Boggs 1999, Burnard 1991, Rogers 1981, Tschudin 1995). Trust as a part of the psychological contract between nurse and patient is difficult to define as it is often an intangible interpersonal process that develops over time (Feltham and Horton 2006). If a therapeutic relationship is to develop, the patient must be able to feel from their first contact that the nurse is worthy of their trust (Sellman 2006, 2007).

Earning a patient's trust is a lengthy process and a warm, friendly and respectful greeting is likely to start the process well. Ensuring the client's pre-ferred name or form of address is used, correctly pronounced, and that friends or family members are also welcomed and acknowledged will help to begin to build an early rapport that may lead to the formation of trust. An introduction, a brief explanation of one's role in the patient's care, maintaining eye contact, an open body posture, appropriate proximity and equal height with the patient may all serve to strengthen the patient's willingness to trust the nurse.

However, these simple techniques need to reflect the true intentions of the nurse. If the verbal message (i.e., what the nurse is saying) does not correspond with or match the nurse's facial expression, posture, or tone of voice the disparity between words and manner will create a sense of unease or even distrust (Antai-Otong 1999). Knapp (1980) notes that we may be able to match our facial expressions and posture with what we are saying but we often fail to control the movements of our hands, legs or feet. So we can very easily 'give away' feelings of, say, anxiety, irritation or boredom, by, for example, clenching our hands, swinging our legs or tapping our feet.

Activity 9.3

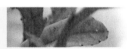

Have a go at saying the sentences below to a partner or while looking in a mirror. Try to match your non-verbal and spoken messages.

- No, you're not disturbing me. It's lovely to see you, please come in.
- I feel very upset at your news, it's so sad this has happened.
- Please don't worry, it was only an old vase – I'm sure I can get another one.

Now repeat the sentences but this time deliberately mismatch your non-verbal behaviour so that there is incongruity between the meaning of the words and the way you deliver them. For example if the last statement is accompanied by an angry facial expression, a rigidly held posture and clenched hands, the reassuring verbal message is likely to be entirely lost. The receiver is likely to retain an impression of the sender's anger in spite of what they say. Try to work out why the non-verbal message is likely to dominate and in this case undermine the sender's verbal message.

Trust is reinforced by the behaviour of the nurse. The nurse who promises to pass on a message or perform a particular task and fails to do so without apology or explanation is likely to lose the trust of a client quickly. The Nursing and Midwifery Council (NMC) gives clear guidelines on the expectations for the behaviour of qualified nurses, including areas of protecting confidential informa-tion, and the need to be trustworthy (NMC 2008). The nurse who breaks a patient's trust not only damages the nurse–patient relationship but also their own standing and the reputation of nursing.

Demonstrating respect, empathy and genuineness

Empathy is the ability to 'step into' the inner world of another person in order to understand their thoughts, feelings, behaviours and meanings.

Rogers (1961, 1981) claims that respect, **empathy** and genuineness are the core conditions for building and maintaining therapeutic relationships. Demonstrating warmth and respect form what he termed unconditional positive regard: that is, accepting others for what they are, not on the condition that they behave in certain ways or because they exhibit particular characteristics.

Respect

Treating people with respect is a fundamental tenet of nursing practice. The way a nurse introduces themself to, and the manner in which a nurse addresses, a patient will convey (or fail to convey) an attitude of respect for the other person. So the nurse who routinely addresses all older patients by their first name or by the moniker of 'pet' or 'dear' (even where that is a local convention) will be failing to respect those patients who would prefer to be addressed in some other way. The routine of asking patients how they would like to be addressed and then making that preference known to other health care professionals is one way in which respect can be shown. To show respect is thus to value and act in accord with the preferences and choices of others, and one way this can be demonstrated is by respectful communication with patients.

Being respectful entails paying close attention to what the client says, ensuring the client understands all aspects of their care, seeking permission or consent and protecting and actively promoting the client's privacy. Being respectful also includes maintaining client confidentiality, promoting choice and accepting different cultural behaviour (Lago 2006).

Case 9.2

Shirley, aged 57, has a long history of mental health problems. She is currently experiencing periods of low mood, with a loss of appetite and insomnia. She tries to describe her thoughts and feelings to Marty, her named nurse. Shirley speaks hesitantly and in little more than a whisper. Marty finds it increasingly difficult to focus on what Shirley is saying and allows himself to lose concentration. His eye contact with Shirley becomes fleeting and he begins to gaze out of the window. He tries to stifle a yawn and once or twice interrupts Shirley by asking about inconsequential details.

Activity 9.4

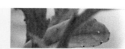

Read Case 9.2 and have a go at answering the following questions:

- How is Marty's behaviour likely to affect Shirley's expression of her thoughts and feelings?
- What might she interpret from his behaviour?
- What effect could this have upon the relationship between them?

Being respectful requires assertiveness. To be assertive involves clear and direct communication of individual needs and, equally important, acknowledgement of the needs of others. When we show respect we are granting the other person's right to be treated with dignity and consideration while at the same time not ignoring or undermining our own needs.

Respect does not require the nurse to agree with the client's perspective or point of view, for respectful disagreement involves stating your point of view, explaining the reasons you hold that opinion and acknowledging that others may have a different or conflicting viewpoint. Respect entails listening attentively, clearly acknowledging differences where they exist and not succumbing to the need to be right at all costs. The nurse who apologises for mistakes, misunderstandings, individual shortcomings and/or unforeseen changes to plans, not only demonstrates professional accountability but also respect for the injured party. Thurgood (2004) notes that clients can be forgiving if the conditions of trust and respect are in place.

Arnold and Underman Boggs describe empathy as 'the ability of a person to perceive and understand another person's emotions accurately and to communicate the meaning of feelings to the other through verbal and non-verbal means' (1999 p. 110). When we mentally put ourselves in the shoes of others, and then verbally convey what it might be like to wear those shoes, we are being empathic. Empathy aids in establishing a therapeutic relationship by conveying a sense of being cared for to the client (Corbett 1995). Balzer-Riley (1996) suggests that it is not empathy by itself that is beneficial, but the intention of the giver and the perception of the receiver. For the client the experience of receiving an empathic response is the experience of feeling a connectedness with the nurse, a feeling of being cared for, understood and accepted as a person. For the nurse, empathy can bring the sense that they are establishing and maintaining a caring relationship in which they demonstrate respect for and acceptance of the client's internal world.

Pike (1990) cautions that empathy is not getting lost in the world of another person: rather it is the imaginative but controlled awareness by the nurse that their feelings are separate from those of the client. In this way the nurse gains a valuable insight into the emotional sphere of the client but is able to maintain a sense of objectivity without being overwhelmed by the client's affective material.

Responding empathically can be broken down into a number of steps:

1. Focusing on the speaker by filtering out as many distractions as possible, paying close attention to both the verbal and non-verbal messages, and recognising any feelings that are being expressed.
2. Being aware of one's non-verbal responses, including facial expression, eye contact and gaze, gestures, posture, proximity and touch.
3. Being aware of one's verbal responses, the choice of words, the tone of voice, volume, articulation, pitch of voice and rate of speech as well as aiming for congruence between verbal and non-verbal communication.
4. Identifying any dominant feelings being expressed by the speaker.
5. Conveying an empathic response by verbally reflecting back the feelings you think you have heard. For example, 'It sounds as if you feel really disappointed that you won't be able to go home today as planned.'
6. Checking to see if your interpretation of the speaker's feeling is accurate. For example 'Have I got that right?' or 'Is that how you are feeling?' Checking allows for feelings to be clarified in a number of ways. If your interpretation

is correct the client will feel relieved that you understand them and are likely to want to expand further. If your interpretation is incorrect the speaker has the opportunity to clarify for you and perhaps for themselves what they mean; 'No, it's not that I'm disappointed I'm not going home yet, I know that I will be going very soon, it's more that I'm anxious about being able to cope when I get there.'

This last step, of checking your interpretation and understanding of the client's feelings, is particularly important. Failing to do this may result in the client experiencing a sense of being told what they are feeling. Far from being understood and accepted, the client is then likely to feel alienated. Empathic responses, in reflecting back the feelings the client expresses, can serve as permission for the patient to voice what they might regard as unacceptable.

Activity 9.5

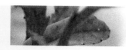

Consider the interaction between Julia, a 49-year-old patient recovering from a partial mastectomy and Lucy, a second-year nursing student.

Julia: I know I shouldn't be thinking like this. Perhaps I shouldn't even be saying this. I know I've got a lovely family. I just feel at times that I haven't got the energy to carry on. Sometimes, I just wish that I could go to sleep forever and not wake up again.

Lucy: Now cheer up, surely it's not as bad as all that!

Julia: I know you think I'm being silly.

Lucy: As you said, you have got a lovely family, very supportive. You are very lucky; you should count your blessings.

- What feelings might lie behind Julia's words?
- How might Julia feel after hearing Lucy's response?
- Is Julia likely to feel able to discuss her feelings further?
- What might lie behind Lucy's attempt to cheer Julia up?
- Try to write out a response that Lucy might give which conveys a more empathic response to Julia's first statement.

Congruence relates to the harmony or consistency in communication messages, for example between verbal and non-verbal means.

Congruence between non-verbal and verbal communication will help to convey to the client a sense that the nurse is being genuine or authentic in their approach. The absence of genuineness is said to lead to sterile application of communication techniques (Arnold and Underman Boggs 1999). Being authentic requires the nurse to be clear about their own beliefs, attitudes, thoughts and feelings. This in turn relates to the need for assertiveness skills, self-awareness and in particular, awareness of personal limitations and some of the difficulties in managing a professional image.

Although much of current nursing literature exhorts the need for genuineness (Arnold and Underman Boggs 1999, Nelson-Jones 2005, Thurgood 2004), little attention has been paid to the difficulties associated with being authentic in clinical settings. The reality of busy clinical areas often means that nurses feel they do not have the time, opportunity or energy to apply Rogerian principles of empathic understanding, respect and genuineness in their all too hurried and fragmented client contact (Norton 2004). Nelson-Jones (2005) acknowledges that inexperience or under-confidence may lead to the presentation of an inauthentic but desperately held professional façade, particularly if the client appears to question the knowledge, authority and previous experience of the professional carer. Perhaps a response which honestly acknowledges areas of inexperience, particularly in not having experienced the same emotions as the client, will be both a genuine response and one which conveys a truthful validation of the uniqueness of the client's emotional experience: a response of *I know exactly how you feel* is likely to be the point at which clients will question, albeit silently, the genuineness of the nurse.

Part 3: Exploring communication and interpersonal skills

As a student nurse you may have been told that it is unprofessional to allow your personal feelings to show, particularly if you feel critical of the client. This suggests a need for a degree of professional detachment seemingly at odds with the requirement to be genuine within empathic responses.

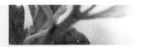

Research focus 9.2

Aranda and Street (1999) explored nurses' concepts of being authentic and the need for flexibility in presenting aspects of themselves to clients in order to respond to their particular needs, for example, to gain greater access to the details of the patient's life or seek greater concordance with treatments. The nurses in the study termed this being a chameleon. They expressed discomfort at changing styles of interaction with clients with its implication of being manipulative and inauthentic (even when the overall goal remained improvement of patient outcomes).

Aranda and Street propose that reconciliation of these tensions is possible through the concept of a nurse–patient relationship governed by intersubjectivity. Intersubjectivity suggests that all human relationships are co-constructed by the participants, that our reactions to others are shaped and formed by their interpretation of us. The circular transactional model of communication previously mentioned (Figure 9.2) illustrates the fluid nature of this process. Shifts in presentation of one's self are not necessarily inauthentic or manipulative; they merely represent individuals' responses to each other as each contributes to the development of the relationship.

The more advanced and complex communication skills

Active listening

Many people mistakenly believe that because they are good talkers they will be good listeners. Stickley and Freshwater (2006) note there is no guarantee that a fluent conversationalist will make a good listener. Here it is useful to distinguish between hearing and listening. Hearing involves the capacity to be aware of and receive sounds. Listening involves both hearing the sounds and interpreting their meaning. According to Gordon (1970), active listening involves trying to accurately understand a speaker's messages and to demonstrate understanding by carefully chosen responses. Requiring the exercise of both receiver and sender skills, active listening is considered an essential skill in creating and maintaining the therapeutic relationship (Arnold and Underman Boggs 1999, Burnard 1998, Nelson-Jones 2005, Stickley and Freshwater 2006).

Burnard (2003) suggests that while social (or phatic) communication can aid in establishing rapport with patients, effective therapeutic communication requires the listener to move on from the phatic stage to what Wright (2006) terms 'deep listening'. For Wright, deep listening necessarily involves setting aside one's own thoughts, listening without judging and attending closely to what is being said. In this sense the effectiveness of the therapeutic conversation depends on the nurse's ability to listen and detect clues that might entail the need for sensitive responses; responses that aim to help the client explore and express their feelings. Active listening requires:

- Presence or attending skills.
- Asking questions.
- Clarifying, restating and paraphrasing.
- Using silence.
- Reflecting feelings.

Presence or attending skills

Presence or attending refers to the ability of the nurse to remain physically, spiritually and emotionally attuned to the client's communication.

Gardener (1992) identifies presence as a therapeutic gift of self and as 'the embodiment of caring in nursing' (p. 193). **Presence or attending** skills convey an unselfish interest in the client; unselfish in the sense that the focus remains on the speaker. Presence refers to the ability of the nurse to remain physically, spiritually and emotionally attuned to the client's communication. Attending calls for the listener to concentrate and focus on what the speaker is saying by trying to suspend any personal thoughts or ideas in order to interpret and understand the other person's perspective.

To be effective, this level of intentional focus must be congruent with non-verbal messages of interest. A still and open posture, a slight lean of the upper body towards the speaker, and direct eye contact will convey the listener's focus and interest. Appropriate facial expressions such as a smile or a frown or a nodding of the head may encourage the speaker to continue. Periodically verbal encouragements such as: *go on* or *please take your time* or short vocalisations, for example, *mm* or *uh-huh* can be given. Attending skills may sound relatively straightforward, even simplistic. However, practice, concentration and a genuine desire to understand the patient is needed in order to ensure that active listening is not 'acting' listening. Over time practice will enable these skills to be incorporated into the nurse's personal communication style and thus become both genuine and subtle.

Asking questions

Open questions are those that require more than mere *yes, no* or other single word response.

Asking questions enables the nurse to find out about the patient. **Open questions** are useful in eliciting clients' thoughts or feelings. Perhaps the most common exception to this is the everyday *how are you?* which, although an open question, is commonly understood as a greeting rather than an enquiry: thus tends to be met with a *fine* or an *OK*-type response. However, it can be easily adapted to become a more open question as it would be, for example, in the enquiry *how do you feel about having surgery tomorrow?* If the invitation to expand is rebuffed by a simple *OK thanks*, it is appropriate to remember that therapeutic questioning should not become interrogation. Therapeutic questioning requires a sensitive and accurate reading of the verbal and non-verbal messages from the client and a willingness to adopt flexible communication strategies based on responses received.

Closed questions are those that require no more that a mere *yes, no* or other single word response.

Closed questions are appropriate when information is needed quickly or in a structured format. Examples of closed questions might be *when did you have your last insulin injection?* or *does the pain get worse on exertion?* A variation of the open question is the focused question which is useful when seeking specific information about a particular subject or issue, for example, *can you tell me more about the pain in your shoulder?* or *can you describe your pain?*

Arnold and Underman Boggs (1999) note a further type of open question, the circular question. Circular questions focus on the interpersonal context in which an illness occurs and are designed to identify family relationships as well as the impact illness might have on individual family members. Questions of this kind can help illuminate the patient within the contexts of family or others involved in their care. An example might be, *who in your family is likely to be most affected by your father's illness?* or *how is your younger sister coping with your mother's diagnosis?* Loos and Bell (1990) suggest that circular questions can be particularly helpful in including the family and others in the care of the client.

Activity 9.6

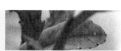

Can you identify which of the following are open questions, which are closed questions, and which are circular questions?

- How do you feel about being discharged from hospital?
- Have you lost weight recently?
- Do you feel overwhelmed by all your visitors?
- How will your partner manage the house and the business without you?
- Do you have any pain?
- Can you tell me if your child lost consciousness?
- What do you feel is the best course of treatment for you right now?
- Can you squeeze my hand?
- Ten milligrams a day – is that your normal dose?
- How will your father view his son's refusal to visit?
- How do you feel about having a different community nurse?

While most of these questions clearly fall in one or other category, others incorporate elements of more than one type. For example, the question, *do you feel overwhelmed by all your visitors?* can be answered as both an open and a closed question. You might find it useful to discuss your ideas about which are open, closed or circular questions with other students on your course.

Clarifying, restating and paraphrasing

Seeking clarification is sometimes necessary if the nurse is to understand the client's message. Using a neutral tone to ask the client to elaborate or explain helps ensure that they do not feel they have to justify or defend their thoughts and feelings. A simple question that asks for clarification, such as, *can you explain that to me?* demonstrates interest in the client, checks the accuracy of interpretation and allows the client to feel that they have been heard.

Restating is the repetition of a small section of the sender's message, often in the form of a query, using the sender's own words. This allows the sender to hear for themselves what they have said and provides the opportunity for them to clarify, amend or be more specific. For example, a client might say: *since my heart attack I just can't get on with the things I want to do. I feel I'm no use to anyone anymore.* In restating the fragment . . . *no use to anyone?* as an enquiry, the nurse provides the patient with an opportunity to expand on what could be a significant point. Restating is a useful technique but it needs to be used sparingly or it can hinder effective communication by interrupting the flow of a client's thoughts

Both clarification and restatement can be counterproductive if the listener's tone of voice is accusatory or demanding. However, restating can be used as a positive affirmation of the client. For example, in response to a client who says, *I think I've done quite well with my exercises*, the nurse might restate the fragment . . . *only quite well?* in a warm tone of voice and thus convey to the client a sense of achievement.

To paraphrase is to attempt to put into different words the core elements of another person's message. Paraphrasing a client's thoughts and feelings should always be done tentatively so that the client can correct any misinterpretations or confirm correct understanding. Accurately paraphrasing can mirror the speaker's material but offers the possibility of being clearer and more succinct than the original messages. There is no single correct way of paraphrasing and much will depend on the listener's own choice of words, but if the message has been accurately heard the client is likely to confirm it, for example, *yes, that's right* or *you've got it exactly.*

Using silence

Using silence as an active listening skill offers the patient time to think, and as Arnold and Underman Boggs (1999) note, allows the nurse to step back momentarily and process what they have heard before responding. A natural anxiety on the part of the nurse concerning how to respond or whether the response is appropriate and helpful to the client may lead to filling silences with unnecessary comments. The length of a silence needs to be carefully judged and much will depend on the client's ability to process information and respond to the nurse.

Ending a silence too quickly may not only give the client insufficient time to formulate their thoughts and responses but may convey to the client the nurse's anxiety or discomfort with the topic. Sharing a silence can convey the nurse is willing to 'be with' the client in the sense of attending or presence, as outlined earlier. Silence may occur for many reasons, and might mean that something has touched the client deeply; respecting the client's silence and sitting without breaking the mood can demonstrate an empathic understanding and acceptance of the client's feelings.

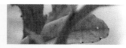

Activity 9.7

When you talk with patients be aware of silences as they arise.

- Ask yourself why did the silence occur?
- Look for non-verbal clues that may help you to form an answer.
- Be aware of how silences make you feel.
- Do you try to break a silence as quickly as you can, and if you do, why?
- Is it easier to let the silence continue with some patients and not with others?
- How do you break silences?
- If you cannot break a silence with words (and most of us are often not as articulate as we would like to be) what non-verbal means of communication might be appropriate?

Reflecting feelings

Reflecting feelings can involve paraphrasing but the focus is more on the client's expression of feeling rather that on the words they use. Nelson-Jones (2005) defines the skill of reflection as 'empathizing with a client's flow of emotion and communicating this back' (p. 104). Reflection involves the skilled interpretation of verbal and non-verbal clues. Emotions are not always verbalised but may be observed as incongruence between the patient's verbal and non-verbal messages. *I'm fine* might be a verbal response to the question of how the person is feeling but the non-verbal clues of a sad facial expression or even tearfulness will probably undermine the verbal message. Reflection tries to capture both the overt and covert messages and reflects them back in an empathetic manner.

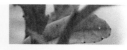

Activity 9.8

In the following piece of dialogue a third-year student nurse, Simon, uses reflection in a sensitive and effective way, enabling Clyde, a 17-year-old patient, to express his feelings.

Clyde: I can't bear all the noise in here.

Simon: You are finding the noise upsetting?

Clyde: It's just that there are so many people around all the time. I can't explain it; somehow it makes me feel alone.

Simon: It sounds like you are feeling lonely. Is that how you feel?

Clyde: I guess so. I feel a bit silly really.

Simon: It doesn't sound silly to me at all. Feeling lonely is very upsetting.

Review the skills discussed so far in this chapter and try to identify other elements of therapeutic communication involved in this exchange. You may find this more productive if you undertake this part of the exercise with another student.

Patients may resist revealing their underlying feelings, but gentle and sensitive use of reflection at a more advanced level may help the patient to articulate and understand for themselves their emotional responses to health-related issues. Egan suggests the following questions may help students to clarify the reflective process at a more advanced level:

- what is this person only half saying?
- what is this person hinting at?
- what is this person saying in a confused way?
- what messages do I hear behind the explicit messages?

(Egan 2002, p. 200)

Listening to self and developing self-awareness

Stickley and Freshwater (2006) assert that before we can listen successfully to others it is important to develop the art of listening to ourself. This involves becoming conscious of the thoughts, feelings, attitudes, beliefs, prejudices and values likely to affect our interactions with others. Nurses are expected to protect the interests and dignity of patients and clients, and to not discriminate against individuals because of, for example, gender, age, race, ability, sexuality, economic status, lifestyle, culture and religious or political beliefs (NMC 2008), but this is not to be confused with an assumption that we are neutral in our manner with each client. Burnard (1992) urges practitioners to 'stay awake' while listening and by this he means being alert not only to the client's messages but also to one's internal concerns.

To be able to accomplish this kind of 'internal listening' the nurse needs to develop self-awareness. Self-awareness is described by Arnold and Underman Boggs (1999) as providing an 'inner frame of reference for connecting emotionally with the experience of another' (p. 69). Nurses can learn about themselves through a process of reflecting upon their motives, feelings, responses and behaviours in relation to others. A specific incident, perhaps initially regarded as negative, for example, an unsuccessful confrontation, or an interaction that could be felt to be more positive, such as a warm and caring interpersonal exchange, can be useful in providing a focus for the nurse to reflect critically upon and record both their strengths and the areas in need of further development (see Chapter 13 for more on reflective practice).

Burnard (2002) suggests a positive correlation exists between the nurse's level of understanding of self and their openness and honesty in interactions with others. By knowing personal prejudices, motivations and current abilities, the nurse is able to increase their capacity for being empathic with clients. Jourard (1991) argues that if nurses are ignorant or afraid of their own self, they are more likely to feel threatened or intimidated by client self-disclosure.

Activity 9.9

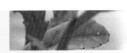

The five questions below are based on those set by Carl Rogers (1958) and are designed to encourage self-awareness in the nurse–patient relationship. Think of a client that you have recently worked with and with whom you feel you have a therapeutic relationship. Work through the questions, applying each to your relationship. You might be tempted to simply answer 'yes' and move on but try to think about each question carefully. You could make short notes exploring how you can demonstrate or illustrate that you are able to answer 'yes'. What areas might still be in need of further development? What steps could you take to start to achieve this?

→

1. Can I *be* in some way which will be perceived by the other person as trustworthy, dependable, or consistent in some deep sense?

2. Can I let myself experience positive attitudes toward this other person – attitudes of warmth, caring, liking, interest and respect?

3. Can I let myself fully enter into the world of their feelings and personal meanings and see these as they do?

4. Can I accept this person as they are? Can I communicate this attitude?

5. Can I maintain separateness from this person and foster separateness in them?

Setting and maintaining personal boundaries in the therapeutic relationship

One aspect of becoming self-aware is the consequence of being more able to notice where aspects of the therapeutic relationship serve the nurse's own needs rather than those of the client's. Notice that the last of the questions above refers to maintaining a sense of separateness from the client. This

Case 9.3

Jan is a mature student nurse and has formed a close relationship with Georgie, aged 11, who has been a patient on the children's unit for several months. Georgie is aware of his poor prognosis but remains cheerful. From time to time he talks optimistically about his future hopes of being a professional footballer.

Jan has two children, one of whom is the same age as Georgie, and finds it difficult to cope with the knowledge that Georgie is likely to die soon. She feels that she needs to spend as much time with Georgie as she possibly can when she is on duty and is aware that she often thinks about him when she is with her own family. Jan has a strong sense of frustration that little can be done for Georgie. She spends extra time with him before and after each shift. As Georgie becomes increasingly frail Jan finds it almost impossible to hide her distress when he talks about which football club he'd like to play for.

Jan's mentor is concerned about the amount of time she is spending with Georgie and has noticed that she seems to resent other nurses being involved in his care. She gently voices her concerns and listens empathically as Jan acknowledges her distress and anxiety about not being able to cope with Georgie's death. She is also able to acknowledge that her emotional involvement with Georgie and his family has led her to think that she has the most important role of all the care team members in being responsible for his care. Her mentor discloses her own similar experience earlier in her career and explains how supportive the care team were in helping each other come to terms with the death of a young patient. Jan and her mentor discuss the nature of empathy and the importance for professional staff of maintaining a sense of separateness or objectivity with a client.

After talking with her mentor Jan was able to relinquish her sense of being solely responsible for Georgie's care and in consequence felt a sense of relief that she was part of a team of professional staff, able to draw on the support and supervision of experienced colleagues.

may at first seem to contradict the call for 'being with' in attending skills of active listening in order to build an empathetic understanding of the client. However, a sense of separateness is essential in the therapeutic relationship and maintained through appropriate emotional distancing or emotional boundary-keeping.

Therapeutic boundaries are behavioural limits that allow for the safe interaction between client and health care professional (Peterson 1992). According to Malone *et al.* (2004) these limits define and protect the space between a health care professional's power and the client's vulnerability. It is the nurse's responsibility (not the patient's) to set and maintain professional boundaries. The nurse should clearly establish the boundaries of the relationship with the patient when the relationship is first established and must be consistent in maintaining them throughout the relationship.

A nurse who is emotionally over-involved with the patient is likely to be meeting their own needs rather than the needs of the client. Over-involvement is likely to show itself with the nurse coming to believe that only they are able to fully understand and care for the client, losing the necessary detachment and objectivity needed in accurate assessment and delivery of care. The over-involved nurse may give more time and attention to one particular client, coming to see them in off-duty hours, discounting the efforts of other health care professionals and performing tasks for the client that they could, and probably should, perform for themselves. The over-involved nurse may agree to keep the client's secrets or may not pass on information that should be shared with the rest of the health care team. They may also disclose intimate information about themselves and about their experiences in the mistaken belief that they are being empathic or seeking reciprocity with clients.

The Nursing and Midwifery Council states that nurses must, at all times, maintain appropriate professional boundaries in relationships with patients and clients, ensuring that all aspects of the care focus on the needs of the patient (NMC 2008). However, it may be others, particularly more experienced staff, who first become aware of the over-involvement of the nurse. Dowling (2006) makes the point that despite a theoretical understanding of the importance of maintaining a therapeutic emotional distance, inexperienced nurses are likely to be less able to maintain an expectation of equal partnership when working with patients, especially patients whose ill-health renders them vulnerable and those who seek dependency upon nursing staff.

Professional boundaries are limits that demarcate the edges of the relationship between the nurse and the client. The parameters of therapeutic boundaries must be embedded in the core conditions of respect, warmth and authentic concern for the client. The development of self-awareness is pivotal in being able to recognise where professional relationship boundaries have become unclear. However, self-monitoring behaviour is an advanced reflective skill that demands honest and unflinching examination of one's motives and behaviours.

Mentor and supervision support is invaluable in helping the nurse discuss and explore the nature of their relationships with clients. Most nurses will be able to recognise the difficulties faced from their own experiences and will be in a position to offer suggestions and support in managing the situation. Hawes (2005) suggests that a culture of nursing colleagues sharing their experiences of the difficulties of managing boundaries needs to be encouraged if junior nursing staff are to feel able to seek advice and support. Gallop (1998) suggests

Therapeutic boundaries are appropriate emotional distances between the nurse and client in order to preserve a sense of separateness and thus allow for the safe interaction between the client and the health care professional.

a simple reflective question can help to initiate the process of self-monitoring; for example *would other nurses or health care professionals think my behaviour with this client appropriate?*

Dowling (2006) suggests that in certain circumstances self-disclosure may be appropriate but this requires an acute sense of self-awareness. A parent of a sick child who asks if the nurse has children of their own may be seeking reassurance that someone who understands the needs of both the child and the parent is nursing their child. When a distressed client probes the nurse with a question to ascertain the nurse's personal experiences of coping with stressful events, the nurse needs to measure self-disclosure carefully as the outcome of sharing may have a positive or a negative effect. Before self-disclosure, a useful technique might be to pause and think: in revealing this information, whose need is being met? If the answer appears to favour the nurse's own needs (perhaps reflecting the need to feel more intimately involved with a client through a sense of shared experience) then the level of disclosure is likely to be inappropriate.

Relationship boundaries may be tested by patients and might take the form of making unreasonable demands of time and attention, or by indicating that they would like a personal, social or sexual relationship with the nurse. Testing boundaries can also include using behaviours that the patient thinks will provoke a particular response from the nurse, for example, asking for confidential information about fellow patients, making crude sexual innuendoes or telling risqué jokes.

The nurse who deals clearly and directly with boundary testing reasserts the professional parameters of the relationship, allowing both the client and the nurse to refocus on goals that relate to the client's health care issues. A clear statement from the nurse of what is considered acceptable behaviour, far from damaging the therapeutic relationship, will serve to strengthen and underpin future interactions in a constructive and positive manner. Indistinct, ambiguous or violated boundaries within the therapeutic relationship mean that the sense of safety and trust as necessary conditions for the development of close professional partnership working will no longer exist.

Barriers to the therapeutic relationship

There are numerous factors that can raise difficulties in the nurse–patient relationship, including:

- nurse or patient anxiety;
- specific communication difficulties;
- low emotional intelligence.

Client or nurse anxiety can be a threat to the therapeutic relationship. Common causes of stress for patients are apprehension about their health status or about their current and future treatment options. Anxiety might also relate to uncertainty about future coping and the effects of their ill-health on others, including family members. Nurses may be anxious if they feel under-confident, unsupported by colleagues, inexperienced, or insufficiently competent. Student nurses have the additional pressure of being assessed, including the need to achieve the NMC standards of proficiency relating to creating, maintaining and disengaging from the therapeutic relationship.

Research focus 9.3

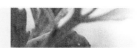

A study by Geanellos (2005) explores the consequences of nurse unfriendliness on client well-being. Findings reveal that nurse unfriendliness, characterised by patients as frostiness, officiousness and apathy gave rise to patients feeling unsafe, unwelcome, anxious and unprotected.

Anxiety can disrupt and seriously detract from the quality of the therapeutic relationship. Nurse–patient communication is likely to be stilted, superficial and hurried. Concentration is more difficult and active listening and attending are problematic for the anxious nurse. Anxiety will undoubtedly inhibit the degree of warmth and level of genuineness shown to the client.

Patient anxiety may result in a need for repeated reassurance from the nurse. When such reassurance is given but fails to provide the comfort sought, the nurse may feel increasingly unable to meet the client's needs and may begin to avoid further contact. In this situation, decreasing patients' anxiety levels is essential if the therapeutic relationship is to flourish, and for patients with severe levels of anxiety, psychiatric and medical interventions may be necessary. Arnold and Underman Boggs (1999) recommend that in mild to moderate levels the nurse can adopt a number of strategies to assist the client. These include:

- Active listening to show acceptance.
- Honesty: answering all questions at the client's level of understanding.
- Clearly explaining procedures, surgery and policies and giving reassurance based on evidence-based practice.
- Acting in a calm, unhurried manner.
- Speaking clearly and firmly (but not loudly).
- Encouraging clients to explore their reasons for anxiety.
- Using play therapy with dolls, puppets, games and drawing for young clients.
- Using therapeutic touch, giving warm baths, relaxing music.
- Teaching breathing and relaxation exercises.

Anxiety levels for the nurse may be reduced by seeking support from mentors, other staff, course and personal tutors, peers and friends. Perhaps the most effective intervention is the one in which the nurse realises that support networks are readily available. Wilkinson (1991) suggests that the nature of the support on offer is a key determinant of a nurse's facilitative communication behaviour. Smith (1992) noted that when nurses feel appreciated and supported emotionally by senior staff not only do they have a role model for sensitive and empathic patient care but they also feel able to care for patients in the same way. Chant and colleagues (2002) agree, and suggest that poor support systems and an occupational or ward culture of task-orientated dominance that excludes or diminishes the importance of individualised support for nursing staff has a direct and negative correlation on the quality and standards of care for patients.

Specific communication difficulties can arise with different client groups with different needs and abilities. A detailed exploration of the needs of all client groups cannot be undertaken in a chapter of this length, and only general comments are offered here.

For clients with limited cognitive ability and/or impaired communication the nurse must strive to deliver verbal messages using uncomplicated language in short sentences, containing a single subject or topic in each sentence. Ample time needs to be given and open questions, occasionally repeated and rephrased if necessary, will allow the client an opportunity to understand interactions and formulate a response. Frequently checking the client's level of understanding by using clarification through repeating, restating and asking for further explanation, is also likely to be effective.

It may be appropriate for nurses to talk with carers or advocates, particularly if the client's ability to communicate is severely limited; however the individual client should not be ignored or excluded and must be addressed directly during conversation and discussion (Godsell and Scarborough 2006). For clients with sensory impairments, face-to-face communication where the nurse's face can be clearly seen is likely to maximise the client's understanding of what is being said. Increasing the speech volume may be necessary but clear articulation and unhurried speech is likely to be equally or more effective. Para-verbal and non-verbal means of communication can enhance or, if necessary, replace limited verbal exchanges. Touch, body positioning and proximity together with explicit attending skills will help to convey the qualities of genuine interest, warmth and respect for the client.

Pictures, photographs and sign language, known as augmentative and alternative communication systems (AACs), can be used to enhance or supplement verbal communication. Picture boards, simple line drawings or objects can provide easy yet effective methods of communication. Other resources such as leaflets and books with symbols, signs and pictures to explain medical procedures are becoming increasingly available in clinical areas.

Emotional intelligence

Emotional intelligence requires an advanced level of self-awareness; emotional intelligence includes the wider and complex human skills of empathy, motivation, self-control and adeptness in relationships.

In recent years the important role **emotional intelligence** plays in effective nurse–patient communication has been recognised (Cadman and Brewer 2001, Evans and Allen 2002, McQueen 2004). Emotional intelligence is defined as 'a core aptitude related to one's ability and capacity to reason with one's emotions, especially in relation to others' (Freshwater and Stickley 2004 p. 92). Superficially this may be interpreted as an advanced level of self-awareness; indeed being self-aware is part of emotional intelligence. However, emotional intelligence encompasses other complex human skills of relationships including empathy, motivation, self-control and adeptness. It is argued that emotional intelligence can be extended and developed through training and that it should be at the heart of education for nursing (Cadman and Brewer 2001, Freshwater and Stickley 2004, McQueen 2004).

Goleman (1998) suggests it is emotional intelligence that determines an individual's capacity to develop the skills or competencies related to the following five elements of effective communication:

1. Self-awareness (emotional awareness, the ability to self assess with accuracy, high self-esteem).
2. Self-regulation (the ability to control emotion and impulse, flexibility in handling change, the ability to innovate).
3. Motivation (the need to achieve, need to initiate, optimism).

4. Empathy (understanding and developing others, a willingness to meet others' needs, the ability to 'tune into' individual or groups emotional states).
5. Social skills (persuasiveness, conflict management, leadership skills).

How does emotional intelligence relate to nursing?

Freshwater and Stickley (2004) claim that emotional intelligence is necessary for effective nursing precisely because nurses invariably work with such human emotions as fear, anxiety, sadness, hope, joy, relief and anger. Evans and Allen (2002) and Cadman and Brewer (2001) hold that the ability to manage one's emotional life while interpreting other people's is a prerequisite skill for any caring professional. In addition to empathy (discussed earlier in this chapter), emotional intelligence includes the ability to manage the emotions we experience as a result of nursing others.

Although it is now acceptable for nurses to show their feelings as they empathise with patients, there is clearly a need to control and manage these emotions if the patient is not to be overwhelmed. Omdahl and O'Donnell (1999) differentiate between acceptable and controlled empathic concern on the one hand and unacceptable overwhelming emotion (or 'emotional contagion') on the other. Thus both the type and degree of emotion shown requires self-regulation. This need for self-regulation is particularly important in relation to negative emotional response to, for example, irritation, anger, frustration, or disgust rather than to the many pleasurable emotions associated with nursing practice. A nurse who is unable to exert some control over their negative emotions may not only damage the therapeutic relationship but also the wider professional image of nursing.

Henderson (2001) suggests that emotional involvement of nurses is regarded as a requirement for excellence in nursing practice, contributing to the quality of care as well as to the emotional well-being of both patients and nurses. However, continuous and intense emotional work can be stressful, demanding and exhausting. Benner and Wrubel (1989) suggest that unrelenting work of this nature can adversely affect the physical and psychological health of the nurse, with the potential to lead to burnout. A balance is needed between providing intimate personal attention to patients and recognising personal limitations. Self-regulation and the adoption of coping techniques such as seeking support and supervision as well as a willingness to accept alternative nurse–patient allocation can be beneficial for both the nurse and the patient.

Druskat and Wolff (2001) emphasise the value of emotional intelligence in teamwork. This relates directly to nurses working with other immediate members of the care team including other health care professionals. The complexities of health care provision across hospitals, primary care and the voluntary and independent agencies demands trust, understanding and cooperation. Motivational, social and collaborative working skills are all part of emotional intelligence. The therapeutic relationship is not an isolated entity and directly benefits from the input of all professionals associated with the care of the client. The nurse unable or unwilling to develop and extend their emotional intelligence capabilities threatens to nurse at a mechanistic or task-orientated level and this can be a significant barrier to the richness of the therapeutic relationship.

Disengaging from the therapeutic relationship

By their very nature, therapeutic relationships are time limited; they have a beginning and they have an end. There are no set time limits for therapeutic relationships; some can last for just a few hours, others may continue for months or even years. Student nurse–patient relationships are inevitably governed by the allocated placement time. However, regardless of the length of the therapeutic relationship the same principles apply. The basic principles of disengagement are:

- *Informing*: letting the patient know that the nurse–patient relationship is coming to an end allows an opportunity for the client to acknowledge their feelings on ending the relationship.
- *Maintaining authenticity and boundaries*: it may be necessary for the nurse to restate the professional boundaries required in the nurse–patient relationship, including the need to not make promises to keep in touch or accept invitations for meeting clients once the professional relationship is ended.
- *Acknowledging*: valuing the patient's contribution to meeting their health care goals as well as to the professional development of the nurse.

Some patients develop a close relationship with a particular nurse: when that relationship ends they may experience feelings that lie anywhere in a spectrum ranging from mild disappointment to intense sadness or loss. Arnold and Underman Boggs (1999) draw an analogy between the psychological responses of bereavement and the termination of the therapeutic relationship for both nurse and client. Part of the therapeutic relationship should include the process of preparing the client for ending the relationship by stating when the nurse or patient will to need to say goodbye. It may be appropriate from time to time to remind the client of the temporary nature of the relationship, particularly if there is a sense that the patient may have started to become over-reliant on their contact with the nurse. The first principle of disengagement is that the nurse should ensure that patients are made aware of the approaching end of the working relationship and, if appropriate, provide the time and opportunity for the patient to acknowledge their feelings.

Many student nurses will be familiar with the experience of feeling tempted to make promises of keeping in touch with clients once they have finished their clinical secondment, possibly prompted by the patient's responses to saying goodbye. However tempting, making such promises is often unwise. It is likely to be impractical and making a promise to keep in touch would therefore be inauthentic. It is also likely to be contrary to the maintenance of professional relationship boundaries, as it could herald the change from professional to social relationship parameters. The second principle is that, if necessary, nurses must politely but assertively restate that the nature of the professional relationship is such that it must remain focused on the client's health care needs.

It may also be appropriate for the nurse to express their appreciation of being in the privileged position of working closely with the patient and to thank them for the contribution they have made to the nurse's preparation in becoming a qualified nurse. The partnership process is a collaborative one, but patients may be unaware of their contribution to the nurse's professional development and unaware of the contribution they have made to meet their own health care goals. It might therefore be appropriate for the nurse to acknowledge how far the goals have been met in the form of a short summary to captures these points. Other resources and future plans for meeting health care needs or the maintenance of health gains can also be discussed, for example, future follow-up care arrangements or referrals to other organisations, agencies and health care teams.

Activity 9.10

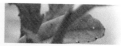

Review the basic principles of disengaging from the nurse-patient relationship and write a short response to the scenarios below.

- You have been working with Ian for a number of weeks and feel that you have established a close nurse-patient relationship. He is aware that today is your last working day on the unit. You have come to say goodbye when Ian says, 'I'd really like to keep in touch. Perhaps you could come round for a drink or a meal? I know that my family would love to see you and I'd like to know how you do on your course.'
- Molly has made little eye contact with you and seems distant in her manner since you talked about the transfer of her care to the community team. You open the subject of her future plans but she interrupts with 'I expect you find it hard to remember anyone, you must see so many different patients all the time. This time next week you won't even remember my name.'

Conclusion

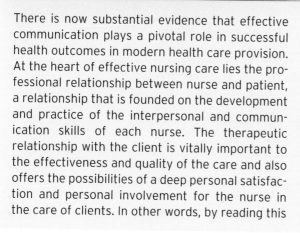

There is now substantial evidence that effective communication plays a pivotal role in successful health outcomes in modern health care provision. At the heart of effective nursing care lies the professional relationship between nurse and patient, a relationship that is founded on the development and practice of the interpersonal and communication skills of each nurse. The therapeutic relationship with the client is vitally important to the effectiveness and quality of the care and also offers the possibilities of a deep personal satisfaction and personal involvement for the nurse in the care of clients. In other words, by reading this chapter you have had the opportunity to explore some of the basic components of communication and interpersonal skills that you can now employ within caring relationships with clients. In acknowledging the importance of communication you can contribute to effective patient care by demonstrating a willingness to enhance your own communication and interpersonal skills. Harnessing your skills of listening to the self, in the development of self-awareness, and in enhancing your ability to set and maintain therapeutic boundaries can help you to overcome barriers to effective therapeutic relationships.

Suggested further reading

Arnold, E. and Underman Boggs, K. (1999) *Interpersonal Relationships, Professional Communication Skills for Nurses* (3rd ed.), London: W. B. Saunders.

Deering, C. and Cody, D. (2002) Communicating with children and adolescents. *American Journal of Nursing* **102** (3), 34-41.

Godsell, M. and Scarborough, K. (2006) Improving communication for people with learning disabilities. *Nursing Standard* **20** (30), 58-65.

Hawes, R. (2005) Therapeutic relationships with children and families. *Paediatric Nursing* **17** (6), 15-18.

Lago, C. (2006) *Race, Culture and Counselling*. Milton Keynes: Open University Press.

McCabe, C. (2004) Nurse-patient communication: an exploration of patients' experiences. *Journal of Clinical Nursing* **13** (1), 41-49.

Miller, L. (2002) Effective communication with older people. *Nursing Standard* **17** (9), 45-50.

Perry, J., Galloway, S., Bottorff, J. and Nixon, S. (2005) Nurse-patient communication in dementia: improving the odds. *Journal of Gerontological Nursing* **31** (4), 43-52.

References

Antai-Otong, D. (1999) It's not what you say, its how you say it. *American Journal of Nursing* **99** (8), 24–26.

Aranda, S. K. and Street, A. F. (1999) Being authentic and being a chameleon: nurse–patient interaction revisited. *Nursing Inquiry* **6** (2), 75–82.

Arnold, E. and Underman Boggs, K. (1999) *Interpersonal Relationships, Professional Communication Skills for Nurses* (3rd ed.). London: W. B. Saunders.

Attree, M. (2001) Patients' and relatives' experiences and perspectives of 'Good' and 'Not so good' quality care. *Journal of Advanced Nursing* **33** (4), 456–466.

Balzer-Riley, J. W. (1996) *Communications in Nursing* (3rd ed.). Missouri: Mosby.

Benner, P. and Wrubel, J. (1989) *The Primacy of Caring*. London: Addison-Wesley.

Booth, K., Maguire, P. and Hillier, V. (1999) Measurement of communication skills in cancer care: myth or reality? *Journal of Advanced Nursing* **30** (5), 1073–1079.

Burnard, P. (1991) Acquiring minimum counselling skills. *Nursing Standard* **5** (46), 37–39.

Burnard, P. (1992) *Counselling: A guide to practice in nursing*. Oxford: Butterworth-Heinemann.

Burnard, P. (1998) Listening as a personal quality. *Journal of Community Nursing* **12** (2), 32–34.

Burnard, P. (2002) *Learning Human Skills: An experiential guide for nurses*. Oxford: Heinemann.

Burnard, P. (2003) Ordinary chat and therapeutic conversation: phatic communication and mental health nursing. *Journal of Psychiatric and Mental Health Nursing* **10** (6), 678–682.

Cadman, C. and Brewer, J. (2001) Emotional intelligence: a vital prerequisite for recruitment in nursing. *Journal of Nursing Management* **9** (6), 321–324.

Chant, S., Jenkinson, T., Randle, J. and Russell, G. (2002) Communication skills: some problems in nursing education and practice. *Journal of Clinical Nursing* **11** (1), 12–21.

Corbett, T. (1995) The nurse as a professional carer. In Ellis, R. B., Gates, R. J. and Kenworthy, N. (eds), *Interpersonal Communication in Nursing: Theory and practice*, Edinburgh: Churchill Livingstone, pp. 91–107.

Courtney, R., Ballard, E., Fauver, S., Gariota, M. and Holland, L. (1996) The partnership model: working with individuals, families and communities towards a new vision of health. *Public Health Nursing* **13** (3), 177–186.

Dickson, D. (1999) Barriers to communication. In *Interaction for Practice in Community Nursing*, Long, A. (ed.). Basingstoke: Macmillan, pp. 84–132.

Dowling, M. (2006) The sociology of intimacy in the nurse–patient relationship. *Nursing Standard* **20** (23), 48–54.

Druskat, V. U. and Wolff, S. B. (2001) Building the emotional intelligence of groups. *Harvard Business Review* **79** (3), 80–90.

Dunn, B. (1991) Communication interaction skills. *Senior Nurse* **11** (4), 4–8.

Egan, G. (2002) *The Skilled Helper: A problem-management and opportunity-development approach to helping* (7th ed.). Pacific Grove, CA: Brooks/Cole.

Ekman, P., Friesen, W. V. and Ellsworth, P. (1972) *Emotions in the Human Face*. New York: Pergamon Press.

Evans, D. and Allen, H. (2002) Emotional intelligence: its role in training. *Nursing Times* **98** (27), 41–42.

Faulkner, A. (1998) *Effective Interaction with Patients*. London: Churchill Livingstone.

Feltham, C. and Horton, I. (2006) *The Sage Handbook of Counselling and Psychotherapy*. London: Sage.

Freshwater, D. and Stickley, T. (2004) The heart of the art: emotional intelligence in nurse education. *Nursing Inquiry* **11** (2), 91–98.

Gallant, M. H., Beaulieu, M. C. and Carnevale, F. A. (2002) Partnership: an analysis of the concept within the nurse–client relationship. *Journal of Advanced Nursing* **40** (2), 149–157.

Gallop, R. (1998) Post discharge social contact: a potential area for boundary violation. *American Psychiatric Nurses Association* **4** (4), 105–110.

Gardener, J. (1992) Presence. In *Nursing Interventions: Essential nursing treatments* (2nd edn), Bulechek, G. and McCloskey, J. (eds) Philadelphia: W. B. Saunders, pp. 191–200.

Geanellos, R. (2005) Undermining self-efficacy: the consequences of nurse unfriendliness on client wellbeing. *Collegian* **12** (4), 9–14.

Godsell, M. and Scarborough, K. (2006) Improving communication for people with learning disabilities. *Nursing Standard* **20** (30), 58–65.

Goleman, D. (1998) *Working with Emotional Intelligence*. London: Bloomsbury.

Gordon, T. (1970) *Parent Effectiveness Training: The tested way to raise responsible children*. New York: Wyden.

Hall, E. T. (1966) *The Hidden Dimension*. New York: Doubleday.

Hargie, O., Saunders, C. and Dickson, D. (1994) *Social Skills in Interpersonal Communication*. London: Routledge.

Hawes, R. (2005) Therapeutic relationships with children and families. *Paediatric Nursing* **17** (6), 15–18.

Henderson, A. (2001) Emotional labour and nursing: an under-appreciated aspect of caring work. *Nursing Inquiry* **8** (2), 130–138.

Holland, K. and Hogg, C. (2001) *Cultural Awareness in Nursing and Health Care*. London: Arnold.

Jourard, S. (1991) *The Transparent Self*. New York: Van Nostrand Reinhold.

Knapp, M. L. (1980) *Essentials of Non-verbal Communication*. New York: Holt, Rinehart & Winston.

Lago, C. (2006) *Race, Culture and Counselling* (2nd ed.). Milton Keynes: Open University Press.

Langewitz, W. A., Eich, P., Kiss, A. and Wossmer, B. (1998) Improving communication skills – a randomised controlled behaviourally orientated intervention study for residents in internal medicine. *Psychosomatic Medicine*, **60** (3), 268–276.

Liberman, R. P., King, L. W., DeRisi, W. J. and McCann, M. (1975) *Personal Effectiveness: Guiding people to assert themselves and improve their social skills.* Champaign, IL: Research Press.

Loos, F. and Bell, J. (1990) Circular questions: a family interviewing strategy. *Dimensions of Critical Care Nursing* **9** (1), 47.

Lubbers, C. and Roy, S. (1990) Communication skills for continuing education in nursing. *Journal for Continuing Education for Nursing* **21** (3), 109–112.

Macleod Clark, J. (1988) Communication the continuing challenge. *Nursing Times* **84** (23), 24–27.

Mallett, J. and Dougherty, L. (2000) *Manual of Clinical Procedures* (5th ed.). London: Blackwell Science.

Malone, S. B., Reed, M. R., Norbeck, J., Hindsman, R. L. and Knowles, F. E. (2004) Development of a training module on therapeutic boundaries for mental health clinicians and case managers. *Lippincot's Case Management* **9** (4), 197–202.

McQuail, D. and Windahl, S. (1981) *Communication Models for the Study of Mass Communication.* New York: Longman.

McQueen, A. (2004) Emotional intelligence in nursing work. *Journal of Advanced Nursing* **47** (1), 101–108.

Nelson-Jones, R. (2005) *Practical Counselling and Helping Skills* (5th ed.). London: Sage.

Nichols, K. (1993) *Psychological Care in Physical Illness.* London: Chapman Hall.

NMC (Nursing and Midwifery Council) (2004) *Standards of Proficiency for Pre-registration Nursing Education.* London: NMC.

NMC (2008) *The Code: Standards of conduct, performance and ethics for nurses and midwives.* London: NMC.

Norton, K. (2004) The therapeutic milieu. In *The Art and Science of Mental Health Nursing*, Norman, I. and Ryrie, I. (eds). Milton Keynes: Open University Press, pp. 241–264.

Omdahl, L. and O'Donnell, C. (1999) Emotional contagion, empathic concern and communicative responsiveness as variables affecting nurses' stress and occupational commitment. *Journal of Advanced Nursing* **29** (6), 1351–1359.

Peplau, H. E. (1991) *Interpersonal Relations in Nursing: A conceptual framework of reference for psychodynamic nursing.* New York: Springer. (First published in 1952.)

Peterson, M. (1992) *At Personal Risk: Boundary violations in professional-client relationships.* New York: W.W. Norton.

Pike, A. W. (1990) On the nature and place of empathy in clinical nursing practice. *Journal of Professional Nursing* **6** (4), 135–140.

Price, B. (2006) Exploring person-centred care. *Nursing Standard* **20** (50), 49–56.

Raeburn, J. and Rootman, I. (1998) *People-Centred Health Promotion.* New York: Wiley.

Rogers, C. R. (1958) The characteristics of the helping relationship. *Personnel and Guidance Journal* **37** (1), 6–16.

Rogers, C. R. (1961) *On Becoming a Person: A therapist's view of psychotherapy.* Boston: Houghton Mifflin.

Rogers, C. R. (1981) *Client-Centred Therapy.* London: Constable.

Sellman, D. (2006) The importance of being trustworthy. *Nursing Ethics* **13** (2), 105–115.

Sellman, D. (2007) Trusting patients, trusting nurses. *Nursing Philosophy* **8** (1), 28–36.

Smith, P. (1992) *The Emotional Labour of Nursing. How nurses care.* Basingstoke: Macmillan.

Stickley, T. and Freshwater, D. (2006) The art of listening in the therapeutic relationship. *Mental Health Practice* **9** (5), 12–18.

Thorsteinsson, L. S. C. H. (2002) The quality of nursing care as perceived by individuals with chronic illnesses: the magical touch of nursing. *Journal of Clinical Nursing* **11** (1), 32–44.

Thurgood, M. (2004) Engaging clients in their care and treatment. In *The Art and Science of Mental Health Nursing*, Norman, I. and Ryrie, I (eds). Milton Keynes: Open University Press, pp. 649–664.

Timmins, F. C. (2004) Improving communication in day surgery settings. *Nursing Standard* **19** (7), 37–42.

Tschudin, V. (1995) *Counselling Skills for Nurses* (4th ed.). London: Bailliere Tindall.

Wilkinson, S. (1991) Factors which influence how nurses communicate with cancer patients. *Journal of Advanced Nursing* **16** (6), 677–688.

Wilkinson, S., Roberts, A. and Aldridge, J. (1998) Nurse–patient communication in palliative care: an evaluation of a communication skills programme. *Palliative Medicine* **12** (1), 13–22.

Wilkinson, S., Bailey, K., Aldridge, J. and Roberts, A. (1999) A longitudinal evaluation of a communication skills programme. *Palliative Medicine* **13** (4), 341–348.

Wright, S. (2006) The beauty of silence. *Nursing Standard* **20** (50), 49–56.

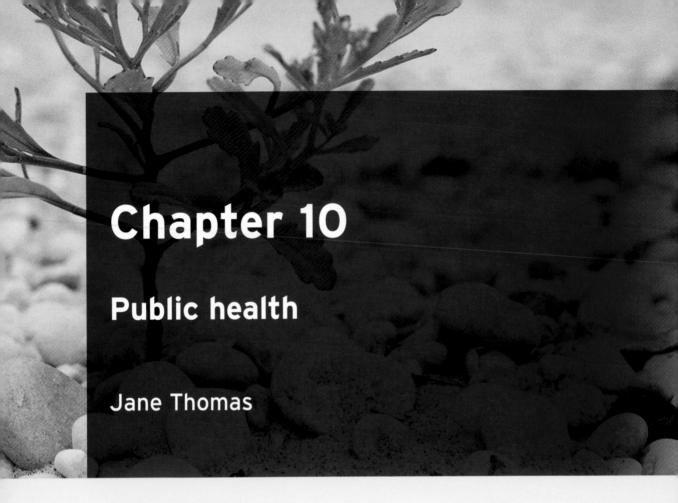

Chapter 10

Public health

Jane Thomas

Learning outcomes

After reading and reflecting on this chapter, you should be able to:

● Define public health and health promotion;
● Explain the origins of public health and the emergence of the 'new' public health;
● Discuss the historical medical dominance of public health in relation to current changes in this area;
● Identify the 10 areas of public health practice;
● Discuss the relevance of public health to nursing.

Related NMC Standards of Proficiency for Pre-registration Nursing Education (NMC 2004a)

- Consult with patients, clients and groups to identify their need and desire for health promotion advice.

- Provide relevant and current health information to patients, clients and groups in a form which facilitates their understanding and acknowledges choice/individual preference.

- Provide support and education in the development and/or maintenance of independent living skills.

- Seek specialist/expert advice as appropriate.

- Contribute to the application of a range of interventions which support and optimise the health and well-being of patients and clients.

Introduction

Public health is an integral part of nursing practice. The daily work of nurses involves aspects of public health even if this is not always recognised as public health work. This chapter helps to illustrate the myriad ways in which nurses engage with public health work in both specialist and non-specialist environments.

The chapter is divided into three parts.

In Part 1, an overview of the range of public health work that goes on in everyday nursing is offered together with a brief explanation of some of the more common public health terms.

In Part 2, an explanation of the importance of public health is offered together with illustrations of how nurses influence the way the public think about health. Awareness of the influence you have in your everyday contact with patients, their families and other members of the public is a starting point for recognising the responsibilities that come with the title of registered nurse. Recognition of this important part of the nursing role allows you to begin to think more deeply about the influence you have and how you might go about being a positive role model in public health.

In Part 3, some of the history of public health is offered before beginning an exploration of some of the more specialised roles of public health within the overall framework of nursing practice. Some of the barriers to effective public health work are acknowledged and some attention is given to the potential future role of nurses in the public health arena.

Part 1: Outlining public health

Case 10.1

Jasmine is a second-year student nurse. On a typical day in practice she washes her hands (often), she encourages healthy eating, she offers reassurance on a variety of health-related topics, she provides advice on lifestyle choices, and she responds to questions about the effects and side effects of drugs or other treatments.

Jasmine is studying to be a mental health nurse, but you cannot tell this merely from the activities listed above. She might just as easily be studying to be a children's nurse, a learning disabilities nurse, or an adult nurse; and she could be working in a hospital or a community setting. Hand washing, encouraging healthy eating, offering reassurance on health-related issues, providing advice on lifestyle choices and answering questions about medications and treatments are all ways in which nurses engage with public health.

These activities are a common aspect of nursing. Of course, the detail will be different within each branch, for example:

- A learning disabilities nurse might help residents of a group home to choose their evening meal.
- A children's nurse might help a young child to learn how to brush her teeth.
- An adult nurse might advise on dietary choices for someone recovering from a heart attack.
- A mental health nurse might encourage an individual to practice relaxation techniques.

Nurses do these sorts of things as part of their everyday nursing practice, and each activity contributes in one way or another to the health and well-being of individuals and/or groups. These types of contribution form part and parcel of what public health is all about. Thus public health is an essential part of nursing, even if it not all nurses recognise it. This makes public health relevant to all nurses in all branches wherever and whenever nursing takes place. This is why you need to know about public health, and why you should read this chapter.

You will already know that knowledge for nursing is drawn from a wide range of different subject areas. Public health knowledge also comes from a number of different subject areas and adds in its own way to the body of professional nursing knowledge. This chapter offers an explanation and exploration of a number of the core concepts of public health. Some of these concepts contribute to all branches of nursing while others have more specific relevance, and this chapter should help you to understand the relevance of public health to your current and future nursing practice.

Public health is difficult to define. It tends to be understood as an umbrella term for a range of activities undertaken by a number of different professionals who come together to study and/or influence health and patterns of disease. Some of the disciplines that contribute to public health are medicine, **epidemiology**, psychology, sociology, health promotion, nursing, social policy, health information, economics and anthropology. From a nursing perspective, public health is wide-ranging and involves nurses in a variety of ways including aspects of lifestyle choices, social change, environmental issues, empowerment and balancing **health intelligence** and lay knowledge. Traditionally, the focus has been on activities related to disease, particularly communicable disease, and priorities are determined by mortality and morbidity information. More recently public health attention has turned towards demographic trends, health improvement and non-communicable disease. There is also a growing awareness of socio-economic and social influences on health status. Public health priorities are identified on account of their impact on health or resources, their suitability for intervention and their public profiles.

Public health 'is the science and art of preventing disease, prolonging life and promoting health through the organised efforts of society' (Acheson 1988, p. 1).

Epidemiology involves the study of how, when and how often disease spreads, and of the factors that contribute to health and disease among populations.

Health intelligence is a term used to express the idea of collecting information about health which can come from a number of sources and in a number of forms.

Public health or health promotion

'**Health promotion** is the process of enabling people to increase control over, and to improve, their health' (WHO 1986).

The way that the two terms 'public health' and '**health promotion**' are used can be confusing. Naidoo and Wills (2005) suggest both terms should continue to be used and that it may be appropriate to combine them in the form of a single term. Thus you may see it expressed as 'health promotion/public health' or as 'public health and health promotion', and it is always useful to combine both terms when searching the literature. As Naidoo and Wills note, retaining the two terms acknowledges their different historical origins rather than their current differences (health promotion developed from a focus on individual behaviour whereas public health arose out of what used to be called public health medicine). For the purposes of this book you need to know that the terminology of new public health has been adopted, where public health is understood as the overarching discipline within which health promotion is recognised as one of the contributing activities.

Part 2: Explaining public health

Why public health is important for nurses

Promoting health has long been recognised as a part of what nurses do and it continues to be the main public health focus for pre-registration nursing students. However, nurses have been involved in broader aspects of public health in one way or another at least since the time Florence Nightingale unpacked her bags at Scutari. Nightingale recognised the harm that could result from patients being nursed too close together and thus illustrated an early awareness of the need to control and prevent the spread of infectious disease. She also kept meticulous records that provided information to show patterns of disease and recovery (an early example of gathering health intelligence). Public health continues to be part of everyday nursing practice. Health visitors, community nurses, school nurses and infection control nurses are among those that have an obvious and clearly defined public health role, but as suggested in Part 1 of this chapter, all nurses have a part to play in public health, even if this role is not always readily acknowledged or easily understood.

Case 10.2

Linda Wilson is a busy housewife and mother. She has recently been diagnosed with diabetes and is adjusting to her insulin regime. Linda has always been of heavy build and is worried that the more structured eating regime required now will add to her weight. She has been given a lot of information about healthy eating and diabetes but has yet to find time to read it.

Linda enjoys preparing food for the family and often 'finishes off' any food the children leave. She takes an interest in the healthy diet information the children bring home from school but time and cost lead her to stick to what she knows. She knows that she, her husband and her children are overweight. She worries when she reads about childhood obesity in the newspapers and sees features on TV. She would like to set a good example to the children but worries that the diabetic regime would not suit that. Linda feels that she is 'always on the go' and can't understand why she never loses weight. She has been unable to establish a pattern of exercise beyond walking the children to school.

Linda is the type of client you might meet in a number of different practice settings, such as the diabetic clinic of an outpatient department, an accident and emergency department, a local health centre, or an acute medical or surgical ward. Her situation illustrates many of the issues that currently challenge public health: the steady increase in lifestyle-related health problems such as diabetes; the role of the media and its influence on health behaviour; lifestyle issues such as diet and exercise; the link between poverty and problems such as obesity; the health status of individuals and so on. She benefits from health advice from her general practitioner and practice nurse as well as from the school health service through her children. For Linda, and for any nurse advising her, there is a range of options available if she is to establish a balance in her diabetes and develop a healthier lifestyle. This will inevitably require Linda to make changes in some of her behaviours related to, for example, diet and exercise and it provides the opportunity for the promotion of health through health education.

Activity 10.1

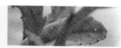

Think about the health care settings you have experienced and try to identify examples of public health activities undertaken by nurses.

As you will probably have identified from Activity 10.1 there are numerous examples of public health activities that take place in everyday nursing practice. For example, during a single working day a nurse might be asked about, amongst other things, giving up smoking, the effects and side effects of medications, holiday vaccinations, benefit entitlements, children's immunisations and advice on lifestyle, all in addition to the usual role of assessing, planning and delivering nursing care. Patients also commonly ask for reassurance about malignant disease and its causes, screening and prognoses, as well as health scares and 'miracle cures' as reported in the media. These issues combine to form part of what makes up the concept of public health and nurses have a major contribution to make.

Public health embraces a whole range of issues that contribute to health or illness and is concerned with, for example, population and individual issues, lifestyle changes and epidemics and health promotion and health protection, all in relation to both individuals and groups. Nurses have a key role to play in this because of the one-to-one patient contact and because of the unique relationship with patients in primary, secondary and tertiary care. Being in direct contact with the public on issues of public health puts a lot of responsibility on the nurse. Members of the public often expect nurses to have enough knowledge and skills to advise and support them across a vast range of health issues, although it is not clear how reasonable these expectations are.

Environmental health officer is a local government role that has developed considerably in recent years to align with public health. Areas of interest include food hygiene, safe environments and health protection.

Public health in the UK currently includes diverse professional groups such as nurses, health promoters, **environmental health officers**, epidemiologists, health statisticians, pharmacists, health researchers, therapists, dieticians, doctors and midwives. Within nursing, amongst those with whom public health nurses work are cardiac rehabilitation nurses, school nurses, occupational health nurses, respiratory and diabetic specialist nurses. Each of these has a specific profile that relates either wholly or partly to public health work. While each has a contribution to make, interdisciplinary and interprofessional working has become a necessity within the sector as the need to build professional alliances and develop innovative practice is increasingly recognised (for more information on interprofessional working see Chapter 5).

As illustrated above, public health is a broad concept, embracing a range of activities related to nursing and beyond. It includes infection control, disease and accident prevention, health promotion, health protection, health improvement and quality issues in the provision of care and service. It has relevance to the practice of all nurses, whether working with individuals, groups, communities or populations. Many elements of daily nursing practice, such as infection control precautions, notification of infection, statistical reporting and observing policies involve the application of public health practice. Many nurses working in the community have explicit and direct links to public health roles including for example, midwives, school nurses, occupational health nurses, some managers and some educationalists. With such a wide-ranging remit it can be difficult to understand the scope and extent of public health in relation to nursing. It is hoped that by reading this chapter you will be better able to understand public health and to see how it links to your current and future practice.

Health promotion in nursing practice

Activity 10.2

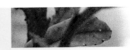

Sabrina works on a busy cardiac unit in a general hospital. Her role involves caring for patients recovering from acute cardiac episodes and most need to consider lifestyle change as part of their recovery. She has an interest in health promotion which (as you now know) forms part of public health practice.
    Have a go at answering the following questions before reading on.

- What type of lifestyle issues would be relevant for Sabrina to address with patients?
- What methods might she use to promote health?
- Who might her target audience be?
- What approaches might be appropriate?

Lifestyle issues

The lifestyle issues for people who have cardiac problems are well documented and include the need to take regular exercise, eat a healthy diet, reduce or give up smoking, reduce alcohol consumption, avoid substance misuse and try to avoid stressful situations.

Sabrina's methods

Many surviving cardiac patients are keen to make changes in their lifestyle in order to reduce their chance of repeat heart problems (even if in the long term most do not make permanent lifestyle changes). So these types of patients are likely to be receptive, at least in the short term, to advice given to them by health care professionals. Typically, a cardiac unit will be awash with information leaflets on promoting healthy eating, taking regular exercise, giving up smoking and moderating alcohol consumption. So a large part of the 'how' of health promotion here involves health education. Cardiac nurses spend a lot of time with patients re-enforcing the message of the need for permanent lifestyle changes to avoid future heart problems. Sabrina might also be able to refer patients to support groups and rehabilitation programmes where exercise regimens can be tailored to the individual needs of patients.

Research focus 10.1

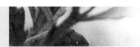

An example of the problems of changing lifestyles is found in the work of Lawlor and Hanratty (2001). Their work looked at the effect of advice regarding physical activity in primary care. They found that it was difficult for patients to make long-term changes on the basis of such advice. Studies in other areas of lifestyle have been more successful, for example, Law and Tang (1995) found more lasting results in relation to smoking. A number of factors play a part in the longevity of lifestyle change and research studies can help us to understand the significance of these for practice.

Sabrina's target audience

Clearly the patient is the primary focus of Sabrina's health promotion activities, and rightly so. However, few individuals can make changes to their lifestyles without it affecting a number of other people. For example, the 48-year-old male who wants to change his diet to eat healthily will need an enormous amount of willpower to make a permanent change if other members of his family continue a regular diet of burgers, chips, chocolate, crisps, doughnuts and other foods high in salt, sugar and saturated fats. This illustrates the point that for health promotion to be successful it needs to do more than merely take aim at individuals.

Sabrina's approaches

These might be thought about in three phases: short, medium and long term. In the short term there are the medical interventions and the immediate changes in behaviour. Sabrina will need to focus on helping patients to understand the

Concordance has replaced the term compliance. Concordance is preferred as it implies patient involvement in agreement to follow the requirements of a treatment regimen.

need for **concordance** with treatment. This will include giving information about the effects and side effects of prescribed medications and about when to seek further medical advice or assistance. Sabrina will also work to help patients understand the need to build up their activities gently, and to know when to slow down or stop during the initial stages of their cardiac rehabilitation programme.

In the medium term Sabrina will focus on providing information, education and advice about what constitutes a healthy diet, what foods to avoid and the importance of regular exercise. She will also stress the importance of making these sorts of lifestyle changes permanent in order to reduce the likelihood of recurrence of cardiac problems. For obvious reasons, Sabrina will need to ensure the information is accurate and given in a way that the patient can understand. The patients Sabrina has contact with will reflect the profile of individuals within the community so while some will be readers of broadsheet newspapers others will read the tabloids, some may be unable to read (e.g., might have eyesight problems or may never have learnt to read) and some will struggle with English as their second language. If Sabrina is to help each cardiac patient to understand the implications of their medical condition she will need to be able to communicate effectively with all types of people (for more on communication skills see Chapter 9).

Long-term approaches to health promotion require changes in the general environment in which we all live. For example, even in the case of a person who wants to make lifestyle changes, it will not matter how much health education they receive if they cannot get to a shop that sells fresh fruit and vegetables.

It is tempting to think that health promotion is just about giving people accurate information and leaving them to make the right choice. If only it were so easy! Public health in general and health promotion in particular is complicated and there are all sorts of reasons why people do not always behave in ways that contribute to their own health, or to the health of others. We will say something about the factors that affect the way people behave in relation to their own health later (see Part 3 of this chapter).

Public health with vulnerable groups

Activity 10.3

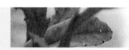

Sanjay works in a community home supporting clients with learning disabilities. The group is made up of six clients – four females and two males. The youngest client is aged 20 and the oldest is 51. Two residents are in a long-term relationship and one other has a girlfriend living elsewhere. Four of the residents are engaged in sheltered work but two are unable to do so due to health problems.

Have a go at answering the following questions before reading on.

- How might Sanjay achieve health improvement with this client group?
- Using the example of food hygiene, consider Sanjay's contribution to health protection.
- How could Sanjay's preventative practice help his clients?
- What knowledge and skills would Sanjay need to work with these clients?

Health improvement

There is a range of areas that Sanjay might focus on in order to assist the residents improve their health including: drug concordance, nutrition and diet, alcohol and smoking, and sexual health and contraception.

Health protection

Safe food-handling is an essential component of safe and effective practice for all nurses. It is even more important for Sanjay because the residents of this group home are likely to be vulnerable to poor food hygiene. If only one member of the home has unhygienic habits it can create a danger for all the residents. So Sanjay will be able to contribute to health protection for the group by taking a lead in promoting good practice in food hygiene. This will involve aspects of personal and kitchen hygiene (e.g., effective hand washing); food storage (e.g., keeping raw and cooked meats separate); and thorough cooking (e.g., ensuring frozen food is properly prepared and cooked).

Prevention

Prevention involves some kind of intervention designed to stop something from happening, directly or indirectly. It requires knowledge, skills and attitudes and may encompass health education and protection. Examples include contraception, immunisation, avoiding stress, and anger management.

Knowledge and skills

It should be clear by now that if Sanjay is going to be effective in health improvement and protection he will not only need to be knowledgeable about the things identified as important for his particular area of practice but will also need to be skilled in encouraging and enabling this specific client group to adopt healthy rather than unhealthy behaviour. So Sanjay will need knowledge of, amongst other things, nutrition, food preparation and hygiene, workplace safety, sexual health and contraception, and alcohol and drugs. He will also need to have the skills to communicate effectively with people with different communication abilities and be able to facilitate learning for individuals of varying intellectual capacities (for more about communication skills see Chapter 9; for more about learning and teaching see Chapter 11).

Hospital-based public health

Activity 10.4

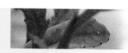

Marte is a staff nurse working in a mental health facility. She works on Forsythia Ward, an 18-bedded unit where most patients have long-term problems. Some patients spend long periods in supportive care environments, including acute hospital care, and depend on that infrastructure. The ward includes some rotational respite beds so Marte also has a changing group of clients who have home carers and so have different needs and challenges. In this group her care is focused not just on the client but on the carers too.

Have a go at answering the following questions before reading on.

- What contribution might Marte make to public health?
- Identify three priority issues that she could address with this client group.
- What barriers may prevent Marte from working productively with her client group?
- What are the advantages of working in this setting?

Contribution

The contribution nurses make to the mental well-being of individuals and groups is often overlooked. Nevertheless, the link between physical and mental health is widely recognised and there is growing acceptance of the idea that physical health actually depends on mental health (Naidoo and Wills 2005, WHO 2005). There is some recognition of the psychological needs of patients in general health care environments: providing information as a way to reduce anxiety in pre-operative patients is one example of the contribution adult and children's nurses make in this respect (although providing information may increase anxiety in some patients). Mental health nurses make a much more obvious contribution in respect of people with mental health problems as well as to their relatives and carers. Indeed some might say that this is the point of mental health nursing or, to put this another way, mental health nursing can be said to have public health at its very core.

Thus Marte's contribution to public health is both general and particular. The general contribution stems from her everyday work but her particular contribution might involve, amongst other things, health intelligence (including, for example, the collection of data on inpatient stays and notifiable health problems), health protection (the application of policies to assist in the proactive management of health problems) and health promotion and prevention.

Priority issues

There are a number of priority issues that Marte might focus on depending on the nature of the particular mental health problems of the clients on Forsythia Ward. She might, for example, focus on identifying patients at risk of suicide, following the National Suicide Prevention Strategy (DH 2002), or she might focus on **empowerment**, stress management, safety, or lifestyle issues (such as diet, smoking reduction or cessation, alcohol and drug use and abuse, or exercise).

Empowerment involves assisting individuals to make independent decisions and so to take control of their lives. In public health terms this relates to enabling people to make autonomous and informed health-related choices.

Barriers

Barriers are factors that impede or prevent effective action. For example, institutionalisation, lack of cooperation from colleagues, lack of commitment of colleagues/families can all impede Marte in her public health work with this group of clients.

Advantages

One advantage is that Marte has everyday contact with each client on the ward so they are, so to speak, something of 'a captive audience'. This enables Marte to build relationships over time with the clients as well as with their relatives and carers, which can help Marte to identify priorities for health improvement activities within a supportive environment.

Outbreak of *E. Coli*: management of an infectious source

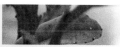

Activity 10.5

Betsan is a practice nurse. Three patients from the practice have been identified as having *E. Coli*, a form of food poisoning notifiable under public health regulation. Two of the patients are children attending the local primary school and the third is an 84-year-old lady. There are seven other cases within a five-mile radius and the public health emergency response team have identified the source of the outbreak as infected meat, sold at the local market.

Have a go at answering the following questions before reading on.

* What role might Betsan have in dealing with patients about the *E. Coli* issue?
* What issues/topics might she cover?
* Who would she liaise with on this public health problem?
* What information sources could she use?

Role

News of an outbreak of an infectious form of food poisoning (such as the one described here) travels quickly around a community. Local people will soon know about it, it may become a story in the local news media, and it may even make national headlines. As a result Betsan may find she becomes besieged with requests for information and advice, particularly from patients registered with the practice. Thus Betsan will need to act as both health educator and care advisor. She is also likely to have a significant role in relation to the collection and testing of samples of faecal matter in conjunction with the local pathology department.

Topics

Betsan will need to provide information on personal hygiene (particularly the importance of effective hand washing) and food hygiene (including food handling) and she will need to be able to offer advice on care for those suffering from food poisoning.

Liaison

Betsan will need to liaise with a range of different professionals including general practitioners, school nurses, members of the local public health team, pathologists and local government officers (in particular, environmental health officers).

Information services

Betsan will be able to access information from a range of sources (e.g., the health protection agency, NHS Direct, the Internet, leaflets and clients themselves) and work with a range of personnel including specialist colleagues (e.g., environmental health officers and pathologists).

Public health in industrial settings: risk management

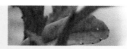

Activity 10.6

Kamaria is an occupational health nurse working in a factory where cleaning products are made. Her role involves monitoring the health of the workforce, maintaining health and safety awareness and health promotion.

Several incidents of exposure to noxious substances have attracted attention at the factory in the past two years. Two cases involved workers; one a case of accidental spillage when not wearing protective clothing and the second a case of inhalation of fumes caused by the interaction of substances in a storage area. The Health and Safety Inspectorate are investigating both cases.

The third, more recent, case involves a youth who accidentally came into contact with fluids stored securely in the yard area while trespassing at night. Local environmental health officers in collaboration with the police and safety agencies are investigating the incident. The factory owners are cooperating fully and want Kamaria to participate in the public health aspects of maintaining workers' health.

Have a go at answering the following questions before reading on.

- How might Kamaria be involved?
- What are the key aspects?
- What approaches could Kamaria use?
- How might Kamaria organise her intervention?

Involvement

Kamaria is likely to be involved in a number of different ways. In terms of health promotion she will help in educating the factory workforce about the dangers of working with or near noxious chemicals. She may be the first point of contact for employees who are exposed to the chemicals, providing care and ongoing support. She may also become involved with the media, and she will probably contribute to the development of a factory-wide action plan to reduce the likelihood of future incidents of exposure to noxious chemicals.

Key aspects

Kamaria will need to be knowledgeable about the Control of Substances Hazardous to Health (COSHH) regulations, the care and maintenance of safety equipment, good hygiene practice and first aid, particularly in relation to noxious chemical exposure.

Approaches

Kamaria will need to take a number of different approaches if she is to contribute to the way risk is managed in the factory. By providing education she can aim not only to help change the way people behave in relation to noxious chemicals but also to empower individuals to take control of risk management for themselves.

Organising interventions

Kamaria will need to be proactive if she is to make a contribution to the health and well-being of everyone associated with the factory. Given that the factory owners are supportive of her role it should be possible for Kamaria to set out a plan of action on helping manage risk across the organisation. She could engage with labelling products and stored chemicals, and with an information campaign in the local press to remind the public that this workplace is dangerous and not for public access.

She could stage health education sessions for the workforce on:

- safe storage and handling of substances;
- the importance of wearing protective clothing;
- first aid if accidental exposure occurs.

She might also get involved in spot checks to ensure that protective measures are being taken, which could form part of team-building by praising or rewarding the staff who take the risks seriously and respond accordingly.

Public health and nursing

Each of the above examples illustrates ways in which nurses engage with public health. As you might expect health promotion looms large but as each scenario suggests, it is not always easy to separate health promotion from other aspects of public health. This is why public health is now understood as reflecting a broad idea of the factors that contribute to the health and well-being of individuals and communities; and it is why nurses are seen as well placed to make a significant contribution. As a result:

1. Public health has a place in pre-registration nurse education in the form of evidence-based practice, health needs assessment, infection control, risk and crisis management, health protection and improvement and quality issues;
2. More areas of nursing are developing an awareness of public health and working with other disciplines on public health targets and population health; and
3. It is now possible for nurses with a particular interest in public health to become registered as specialist community public health nurses and to work alongside specialists in the field from diverse disciplines.

Part 3: Exploring public health

Along with the recognition of public health as an important aspect of nursing comes a responsibility for each nurse to engage with other professionals to enhance and advance the public health agenda (Baggott 2000). Nurses are well placed to make a very real contribution to public health because of their versatility, their wide range of public contact and because of their nursing knowledge, clinical experience and health assessment skills. This potential has been recognised by the Standing Nursing and Midwifery Advisory Committee (SNMAC 1995) and has become increasingly relevant as more and more practitioners, whatever their area of work or specialism, recognise the public health aspects of their daily practice. Craig and Lindsay (2000) have outlined the general nature of the nursing contribution, although they are clear that no one area of nursing can claim the connection exclusively or in isolation. They specifically identify the need for more information and training to equip nurses to fulfil their potential to contribute to public health. This is particularly important as public health is developing quickly with a multidisciplinary focus.

A little bit of history

Public health in the UK began to develop following the 1834 Poor Law Amendment Act and was influenced by the work of Edwin Chadwick, culminating in the first Public Health Act of 1848. Historically, there have been two main thrusts of public health, preventative interventions (including broad improvements in social conditions) and the provision of curative health services (see Figure 10.1).

The social reforms of the nineteenth century provided a series of preventative interventions that laid the foundation for improvements in the general level of health and well-being of the population. During the twentieth century, and particularly after the formation of the National Health Service in 1948, health care provision became increasingly dominated by a focus on curative services for individuals with only minor attention given to preventative interventions. Now, in the early part of the twenty-first century, the recognition of the need to ensure a balance between preventative and curative services is finding a voice in policy statements and in practice. Modern (or new) public health favours a population-based approach in which health promotion, health improvement

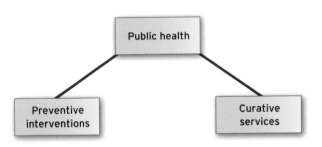

Figure 10.1 The two traditional thrusts of public health.

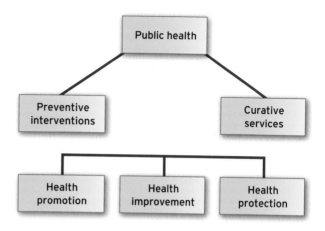

Figure 10.2 The new public health.

and health protection lie alongside each other in the attempt to straddle the traditional preventative/curative division (see Figure 10.2).

Skills for public health

If you have done the activities in Part 2 of this chapter you may have recognised already some of the skills that you will need if you are to engage with public health in ways that are appropriate to wherever you find yourself working as a registered nurse. The good news is that many of these skills are the same skills you need for safe and effective nursing practice, so engaging in public health does not necessarily require you to acquire a new set of special skills. However, if you decide to work in a nursing role that has public health as a primary focus, or if you decide to seek specialist community public health nursing registration, you will need to develop expertise in these skills.

Activity 10.7

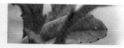

Review the information that follows Activities 10.2 to 10.6 inclusive in Part 2 of this chapter. Identify what skills the nurse needs in each case.

The chances are that in doing Activity 10.7 you will have identified some skills that are common across the cases. Perhaps the three most striking common aspects of the public health role are:

1. Knowledge
2. Communication
3. Education.

Knowledge

In each scenario the nurse needs to know what they are talking about. If Sanjay and Betsan are to be effective in encouraging good personal and kitchen hygiene among their respective client populations they need to know what good practice in personal and kitchen hygiene actually requires. They need to know about effective hand washing, they need to know why it is necessary to store raw meat away from cooked meat as well as how to do this effectively, and they need to know how pathogenic organisms spread as well as the ways in which poor personal hygiene contributes to outbreaks of food poisoning.

Similarly, Sabrina needs up-to-date knowledge about cardiac rehabilitation protocols and treatment regimens, while Kamaria needs a working knowledge of the control of substances hazardous to health (COSHH) regulations, and Marte may need to know what is currently available for people who want to give up smoking.

In each case the nurse needs to be knowledgeable and this knowledge needs to be accurate and based on current best evidence. Many people become cynical about, for example, the possibility of healthy eating when faced with the conflicting information that arrives with their daily newspapers. The influence of the media on public perception about public health and health promotion should not be underestimated, so as a nurse you need to be well informed (and this usually means better informed than the newspapers) about the topic and able to explain what the evidence suggests at this time, while acknowledging new evidence might lead to different advice in the future. This can be a difficult message to get across and it points to the second of the common aspects of public health as identified above.

Communication

In each scenario the nurse needs to be able to communicate effectively with a range of different individuals and groups. Sanjay needs to be able to communicate effectively with people who have varying degrees of cognitive and/or physical abilities, Sabrina needs to be able to explain the implications of living with cardiac disease to individuals (and their families) with widely differing understandings of normal and abnormal physiology (in this case how the heart works and what happens when it goes wrong), and Marte will need a range of strategies to ensure she can be heard by those suffering psychotic episodes. Kamaria will be communicating with factory workers and managers as well as with officials (police, safety officers and environmental health officers) and perhaps members of the public. Similarly, Betsan will be communicating with a range of individuals including patients registered with the practice, school children, local government officials and members of the general public. In addition, Kamaria and Betsan may find themselves fielding and responding to media enquiries.

While there are some common key skills of communication (see Chapter 9) there are significant differences in applying these skills in different situations and specific techniques may be needed for particular audiences. For example, getting your message across in media size 'sound bites' for general consumption requires a very different approach than that needed when confronted with 120 young children in a primary school assembly. So when liaising with officials, Kamaria and Betsan will need to use different terminology to that needed when working with health care colleagues and different terminology again when talking to the general public or the media. While perhaps less dramatic, Marte, Sanjay and Sabrina also need to be able to adapt their language and approach depending on the particular individuals or groups they are trying to communicate with at any given time.

This capacity to adapt the message to the audience applies equally to all other aspects of nursing if a nurse is to be able to communicate effectively. The skill needed to do this should not be underestimated and is a skill that takes on even more importance when one of the aims of communication involves education, the third common aspect of public health as identified above.

Education

There are elements of education in each scenario as in each case the nurse has a role in facilitating learning and, as noted with communication above, the nurse needs to be able to adapt their skills to meet the needs of particular learners. For Sanjay this is further complicated because the residents are acknowledged as having learning difficulties: knowing how each of the residents learns best is crucial if they are to develop and retain good hygiene habits. Knowing how people learn best will be helpful in all cases although it is not always possible (nor necessarily desirable) to individualise learning in all circumstances.

When Kamaria or Betsan provide information via the media they will be attempting to educate the public but will need to concentrate on only one or two key messages. This means that they will need to both identify the most important aspects of the situation and be able to articulate those aspects in ways that are accurate, legitimate and believable. Given the media tendency to sensationalise, this might be a difficult task, especially as the public is known to have a healthy scepticism about official pronouncements on health scares.

Facilitating learning is a fundamental aspect of nursing practice. By way of example, nurses help people to learn how to manage their medications, how to care for their indwelling catheters, how to live with long-term conditions (e.g., diabetes, chronic pain), and how to recognise when they need to seek further medical, or non-medical, advice. Nurses also help families to adapt to living with the changing health-related circumstances of one or more of their members, as well as supporting a variety of different learners (nursing and/or other health and social care students, new members of staff, unqualified staff undertaking national vocational qualifications and so on). Nurses also facilitate their own learning in respect of what they need to know in order to remain a safe and effective practitioner beyond the point of qualification.

As Sabrina recognised (see Activity 10.2), merely supplying information does not necessarily mean that the person will learn something. For learning to take place, the learner (in this case the patient and their family) must understand the information in a way that makes sense to them in their particular situation. It is the facilitation of this process of understanding that nurses engage with when they attempt to enable individuals to, for example, learn to live with their newly diagnosed diabetes.

The skills involved in being knowledgeable, communicating and facilitating learning are many and varied and you will find some information about these skills elsewhere in the book (see Chapter 11). For now the main point is to recognise that public health is a core part of nursing practice, and the skills and knowledge necessary for safe and effective nursing practice are the same skills that enable nurses to make an effective contribution to public health.

Public health nursing as a specialism

Public health nursing is a distinct specialism and has been defined as 'the synthesis of the art and science of public health and nursing' (Minnesota Department of Health 2001). Although constructed with reference to the American public health nursing model, the essential tenets of the Minnesota model translate well into the UK context.

The Minnesota model combines elements from both public health and nursing. Public health contributes a population-based approach with a focus on health promotion and prevention, a grounding in social justice and an emphasis on the greater good. It is driven by epidemiology and in turn organises community resources and long-term community commitments. From nursing the approach draws on independent action within relationships based in an ethic of caring, sensitivity to diversity, a holistic focus and respect for all.

This combination draws together key issues from public health and nursing, and offers a holistic perspective spanning the range from an individual to societal approaches. Thus public health nursing practice:

- Is based on the values of social justice, compassion, sensitivity to diversity, and respect for the worth of all people, especially the vulnerable.
- Derives its authority for independent action from legislation.
- Focuses on entire populations.
- Reflects community priorities and needs while seeking to maintain established caring relationships within communities, families, individuals and systems.
- Promotes health through strategies driven by epidemiological evidence.
- Seeks collaboration with community resources to achieve those strategies (although it will work independently if necessary).
- Encompasses mental, physical, emotional, social, spiritual, and environmental aspects of health.

Public health nursing in the UK

The NMC describes specialist community public health nursing:

> *Specialist community public health nursing aims to reduce health inequalities by working with individuals, families, and communities promoting health, preventing ill health and in the protection of health. The emphasis is on partnership working that cuts across disciplinary, professional and organisational boundaries that impact on organised social and political policy to influence the determinants of health and promote the health of whole populations.*

(NMC 2006)

Since 2004 in the UK, nurses who are able to demonstrate the necessary competencies can register with the NMC as 'specialist community public health nurses'. Thus the NMC Register now has three parts: one for nurses; one for midwives; and one for specialist community public health nurses. For many this registration on what is referred to as the 'Third Part of the Register' follows a period of graduate or postgraduate study leading to an NMC-recognised qualification in public health nursing. Nurses working in public health who do not hold a NMC-recognised public health qualification can apply for specialist community public health nursing registration through the development of a portfolio of evidence demonstrating achievement of the NMC Standards of Proficiency for Specialist Community Public Health Nurses (NMC 2004b).

The standards of proficiency relate to practical and theoretical learning in specialist community public health nursing. Safe and effective public health nursing practice is underpinned by theoretical knowledge that informs practice and is in turn informed by that practice. This includes risk assessment, developing effective relationships, dealing with conflicting priorities and using different theories and perspectives. Specialist community public health nurses work with and respond to the changing and developing health needs of the public and communities. Practice is informed by evidence and professional development and public health nurses need to have the capacity not only to adapt to change but to identify the need for change and, where appropriate, initiate and lead change.

As such, nursing is playing an increasing part in the development of public health alongside other professions within health care from medical staff to therapists, pharmacists to statisticians, environmental health officers to epidemiologists and academics. However, development is also influenced by other factors such as the media, which plays a significant part in public health in terms of attitude formation and is an important source of health information. Harrabin and colleagues (2003) have identified potentially problematic effects in the relationship between public health and policy resulting from media influence. Media interest in health is functional so the portrayal of health issues is often negative or sensational, ignoring the less dramatic or high-tech topics. An example of this is the MMR vaccination programme. The media took up parental concerns in response to research at an early stage. The research was generalised and presented as more significant than was actually the case. This had the effect of stimulating parental concern, contributing to a marked reduction in the numbers taking up this vaccination. Recovery in vaccination rates continues to be slow despite the fact that the risk has now been shown to be minimal.

The language used by the media can be emotive, emphasising the potential harm in a situation or playing to the natural fear people feel regarding health, illness and the health service. Many staff involved in public health work spend a great deal of time and effort working to lessen these fears and to provide realistic and accurate information and advice. Harrabin and colleagues (2003) suggest the need for an informed exchange between the media and health (policy-makers, managers and practitioners) on the grounds that such arrangements would be of greater benefit to the public in the long term. Of course, the media tends not to have public health as its primary concern so any such arrangement might be difficult to initiate or sustain.

New public health

'New public health' is characterised by understandings of the relationship between health and lifestyle, the need to invest resources, policy, programmes and services in healthier ways of living and better environments. Craig and Lindsay (2000) propose that nursing and public health come together through the notion of the 'new public health' movement. They concur with Ashton and Seymour's (1988) view of the new public health movement as one in which health is viewed as a function of lifestyle and environment (influenced by biology and care provision) and the social aspects of health. This is important because it governs the way in which we respond to those influences. Approaching the 'problem', if one is identified, may be best from a policy or strategy perspective or it may require a 'grassroots' approach, working from the basics. Current approaches are characterised by terms such as bottom-up (referring to the emphasis of action originating from practice or the population) or top-down (referring to strategists, policy-makers and authority) or as upstream or downstream (see Box 10.1).

Box 10.1   Upstream versus downstream

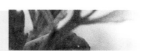

Imagine you come across a person drowning in a river. You jump in and pull them to safety only to find a second drowning person coming down the same river. You save the second person only to find a third in need of rescue, then a fourth and fifth and so on. Such a process demands a great deal of your time and energy and if it continues, no matter how hard you try you will never be able to save everyone. You might enlist a passer-by to help but even as you take turns in saving the poor souls floating down the river, and even as you get further offers of help, you have a never-ending situation with several people constantly occupied in responding to an ongoing problem.

However, if you make the time to think about it you might start to wonder what is causing so many people to fall into the river in the first place. Assuming you can organise a rota with enough people to continue rescuing drowning individuals, you might venture 'upstream' to try to find out what is going on. Imagine you find people trying to cross a partly submerged bridge only to be swept away by the current. Now that you have identified the root cause of the problem you can try to do something about it. In this case you might work with the local people to raise the bridge above the waterline to make it safe to cross. With few, if any, people now falling into the river the effects downstream will be dramatic and might result in a need only for the strategic placing of an emergency lifebelt.

In this analogy being downstream rescuing drowning people represents a health intervention that reacts to the unfortunate and obvious outcomes of a deeper, more fundamental problem (so it is a reactive approach), whereas in the attempt to be 'upstream' new public health aims to repair the broken bridges of health by taking a preventive and more proactive approach.

The development of public health in the UK and beyond

The **World Health Organization** (WHO) is a global institution, structured on a continental basis. The UK is part of WHO Euro – the European section.

Major public health development has occurred in recent years on a global scale orchestrated by the **World Health Organization** (WHO) which works to improve health across continents and countries by involving local populations and by providing supporting expertise. In the UK the development of public

The **Acheson Report** (1988)
The 1988 Report produced
by Lord Acheson that led to
the establishment of annual
reporting on the state of the
public health and the role of
the Director of Public Health
in all areas of the UK.

health has been influenced by the Acheson report. The **Acheson Report** (Acheson 1988) specifically sought to use the term 'public health medicine' rather than 'community health', reflecting the medical dominance and disease focus of the time. The report recommended the appointment of Directors of Public Health in each Health Authority to lead the specialism by establishing working priorities, planning and evaluating strategy, policy development and the control of communicable diseases.

Lucas and Lloyd (2005) have explored the long-standing medical dominance in public health and the differential between the effects in the UK and America. They have identified the American educational approach as more multidisciplinary and note that the pace of change away from medical dominance in the UK has been slow. The development of public health has been a gradual process following the publication of the Acheson report for a number of reasons to do with structure and funding. There has been an increased interest since the emergence of the 'new' public health that emanated from work in the UK by Ashton and Seymour (1988) and the **Ottawa Charter** (WHO 1986). This increased interest has been fuelled by theoretical debate, resource pressures and policy drivers and has had the effect of accelerating the development of public health. Changes in public perceptions and media pressure have also had an effect in identifying shortcomings and unmet needs and thereby stimulated public awareness. These factors have combined to create the momentum for change currently evident in public health.

The **Ottawa Charter** is a
strategy for global health
promotion, produced by the
WHO at Ottawa, Canada in
1986. The Charter champions
five principles: (1) strengthen
community action; (2) develop
personal skills; (3) build healthy
public policy; (4) create
supportive environments; and
(5) reorient health services,
together with three modes
of action: (1) enabling; (2)
mediation; and (3) advocacy.

Baggott (2000) recognised the pattern of variation in the dominance (or otherwise) of public health within health care and in the approaches taken to it over time, while Bunton and MacDonald (2002) identify the shift from a social towards an environmental focus as part of the new public health of the late twentieth century. This is reflected in the WHO (1985) Health for All strategy in health improvement that has endured as a set of guiding principles, but the emphasis has developed more towards environmental aspects, inequalities and sustainability. The concerted development of public health on a more international basis in line with Health for All has been helped by initiatives such as **Healthy Cities**. This work was based on WHO principles of reorienting health services towards primary care, promoting public participation and partnerships and improving the health of those most in need.

The **Healthy Cities** initiative.
A European (WHO Euro)
initiative designed to facilitate
the development of health
promotion in urban
environments. During the
1980s and 1990s, five UK cities
participated in this initiative.

This combined with environmental developments such as Local Agenda 21, which drew local authorities into more integrated planning on environmental issues, and helped to establish a more positive and interactive context for health improvement. The gradual progression of the public health movement across Europe suggests a higher future profile and the potential for more unified health strategies in the long term. The important thing about strategy is that it provides guidance to enable the operational delivery of better health and a framework for action.

The public health context

Public health focuses on individuals and populations, seeking to protect and improve health through surveillance, notification, regulation and jurisdiction. Public health is described by **Skills for Health** as:

- Taking a population perspective
- Mobilising the organised efforts of society and acting as an advocate for the public's health
- Enabling people and communities to take control over their own health and well-being
- Acting on the social, economic, environmental and biological determinants of health and well-being
- Protecting from and minimising the impact of health risks to the population
- Ensuring that preventive, treatment and care services are of high quality, based on evidence and are of best value.

(Skills for Health 2004 p. 6)

This description includes many of the aspects of care and public health with which you have become familiar in nursing. Parts of it may also remind you of the WHO (1986) definition of health promotion in the Ottawa Charter and the Acheson Report.

Skills for Health is a UK organisation established in 2002 working to integrate skills development in the health sector across the four home nations. Current priorities include the development of competence-based development in public health practice.

Activity 10.8

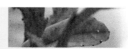

Think about your experience of being a student nurse. Try to identify some of the things you have been told are important considerations in delivering a service to patients and clients in the twenty-first century.

There is a good chance that reflecting on your experiences will lead you to recognise issues such as evidence-based practice, advocacy, interprofessional working, quality assurance and personal responsibility for health. All these issues, in various ways, contribute directly to the purposes of public health. Most are addressed elsewhere in this book so here the focus is on personal responsibility for health.

Personal responsibility for health

There is an often unarticulated and sometimes unacknowledged set of beliefs and values that lie behind the idea that we are all responsible for our own health. The idea is so powerful and so pervasive that it can be difficult for nurses (as well as other health and social care professionals, policy-makers, government spokespersons and so on) to understand why individuals fail to adopt healthy lifestyles. As pointed out in Chapter 2 of this book, this view can lead us to blame some people for their illnesses and might lead us to think that they should wait longer for treatment (or even that they should be denied treatment altogether) on the NHS. For example, in a busy accident and emergency department, the drunk teenager whose fractured fingers resulted from punching a wall on the way home from the pub might not seem to the staff to be as deserving of their attention as the innocent victim of a stabbing. Similarly we might agree with the idea that a person who refuses to give up smoking should not take precedence over the non-smoker on the waiting list for heart bypass surgery (we might even think that they should not be offered surgery at all unless they stop smoking). However, to take such a view is to discriminate on the grounds of desert (i.e., some people are more deserving than others) and echoes the discredited basis of the eighteenth-century poor law with its notion of a deserving and an undeserving poor.

The basis of this discriminatory view comes from a particular perspective about personal responsibility for health that goes something like this:

- There is a lot of easily available health information.
- A great deal of this information is uncontroversial (for example, few people seriously doubt that smoking, eating a diet high in saturated fats, or drinking excessive amounts of alcohol will have a detrimental effect on the health of an individual).
- Any reasonable person will choose to follow a healthy lifestyle.
- Anyone who does not is to blame for their own ill health.

This view is sometimes unintentionally reinforced by attempts at health promotion. For example, if Sabrina (see Activity 10.2) were to take the view that once a person understands the dangers of not making healthy lifestyle choices they are foolish to continue to eat a diet high in salt, sugar and saturated fats, consume excessive amounts of alcohol and lead a sedentary lifestyle; and therefore to be blamed for their future ill health. If only it were so simple!

Some of the limitations of this view can be quickly outlined.

1   It takes little account of individual genetic make-up or inherited features

While we all share a common physiology there remain differences in individual physiological responses to threats to health. Not everyone who smokes will develop a life-threatening smoking-related illness (most people claim to know of someone who smoked 20 cigarettes a day for 70 years without ill effect). Not everyone who comes into contact with a pathogenic organism will contract the disease, and even while those that do will exhibit some common symptoms (that is, after all one of the bases for disease classification) each infected person will suffer some symptoms worse than others. Also, not every cardiac patient who returns to an unhealthy lifestyle will do as badly as we might expect.

2   It takes little account of the social situation of individuals

As pointed out earlier, the person who lives in an environment where healthy lifestyle choices are difficult to make is less likely to make permanent (or even temporary) changes. Those without ready access to fresh fruit and vegetables will find it harder to change their diet; those whose social life consists of 12 pints-a-night and a takeaway on the way home may find unpalatable the choice between on the one hand eating healthily but losing any form of social life and on the other continuing the unhealthy eating but retaining friends. Put this way, it is not so hard to understand why some people decide against adopting a healthier lifestyle. To assume that individuals will want to extract themselves from their social situation just to follow the health promotion advice of health care professionals is to fail to understand that not everybody values their health equally.

3   It assumes a specific (professional-oriented) view of 'reasonableness'

When health care professionals talk about people being reasonable (or unreasonable), what they often mean is reasonable as defined from a professional perspective steeped in a particular set of values and beliefs about health. Health advice comes from what might be described as an educated and well-informed section of society that does not reflect the diversity of the general population. Arguably, being 'reasonable' in the sense that a reasonable person does not take unnecessary risks with their health can be paternalistic, for it is rather like being told what to do by those who think they know best. Yet health care professionals themselves are often guilty of taking risks with their health. Skiing, bungee jumping, playing rugby, horse riding and driving might seem more respectable pastimes than smoking, drinking or recreational drug use but they all contain elements of risk to the health of participants. The cost to the health service of sporting injuries is significant and yet headlines suggesting skiers should not receive treatment because their injuries are self-inflicted, or that rugby-playing injuries are an unjustified drain on limited health care resources, are noticeable by their absence.

4   It takes little account of people's individual goals or priorities

Similarly, the idea that health has a specific value or that it should be a high priority 'good' reflects a normative belief (a belief about how things ought to be) rather than an empirical fact (how things really are). Not everyone places their own health above other considerations in their lives. Parents may place the health and well-being of their children over and above their own. Many individuals simply do not believe they will suffer ill effects from unhealthy lifestyle choices, and some (particularly young) people believe themselves to be invulnerable or invincible, or that ill health is something that happens only to other people. Others still may merely think that if they are to suffer ill health it will happen so far in the future as to not be worth worrying about just now. Indeed, health care workers are not immune from this: how else can we explain the fact that some health care workers smoke, drink to excess and eat diets high in salt, sugar or saturated fats?

5   It takes little account of wider considerations

No one would argue with claims about the positive health effects of good sanitation, clean air and clean drinking water. Neither would many argue with the benefits of public health policies such as the compulsory wearing of seat belts or crash helmets. Yet when we advise individuals about ways they might make healthier lifestyle choices we often ignore the powerful influence of factors individuals can do little, if anything, about. The food industry remains a powerful influence and even if our local supermarket offers us choice it is not always easy to understand which products constitute healthy options. Low fat, low salt or low sugar products might not necessarily be healthy options (it all depends on what else they contain).

6   It assumes a common view about risk-taking

Each of us views risk differently. For some the idea of climbing Everest is a complete non-starter because it is just too risky, for others it is the risk itself that makes the idea attractive. The point is that we each have a different view not only about what constitutes risk but also about how much risk we are prepared to take. For our mountaineer, the risk of not rock climbing may be a life bereft of meaning or a risk of death by boredom, and this would compromise her or his well-being. For some, the risk of future ill health is insufficient motivation for changing current behaviour, particularly if that behaviour is pleasurable.

This is a brief overview of some of the difficulties of a simplistic view of health promotion. For a more detailed discussion see, for example, Naidoo and Wills (2005).

Reflection and public health

Reflection can be useful in enabling nurses to assess their beliefs, values and approaches to practice in general and to public health in particular. Reflection is an intrinsic part of nursing practice but has only recently been recognised as an important element of health promotion. Fleming (2006) has explored the value of reflection in relation to his preventive work on managing aggression in occupational settings. While this is a highly specialised area of intervention, he emphasises the way in which reflection can improve practice. To enable health promotion practitioners to engage in reflection in a planned and coherent manner, Fleming (2006) has developed a Typology for Reflective Practice (see Figure 10.3) which focuses on three domains of practice, the role of self (individuals and teams), the influence of the planning context (socio-economic and other environmental and political factors) and issues related to the process of planning/delivery of programmes. Other domains of public health practice could be replaced or inserted, linking your understanding of reflection in general to the specifics of public health. Reflection is a transferable skill and nurses can use it in their daily practice, in health promotion and to help others to understand public health.

The purpose of public health

Skills for Health state that the purpose of public health is to:

- Improve the health and well-being of the population.
- Prevent disease and minimise its consequences.

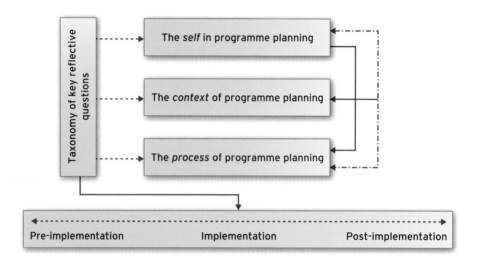

Figure 10.3 Typology for reflective practice.
Source: After Fleming (2006).

- Prolong valued life.
- Reduce inequalities in health.

Skills for Health (2004 p. 6)

Thus the range of activities that fall within the remit of public health practice has extended from the traditional medical model based on epidemiology and disease prevention to more integrated and proactive models combining health statistics and projection, health education, health improvement, harm reduction and health protection. The issue of competence, skill and knowledge development and practice standards engendered by Agenda for Change (DH 2004a) and the Knowledge and Skills Framework (DH 2005) has been addressed in public health. The development of the National Occupational Standards for Public Health practice (Skills for Health 2004) demonstrates with clarity the areas of practice within the specialism. The ten areas of public health practice are:

1. Surveillance and assessment of the population's health and well-being
2. Promoting and protecting the population's health and well-being
3. Developing quality and risk management within an evaluative culture
4. Collaborative working for health and well-being
5. Developing health programmes and services and reducing inequalities
6. Policy and strategy development and implementation to improve health and well-being
7. Working with and for communities to improve health and well-being
8. Strategic leadership for health and well-being
9. Research and development to improve health and well-being
10. Ethically managing self, people and resources to improve health and well-being.

Skills for Health (2004 p. 6)

As you can see these ten areas of public health are consistent with the general aims of nursing, and most nurses will be contributing to one or more of these ten areas of public health whenever they are engaged in nursing practice.

There are differences in public health provision across the UK. In England, Primary Care Groups replaced general practitioner (GP) fund holders and other commissioning arrangements with a view to gaining Primary Care Trust status over time. In Wales, Local Health Groups were set up to plan and commission services and subsequently became Local Health Boards. In Scotland, local health co-operatives involving GPs were formed under Primary Care Trusts. While the mechanisms varied, the policy was similar in that it replaced the GP fund holder with a more inclusive and cooperative health improvement body.

Each of the four UK nations has developed a strategic framework for public health focusing on health improvement with particular emphasis on improving the health of those most disadvantaged. Each nation has devised targets using disease reduction and prevention approaches with a key focus on reducing social exclusion. While the details of the individual strategies and the means for their delivery differ, they share the common aim of seeking to reduce inequalities through health improvement. Devolution has had an effect on policy development and implementation so difference at the strategic and operational level is to be expected and is likely to continue.

The future of public health

Public health policies such as Choosing Health in England (DH 2004b) and Health Challenge Wales (WAG 2004) have contributed to the Shaping the Future project (DH/WAG 2005). This UK-wide project, known as 'Shaping the Future of Health Promotion' was reported in a document entitled *Shaping the Future of Public Health: Promoting health in the NHS* (DH/WAG 2005). The report explores the specialised role of health promotion in health improvement and the potential for health promoters to meet public health needs. It also gives an indication of the need for core disciplines working in public health to take an integrated approach as the new public health takes centre stage in improving the health and well-being of the UK population.

One critical issue for public health relates to the registration of Specialists in Public Health. The registration was introduced for those practitioners who have attained 'specialist' status as a means of monitoring and supporting excellence and continuing professional development at the highest level in public health practice. Specialist status initially attracted the traditional medical specialists in public health when the United Kingdom Voluntary Register was established. This Register differs from the NMC Register in that it has been constructed around a professional grouping rather than by statute. There are similarities insofar as both set entry criteria and confer enhanced professional status, but the public health register does not have statutory status or mechanisms for the regulation of registration (e.g., regular renewal or the authority to withdraw registration). The NMC Register has one section specifically for specialist community public health nurses, enabling them to register their professional qualification. A specialist community public health nurse cannot practise without such registration but does not need to be registered on the UK voluntary public health register, although they can apply at some other time. Since its inception the Register has been developed and now contains categories for Defined Specialists and Generalist Specialists and this has attracted medically and non-medically trained practitioners working at senior levels in public health. As specialist status has developed so has the debate around how to support and classify others working in public health, resulting in discussions around the development of 'practitioner' status. As one of the wide group of public health staff, public health nurses, alongside therapists, pharmacists, environment health officers and others could seek practitioner status in the specialism. The public health career framework provides a conceptual basis for career development in this area (Public Health Resource Unit 2007).

Conclusion

Public health is an important aspect of nursing practice. Wherever and whenever nursing takes place it is likely that it involves some form of public health. Some nursing activity and some nurses will have an obvious and well-developed public health role while others will choose to make public health the focus of their professional careers. However, because the general aims of public health and the general aims of nursing are so closely aligned most nurses will be making a contribution in one way or another to public health. It is worth remembering that public health is part of nursing practice as identified at a minimum within the NMC *Standards of Proficiency for Pre-registration Nursing Education* (NMC 2004a) as follows:

- Consult with patients, clients and groups to identify their need and desire for health promotion advice.
- Provide relevant and current health information to patients, clients and groups in a form which facilitates their understanding and acknowledges choice/individual preference.

- Provide support and education in the development and/or maintenance of independent living skills.
- Seek specialist/expert advice as appropriate.
- Contribute to the application of a range of interventions which support and optimise the health and well-being of patients and clients.

The dynamic specialism of public health is likely to continue to develop in response to perceived public health needs. The growing prominence of public health and the emerging recognition of its relevance to everyday practice will bring more and more opportunities for nurses to develop their own roles within it. If you now have a clearer understanding of the fundamentals of public health then the aims of this chapter have been met. It is hoped that this understanding will inform your nursing practice and may provide a focus for a stronger interest in the future. However, you should remember that this chapter merely offers an introduction to the complex nature of public health. Should you wish to find out more, look at the list of suggested further reading.

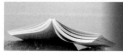

Suggested further reading

Bailey, L., Vardulaki, K., Langham, J. and Chandramohan, D. (2005) *Introduction to Epidemiology*. Maidenhead: McGraw Hill Education/Open University Press.

Davies, M. and Macdowall, W. (eds) (2005) *Health Promotion Theory*. Maidenhead: McGraw Hill Education/Open University Press.

Pomerleau, J. and McKee, M. (eds) (2005) *Issues in Public Health*. Maidenhead: McGraw Hill Education/Open University Press.

Wanless, D. (2001) *Securing our Future Health: Taking a long-term view*. London: Department of Health.

Wanless, D. (2004) *Securing Good Health for the Whole Population*. London: Department of Health.

References

Acheson, D. (1988) *Public Health in England: The report of the committee of inquiry into the future development of the public health function*, CM 289. London: HMSO.

Ashton, J. and Seymour, H. (1988) *The New Public Health: The Liverpool Experience.* Milton Keynes: Open University Press.

Baggott, R. (2000) *Public Health: Policy and politics.* Basingstoke: Macmillan.

Bunton, R. and MacDonald, G. (2002) *Health Promotion: Disciplines, diversity and development.* London: Routledge.

Craig, P. M. and Lindsay, G. M. (eds) (2000) *Nursing for Public Health: Population-based care.* London: Churchill Livingstone.

DH (Department of Health) (2002) *National Suicide Prevention Strategy For England.* London: DH.

DH (2004a) *Agenda for Change – Proposed Agreement.* London: DH.

DH (2004b) *Choosing Health. Making healthy choices easier. Executive Summary.* London: DH.

DH (2005) *The NHS Knowledge and Skills Framework and Development Review.* London: DH.

DH/WAG (Welsh Assembly Government) (2005) *Shaping the Future of Public Health: Promting health in the NHS (Project Report).* London: DH.

Fleming, P. (2006) *Reflection – A Neglected Art in Health Promotion.* Oxford: Health Education Research, Oxford University Press.

Harrabin, R., Coote, A. and Allen, J. (2003) *Health in the News: Risk, reporting and media influence.* London: King's Fund.

Law, M. and Tang, J. L. (1995) An analysis of the effectiveness of interventions intended to help people stop smoking. *Archives of Internal Medicine* **155** (18), 1933–1941.

Lawlor, D. A. and Hanratty, B. (2001) The effect of physical activity advice given in routine primary care consultations: a systematic review. *Journal of Public Health Medicine* **23** (3), 219–226.

Lucas, K. and Lloyd, B. (2005) *Health Promotion: Evidence and experience.* London: Sage Publications.

Minnesota Department of Health (2001) http://www.health.state.mn.us/divs/chs/phn/interventions.html Accessed 9 February 2006.

Naidoo, J. and Wills, J. (2005) *Public Health and Health Promotion: Developing practice* (2nd ed.). Edinburgh: Bailliere Tindall.

NMC (Nursing and Midwifery Council) (2004a) *Standards of Proficiency for Pre-registration Nursing Education.* London: NMC.

NMC (2004b) *Standards of Proficiency for Specialist Community Public Health Nursing.* London: NMC.

NMC (2006) (http://www.nmc-uk.org/). Accessed 18 May 2006.

Public Health Resource Unit (2007) *Public Health Skills and Career Framework.* (http://www.phru.nhs.uk).

Skills for Health (2004) *National Occupational Standards for the Practice of Public Health.* London: Skills for Health.

SNMAC (Standing Nursing and Midwifery Advisory Committee) (1995) *Making it Happen.* London: Department of Health.

WAG (Welsh Assembly Government) (2004) *Health Challenge Wales* (http://wales.gov.uk/hcwsubsite/healthchallenge/?lang=eng).

WHO (World Health Organization) Regional Office for Europe (1985) *Targets for Health for All: Targets in support of the European Regional Strategy for Health for All*. Copenhagen: WHO.

WHO Regional Office for Europe (1986) *The Ottawa Charter*. Geneva: WHO.

WHO (2005) *Promoting Mental Health: Concepts, emerging evidence, practice*. Geneva: WHO.

Chapter 11

Learning and teaching

Derek Sellman and Jane Tarr

Learning outcomes

After reading this chapter you should be able to:

- Recognise that learning and teaching are an integral part of being a registered nurse;
- Develop your own learning capabilities to be an effective learner;
- Identify different approaches to and opportunities for learning;
- Acknowledge the skills, aptitudes and knowledge required to engage in effective learning and teaching;
- Outline factors that contribute to a favourable learning environment;
- Acknowledge the value of self-assessment and self-reflection in enhancing learning;
- Identify barriers to successful learning;
- Discuss the components of effective learning and teaching.

Related NMC Standards of Proficiency for Pre-registration Nursing Education (NMC 2004)

- Use professional standards of practice to self-assess performance.

- Identify and respond to patients' and clients' continuing learning and care needs.

- Demonstrate the ability to transfer skills and knowledge to a variety of circumstances and settings.

- Take action to meet any identified knowledge and skills deficit likely to affect the delivery of care within the current sphere of practice.

- Contribute to creating a climate conducive to learning.

- Contribute to the learning experiences and development of others by facilitating the mutual sharing of knowledge and experience.

Introduction

For a registered nurse, a willingness to facilitate learning is an integral aspect of competent nursing practice. Wherever and whenever nursing occurs, learning is almost certainly taking place. Thus a basic knowledge and understanding of learning and teaching is an essential prerequisite for safe and effective nursing. This chapter helps to articulate the professional obligation for learning and teaching that is made explicit in various Nursing and Midwifery Council (NMC) documents based on the recognition that patients are entitled to a high standard of professional care from registered practitioners.

The chapter is divided into three parts.

In Part 1, we outline some aspects of the topic of learning and teaching, and emphasise the point that the differences between learning and teaching are not as distinct as is commonly thought.

In Part 2, we begin to explain further some important aspects of learning and teaching including the role of the teacher in setting up an environment conducive to learning. We suggest some of the things that make a good or poor teacher and how these things impact upon students' learning. We explain Race's (2006) competency model as a way of assisting in identifying learning needs.

In Part 3, we introduce the idea of individual learning styles and begin to explore some aspects of what makes an effective learner. We also stress the important relationship between effective learning and safe nursing practice.

Part 1: Outlining learning and teaching

Case 11.1

Sarah is a second-year student nurse. On her current placement she notices that many registered nurses do not wash their hands between patients, and of those who do, many used ineffective hand-washing techniques. Sarah has also noticed that quite a lot of nursing staff routinely wear wrist watches, rings with stones, and other assorted adornments that she has been told constitute infection and/or health and safety risks. When she asks her mentor, Steve, about this, he merely shrugs his shoulders and says that he knows they should pay more attention to hand hygiene but the ward is just too busy and anyway the infection rate is no higher here than in any other local practice area.

Those who observe, work with, or are the recipients of nursing care learn a great deal from registered practitioners whether or not these nurses intend to facilitate learning, and regardless of whether this comes from positive or negative experiences. One thing that Sarah has learned from this brief and informal interaction with her mentor is that some registered nurses believe it acceptable not to wash their hands between patients. While there is always room for discretion about whether or not to wash your hands between patients (it depends, for example, on the nature of the contact and whether or not the patient is infectious or in need of protection from infection and so on) the mentor (Steve) demonstrates by his response that in general he knows full well that the staff on the ward should practise effective hand washing.

Both Steve and Sarah might be surprised to find their brief interaction described as educational in nature, but it is clear that Sarah has learned something from Steve so in this sense at least we can describe Sarah as a learner and Steve as a teacher. In fact Steve has learned something from Sarah (at the very least he has been reminded of the importance of hand washing), and in this respect Sarah has been a catalyst for Steve to reconsider one aspect of practice of nurses in this placement. Both aspects of learning here can be described as informal because such learning as occurred did so by chance, and both Steve's and Sarah's teaching can be described as unintentional because neither set out to teach: there were no set learning objectives or outcomes, and no teaching plan. Nevertheless learning and teaching has taken place.

There are, of course, differences between **learning** and **teaching** but these differences are probably harder to describe than you might imagine: while it is superficially attractive to think that 'teachers teach' and 'learners learn' this is a simplistic view. We will say more about this during the rest of the chapter, but for now it is worth noting that there is more that unites than divides learning and teaching. For the purposes of this chapter we take the view that while some roles within educational settings are formal (i.e., student nurses have a formal learning role while mentors, tutors and lecturers have formal teaching roles) learning and teaching is going on all the time in all sorts of situations, most of which would not normally be described as part of the formal educational process. Yet these informal learning and teaching experiences are inevitable and play an important role in learning to become a registered nurse.

While the distinctions are often blurred between learning and teaching, both are central features of nursing practice. To become an effective nurse it is necessary to be both an effective learner and an effective teacher, so it is important to develop your capacities for both. This requires you to recognise not only that you have a preferred way of learning but also that everybody else has a preferred learning style (in other words, not everybody learns in the same way). It also requires an open-minded and flexible approach to both your own and others' learning as well as an ability to engage in a range of different modes of learning and teaching. This is particularly important as you move from the highly structured pre-registration education programme to the often less structured and usually self-directed learning needed for safe and effective practice beyond initial registration.

Learning is a process that we experience throughout our lives although we do not necessarily recognise or understand this. A few moments of reflection can lead us to identify some instances when we learn easily (e.g., recognition of the tune and rhythm of our favourite song) and others where learning is difficult (e.g., completing a self-assessment tax form).

Teaching is a process of sharing one's knowledge, skills, insights, perceptions, values and concepts with another. Teaching can take place in both official/formal settings (e.g., in a classroom) or in classic/informal contexts (e.g., during everyday interactions with others). Teachers themselves will learn from the process of teaching.

Learning in practice

Becoming a registered nurse involves spending time in a variety of different practice settings in the company of a number of different professionals. As a student you will find it easier to adapt (i.e., to learn) in some more than other practice environments. Sacks argues that human beings engage in the process of adaptation to such an extent that it may be necessary to:

> redefine the very concepts of 'health' and 'disease', to see these in terms of the ability of the organism to create a new organisation and order, one that fits its special, altered disposition and needs, rather than in the terms of a rigidly defined 'norm'.
>
> (Sacks 1995 p. xvi)

Adaptation in this sense is the ability to learn to respond to changing environments, and just as patients are generally expected to adapt to their situation and learn to take (at least some) responsibility for their own care and treatment, so students of nursing need to adapt to each new situation and learn to take (at least some) responsibility for their own learning.

When do learning and teaching occur?

Pre-registration nurse education involves a structured programme of learning leading to qualification. Learning and teaching take place all the time in informal as well as formal settings. However, the professional practice of nursing is such that learning and teaching do not cease at qualification, rather there is an expectation that a registered nurse will engage in both processes in order to remain a safe and effective practitioner because the knowledge base from which nursing draws continues to develop. Despite starting as a novice, the student nurse will make a contribution to this development, for example, by asking questions of established and routine practice. The significance on knowledge development of asking questions should not be underestimated: it is through attempts to provide satisfactory answers that insights about what is known and what is not known become apparent. It follows from this that what needs to be learned becomes identified and thus the role of learning and teaching can be seen to occupy an integral part of the role of a nurse.

In this first part of the chapter we have tried to outline some aspects of the scope of learning and teaching as a topic and to make the point that the boundary between learning and teaching is not fixed. While the lecturer is required to teach, there are times when the teacher will learn from you (and if they are learning from you, then you are in some sense teaching). The role of the practice mentor may be to facilitate your learning (which might not be the same thing as teaching) but this facilitation of learning applies equally to others, for example, to patients and their families, to other health care workers, to students of other disciplines and so on. You will also recognise that during your practice placements you sometimes help others to learn, for example, you are engaged in facilitating learning each time you help a patient to manage their take-home medication or whenever you explain your placement assessment paperwork to your mentor.

All this illustrates the point that during your nursing course you will learn all sorts of things in all sorts of ways and in all sorts of situations. Only some of these things will be related directly to the learning outcomes of your programme and only some of this learning will take place in formal settings. You will also be involved in teaching and only sometimes will you be intending to teach (often others will learn from you without you intending to teach them anything). This means that you are constantly surrounded by learning and teaching. Once you recognise this you can use the knowledge and skills you have to facilitate both your own and others' learning to influence the quality of the provision of patient and client care. In other words a basic understanding of learning and teaching is an essential feature of effective nursing practice. In the remainder of this chapter we will explain and explore some of these ideas within the context of nursing practice.

Part 2: Explaining learning and teaching

Case 11.2

Mark is a third-year student nurse on his final placement. He is a bit disappointed when his mentor (Khim) tells him that she wants to work alongside him for the first few days of the placement. Mark feels that Khim ought to recognise his seniority and allow him to get on with his work without being constantly supervised. Mark feels this constant supervision might be appropriate for a first-year student but is unnecessary for an experienced and competent third-year student.

For her part Khim knows that third-year students ought to be able to work on their own but she feels it important to observe for herself what Mark can do and what he cannot yet do, as this will help her to find out what he knows and what he does not yet know. She tries to explain this to Mark, but she senses he thinks she is demanding an unnecessary level of monitoring.

The role of mentor may be relatively easy to articulate but many qualified nurses find it a demanding addition to what they consider their primary role of providing safe and effective nursing care. In fact facilitation of learning is an integral part of being a registered nurse (NMC 2008).

General everyday (i.e., non-nursing) understandings of the idea of mentorship are on the lines that a mentor is someone who encourages, guides and possibly befriends within a relationship that need not be formal or even face-to-face. Writers, artists, musicians, academics and so on sometimes speak of inspirational others as mentors even when they have never met. In this everyday use of the term, a mentor is not allocated but chosen and usually by mutual consent. In nursing the placement mentor role is formalised and is often associated with an assessment function, so much so that many students assume that they will be assessed by their mentor (in some places the role is described as the mentor/assessor role).

In the situation described (Case 11.2 above) both Mark and Khim have expectations of what the mentor relationship entails. Mark thinks he should just be allowed to get on with his work, while Khim thinks she needs to know what he can do and what he knows before he is let loose on the patients. This is perhaps not the best start to their educational relationship. While Mark may well be competent in a wide range of nursing tasks, Khim has a personal and professional responsibility to ensure Mark provides safe and effective care while working under her supervision. This is part of what it means to be a registered and accountable practitioner (see Chapter 1). It is because of this that Khim wishes to be sure that Mark can safely do those things that he says he can do and the only way she can do this is to assess his level of skill and knowledge. Making an assessment of his competencies will also help Khim to devise a planned programme of learning related to Mark's individual learning needs. Merely accepting Mark's word that he can or cannot do something would not provide a secure basis for a programme of learning.

Hence Khim wants to work alongside Mark as much as possible during his first few days because she believes this to be the best way to find out what he knows, how he approaches his work, and how he might best learn during the placement. For his part, Mark is interested in learning and believes he knows exactly what it is he needs to learn. He feels that he does not need to waste time demonstrating (yet again) all the things he knows he can do well. He likes to be left alone to get on with his learning in his own way; that is, doing the things he knows he can do and seeking help when he comes across something new. He finds it difficult to understand why he needs to be watched so much during his first few days on the placement when he has already been 'signed off' in earlier placements as competent in many of these everyday nursing activities.

In this situation even if Mark's claims about what he knows or can do are correct, Khim has no way of knowing this when they first meet. So unless Khim is ready to accept Mark's word for it, she needs to make an assessment of his competencies. In other words, Khim is asking Mark to provide some form of evidence to support his claims about his competences.

Formal and informal learning

There is a tendency to think of learning and teaching as something that happens in formal settings and in relation to specific subjects or for specific purposes. Attending a lecture on infection control or enrolling on a pre-registration nursing course are two examples of what most people would understand as formal education. Yet a few minutes thought about, for example, how you learned to take a patient's temperature should help you to recognise that this learning came about from a combination of:

- Being told how to do it (instruction).
- Watching others do it (observation).
- Having a go at doing it yourself (practice).

Of course, learning rarely flows smoothly from the first to the last of these phases. More often than not a learner will weave in and out of different phases in no particular order, sometimes simultaneously and sometimes only being exposed to one phase long after the others. Often one or more of these phases will have been experienced prior to any involvement in **formal learning**. For example, if previously you worked as a health care assistant you probably

Formal learning is intentional and takes place occasionally; it is often hard work and is time limited. It is frequently an individual intellectual activity based upon effort. It is often reliant upon rewards and tests, and tends to be defined by learning outcomes or objectives.

observed other people taking patients' temperatures, you may have had some practice and you may even have had some formal instruction. In fact, you might have arrived as a student fully competent in temperature measurement. Whatever the case, your previous formal or informal learning will have been different to everyone else's. Yet everyone on the course will have learned something in the new formal learning situation, even if only to confirm existing competence.

Smith (1998) identifies 'two visions of learning: an "official" theory that learning is work and a "classic" view that we learn effortlessly every moment of our waking lives' (Smith 1998 p. vii). The classic view of learning (**informal learning**) suggests that learning is based on self-image and is a social activity that takes place continuously, often at the unconscious level.

In the attempt to improve the educational experience of students there has been a move away from concentrating on the development of different teaching strategies towards a focus on understanding the learning process. Claxton's (2002) concept of 'building learning power' seems particularly well suited to pre-registration nursing programmes because of the emphasis on encouraging students to take control of their own learning by **learning-to-learn**.

Approaches to teaching

If learning takes place in different settings and is reliant upon individuals' self-awareness and self-image, then teachers need to cultivate the 'necessary circumstances and frame of mind for desired learning' (Smith 1998 p. 5). This can be difficult for teachers (as facilitators of learning) because it requires attention to be paid to creating an environment in which learning can take place. In the formal learning environment of a classroom, the knowledgeable teacher encourages in students the development of academic skills (e.g., analysis, synthesis and evaluation). In the formal learning environment of the workplace, the skilled teacher encourages students to apply their knowledge to practical situations. In both settings, part of the role of the teacher is to help the student identify appropriate learning opportunities.

Approaches in **formal learning environments** that encourage discussion and dialogue (e.g., seminars and work-based learning days) are designed to help students build their learning power within a social context. According to Vygotsky (1978), learning is a social process where interaction with peers (especially with more able peers) enables the learner to learn more than they would alone and places emphasis on the **social aspect of learning**. Nursing itself is a social process, so this form of social learning can be readily transferred into the practice setting where the sharing of knowledge between novice and expert can be of benefit to both. The relationships between, for example tutor and student, mentor and student, student and patient, and registered nurse and patient can all provide opportunities to learn.

Informal/classic view of learning. On this view 'Learning is unintentional and it takes place all the time, it is effortless and unbounded, it is a social activity based upon one's self image and is not reliant upon rewards or tests and one can remember most of it!' (Smith 1998 p. 5).

Learning-to-learn is a self-conscious approach to evaluating one's capacity to learn and to develop the skills of self-awareness about how one learns.

The **formal learning environment** is organised and structured to ensure that learning takes place. The considerations and priorities of the teacher in practice are presented for the benefit of the learners.

The **social aspect of learning**: where learning takes place in the company of others through interaction, imitation, observation and conversation. We learn with the help of others and by helping others.

Experiential work-based learning

Learning and teaching occur in the workplace both formally and informally. The more formal aspect of learning in the workplace might be thought of as coaching or mentoring. In a practice setting, a student nurse is normally allocated a **mentor**. Ideally a mentor will be an experienced practitioner who can enable a student to build their learning power as well as a sense of professional identity. The relationship between the novice and the mentor will change over time and each will learn from the other. The level of engagement of the nurse with the social environment that is the work placement will influence their capacity to learn from the experience. As Dewey explains:

> *The social environment . . . Is truly educative in its effects in the degree in which an individual shares or participates in some conjunct activity. By doing his share in the associated activity, the individual appropriates the purpose which actuates it, becomes familiar with its methods and subject matters, acquires needed skill and is saturated with its emotional spirit.*
>
> (Dewey 1916 p. 26)

Thus responsibility for learning is shared between student and mentor in the practice setting, but is affected by the social environment of the workplace which helps to form part of a **learning community** in which everyone's capacity to learn is enhanced. The existence of special interest groups (SIGs) reflects this idea of learning communities in which professionals demonstrate an understanding of the need to continue to learn from the opportunities that emerge from their work with clients. Wenger (2000) describes such groupings as 'communities of practice' that form the basis of social learning. Members of a community of practice come together through pursuit of a joint enterprise, through mutual engagement and through the development of a shared repertoire of professional aspirations. It is suggested that learning is enhanced within such a social community because it generates credibility and energy, members within the group learn about each other in a positive manner and this encourages self-reflection. Such an approach is thought to be useful in developing professional identity and in enhancing the learning of all participants, whether novice or expert.

> *Communities of practice grow out of a convergent interplay of competence and experience that involves mutual engagement. They offer an opportunity to negotiate competence through an experience of direct participation. As a consequence they remain important social units of learning even in the context of much larger systems.*
>
> (Wenger 2000 p. 229)

Becoming a nurse in the twenty-first century requires each student to demonstrate their learning by meeting a set of predetermined learning outcomes attached to the different modules that together make up the pre-registration nursing programme of learning. Meeting the learning outcomes of the course requires you to undertake a range of assessments designed to measure your achievement against each of the learning outcomes; hence success on the

A **mentor** is an experienced practitioner in the workplace who supports trainees in understanding the workplace setting, organises their learning in context and holds overall responsibility for the assessment of their professional practice.

A **learning community** is one where all persons involved engage in developing and enhancing their understanding and insight into the common experience they share.

programme requires success in those assessments. It should be no surprise then that students tend to become 'assessment-driven'. To focus on educational assessment in this way is not necessarily a bad thing, and the effective teacher can design assessment strategies to capitalise on students' concerns with assessments. So here we offer a few words on the nature of educational assessment.

Most individuals think about assessment as part of the latter stages of an educational experience but, without disputing the value of the end-point assessment, we take the view that it is helpful for both learners and teachers to think about assessment as a process that can be used constructively to enhance the learning experience.

Assessment-driven is how educationalists describe those students who focus primarily on finding out just what it is they need to do to pass assignments.

Approaches to educational assessment

It would be unusual to join a programme of learning without experiencing **educational assessment**. Even those who undertake a course for which there is no formal assessment will engage in some form of informal self-assessment regarding what they have or have not learned. As a student nurse you will experience a variety of types of educational assessment ranging from the formal written essay or examination to practice-based competency assessment with other less or more formal tests of your knowledge, understanding and skills. One significant feature of this variety of assessment is that different forms of learning will be less or more effective for particular types of assessment. In other words, to be a successful learner requires that you take a learning approach appropriate to whatever assessment type is set for a given unit of learning. For example, if you are required to write an essay then learning how to present information in an academic style (including how to use and present references) becomes an important skill; and if you are required to produce a portfolio then you need to learn how to demonstrate what you have learned from the material you have accumulated. A portfolio is after all a collection of evidence of learning. This skill of working out which approach to learning best suits a specific assessment is an important part of the development of your capacity for self-assessment that in turn is important preparation for assessing your own learning needs as they relate to the needs of patients and clients.

Educational assessment involves the gathering of a range of forms of evidence of a learner's knowledge, skills, conceptual understanding and values: such evidence is used for different purposes. Formative assessment provides the evidence one requires to be able to teach learners at the right level. Summative assessment summarises the achievement of learners, usually at the end of a period of time. Ipsative assessment is about self-awareness of one's own achievements. Peer assessment is what others perceive one to know.

What makes a good teacher?

There are a number of conditions that make effective learning more likely. Most people know something about these conditions simply because we all have some experience of learning. The following activities are designed to help you recognise that you already know quite a lot about learning and teaching.

Activity 11.1

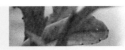

Make a list of the things you think make a good teacher. When you have completed your list, identify the five most important things on your list. Now compare your list with the one we have compiled from nursing students who have undertaken this activity over the years (see List 11.1).

We all know a good teacher when we meet one. Most of us will be able to remember the teacher whose classes we most enjoyed. We will recognise that we learned more from some teachers than others and if we know this it should only require a little thought to identify some of the things that make a good teacher. Some teachers inspire us, others we find boring. Some make learning enjoyable or at least help us to recognise the relevance of whatever subject material they are trying to teach us. The thought of turning up to the classes of some teachers fills us with dread, others we look forward to in anticipation. In an ideal world we think we would want to anticipate eagerly all scheduled classes, although that might just get to be a little bit too intense. One thing that seems to influence students' experience of higher education is the idea, prevalent in the UK, that it is somehow 'uncool' to want to learn or to be seen to be too enthusiastic about learning.

List 11.1 **Common responses of nursing students to the question: what makes a good teacher?**

We have found that student nurses think good teachers:

- are enthusiastic
- are knowledgeable
- are approachable
- are good communicators
- have a sense of humour
- show respect to students
- respond positively to students' questions
- are concise
- are organised
- interact with students
- are challenging
- are flexible with teaching methods
- are supportive
- test students' knowledge and abilites.

We suspect that your list will contain similar things.

List 11.2 **Common responses of nursing students to the question: what makes a poor teacher?**

We have also found that student nurses think poor teachers:

- are too judgemental
- speak in a monotone
- are unclear/lack clarity

- are non-interactive
- knock one's confidence
- are aggressive
- are not open-minded
- set people up to fail
- make people feel stupid.

If we return to the situation between Mark and Khim (Case 11.2) you might be thinking that Khim is not the type of mentor you would want in a final-year placement, yet she is displaying several of the features identified by students (see List 11.1) as things that make a good teacher. She is keen and enthusiastic. She is interested in Mark's progress, she wants to enable him to have a positive learning experience and she wants to help him make the most of his learning opportunities. Like most teachers and mentors, Khim has certain expectations (including the expectation that a student will arrive with some idea about what it is they want to learn) and she responds well to students who are interested in learning.

A good teacher is primarily concerned with developing effective learners. Claxton has identified four ways teachers might talk with learners to help them build learning power, organise learning environments and plan activities. This approach is designed to encourage learners and teachers to develop insight into their own learning processes so that a learning community is created. According to Chambers *et al.* (2004) the approach includes:

- *Explaining* the learning process to learners by informing, reminding, discussing and training.
- *Orchestrating* the resources, environment and activities to support learning to learn through selecting, framing, target-setting and arranging.
- *Commentating* on learners' capacities to learn through informal talk and evaluation through nudging, replying, evaluating and tracking.
- *Modelling* oneself being a learner, encouraging collective commitment to learning through learning aloud, reacting, demonstrating and sharing the experience.

This approach seems particularly relevant for the type of practice-based learning experiences of student nurses and particularly suited to work-based learning in which the placement mentor plays such an important part.

Building relationships within the learning environment

To join a pre-registration nursing programme is to join a group of learners. Together the members of the group can offer each other a valuable learning resource, and the peer learning that occurs in the group may be more valuable to individual students than the normal interactions between student and tutor. Opportunities for discussion, group work, independent learning and study and so on within the programme provide social learning in which student interactions can play a significant role in the learning of all students.

Vygotsky (1978) describes learning as a social collaborative process in which the group can help each individual to learn to do or understand something, and suggests that if you can do something or understand something with help today then you will be able to do it tomorrow without help. He describes this process as the zone of proximal development, the area within which we are able to do new things if we have assistance. Those things that are unknown to us or about which we do not understand are outside of this zone. Tharp and Gallimore (1988) have developed the zone of proximal development into a four-stage process which describes the way in which learning occurs:

Stage 1 – with assistance provided by more capable others: peers, tutors, mentors
Stage 2 – assistance is provided by oneself and the capacity is developed
Stage 3 – the capacity becomes internalised and automatic
Stage 4 – one begins to reflect on the capacity and assist others more clearly.
(Tharp and Gallimore 1988 p. 35)

This framework demonstrates the value of being able to mentor others as part of the process of learning to become a nurse which has become part of the competencies expected of a third-year student nurse. However, it also high-lights the importance of interaction in learning as a social process and thus requires the development of effective communication skills (see Chapter 9). Social learning enables peers to exchange stories of their experiences and as they relate their experiences to each other they are developing a narrative about their own learning process. According to Greenhalgh (2006) using such narra-tives to enhance the quality of health care requires a 'good story' (i.e., one that contributes to the learning of others) which needs to meet the following criteria:

• Aesthetic appeal – the narrative is pleasing to hear and recount; it contains an internal harmony
• Coherence – the narrative is clear and makes a logical whole; it contains a 'moral order' or sense
• Authenticity – the narrative has credibility, based on the experiences of the listeners/readers
• Reportability – the 'so what' value of what is narrated; its significance
• Persuasiveness – the narrative convinces of the tellers' own perspective.
(Greenhalgh 2006, summarised from pp. 9–12)

Work-based learning days seem ideal situations in which stories can provide rich learning opportunities for all or specific learning related to particular con-texts. The sharing of stories in this way can be both a learning and a teaching experience for those involved.

While the relationships between students can be varied and educationally important, relationships developed within the placement can be equally valu-able. As a student you will find yourself working alongside a wide range of individuals with whom you will interact both socially and professionally. In other words you will be engaged in dialogue and conversation with more experienced colleagues. Such relationships may be structured and formal (as exist-ing between mentor and mentee) or unstructured and informal. The discussion between Sarah and Steve (Case 11.1) in relation to hand washing is an example of an informal conversation that resulted in some learning. This type of informal learning is not restricted to the formal type of relationship between mentee and mentor as it is likely that students will learn just as much (if not more) from, for example, health care assistants as they do from those with more obvious recognised qualifications and knowledge. Learning conversations are a recog-nised process of professional development, enabling practitioners to discuss their learning while supporting each other in improving their practice. While Alexander's (2004) exploration of this kind of learning (dialogic teaching) focuses on children, the concept has resonance for adult learning. Dialogic teaching has been defined as including the following characteristics:

- Collective – teacher and learner address tasks together as a group/whole cohort
- Reciprocal – teacher and learner listen to each other, share ideas, consider alternative viewpoints
- Supportive – learners articulate their ideas freely and help each other to reach common understandings
- Cumulative – teachers and learners build on their own and each others' ideas and chain them into coherent lines of thinking and enquiry
- Purposeful – teachers plan and steer talk with specific educational goals in mind.

(summarised from Alexander 2004 p. 27)

This interactive approach to teaching and learning might be found, for example, in a seminar session in higher education or within a learning community in a health care setting.

Race's competence model

Using uncomplicated language, Race (2006) suggests competence can be understood simply as 'can do': to say that someone has competence in a particular task is to say they can do that task. The simple model of competence Race develops from this essential point provides a basis from which to explore the consequences of either knowing or not knowing what it is that one can or cannot do. This is less complicated than it sounds. The following diagrams and explanations should help to explain this.

Race places competence on a north–south axis with consciousness on an east–west axis (Figure 11.1). This provides four quadrants in which it is possible to locate competency in terms of how far a person is aware of the things they can or cannot do.

The competence/uncompetence line (the north-south axis)

Note that Race uses the term *un*competence rather than *in*competence in order to avoid the negative connotations of the latter – think about it: 'incompetence' is often used as a term of abuse.

Race notes there are degrees of competence, which means that for any task it is possible to say how well someone can do that task (this is the equivalent of making an assessment about that person's level of competence). So if you think you are highly competent at communicating, you would place yourself somewhere in the top half of the competence/uncompetence line. The exact point at which you put yourself on the competence/uncompetence line will depend on how highly you rate your competence in communicating. Of course, communication is a complex set of skills so it might be better to be more specific. If you are good at explaining things to patients in words others can understand then you would place yourself close to the competence end of the continuum (e.g., at point X in Figure 11.2). However, if you are not very good

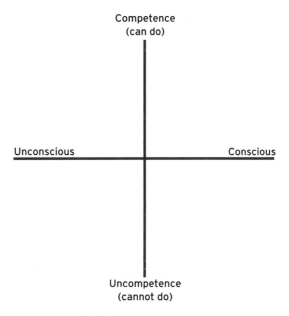

Figure 11.1 The competence model.
Source: Race (2006).

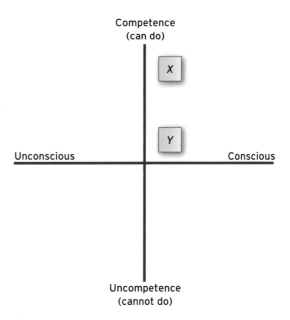

Figure 11.2 Race's competence model showing points of competence where *X* represents a high level of competence in explanation and *Y* represents a low level of competence in active listening.

at active listening then for this skill you would need to locate yourself closer to the uncompetence end of the continuum (e.g., point Y in Figure 11.2). Thus, it is possible to place yourself on the competence/uncompetence line for any and every task that you might undertake.

The unconscious/conscious line (the west–east axis)

The same principle applies to the unconscious/conscious line, only this time with reference to how far you are aware of what you can or cannot do. Of course, everything said so far about the competence/uncompetence line relates to the conscious side (to the right of the line) because you must already know (be conscious of, or aware of) what you can or cannot do in order to locate it on the competence/uncompetence line. You might find this a little confusing but we hope we can clarify this.

The four quadrants

Armed with this information, you should now be able to locate your competence in any specified task in one of the four quadrants (see Figure 11.3) as follows:

- The top right-hand quadrant = conscious competence (knowing what you can do).
- The bottom right-hand quadrant = conscious uncompetence (knowing what you cannot do).

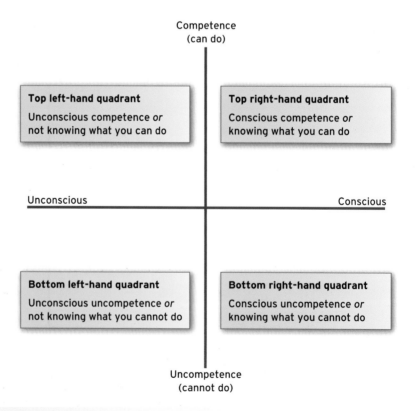

Figure 11.3 Race's competence model showing the four quadrants.

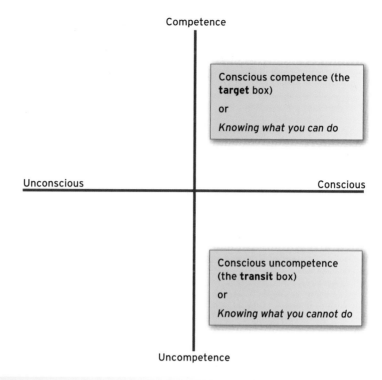

Figure 11.4 The conscious side of Race's competence model.

- The top left-hand quadrant = unconscious competence (not knowing what you can do).
- The bottom left-hand quadrant = unconscious uncompetence (not knowing what you cannot do).

We explain each in turn.

The conscious side of competence

The conscious side of competence includes the two quadrants of 'conscious competence' (*knowing* what you *can do*) and 'conscious uncompetence' (*knowing* what you *cannot do*) (see Figure 11.4).

Conscious competence (the target box)

In this quadrant go all the things you know you can do. Those things you can do very well go somewhere near the top of the box, while those things you can only just about do go near the base. Race calls this the target box because the aim will be to move all the things that you want to be able to do into this box.

Conscious uncompetence (the transit box)

In this quadrant go all the things that you know you cannot do. Some of the things in this box will be things you neither want nor need to do and these can be safely left in this box. You may not be able to ride a horse but if you have no desire to ride a horse then there is no problem about this 'cannot do' thing

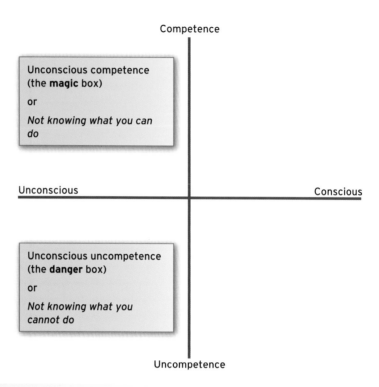

Figure 11.5 The unconscious side of Race's competence model.

being left here. But if you need or want to ride a horse then this will be one of the things you would aim to move into the target box. It is because of this potential for movement that Race calls this the transit box.

The unconscious side of competence

The unconscious side of competence includes the two quadrants of 'unconscious competence' (*not knowing* what you *can do*) and 'unconscious uncompetence' (*not knowing* what you *cannot do*) (see Figure 11.5). Everything on the unconscious side of your competence is invisible to you because as soon as you identify anything you were previously unaware of, it becomes conscious. The implications of this are profound for nursing in general and for learning and teaching in nursing in particular.

Unconscious competence (the magic box)

In this quadrant go all the things you do not know you can do. Once you become aware that you can do any of the things in this box they are no longer invisible to you and so belong in the conscious competence quadrant (the target box). This means that from your perspective your magic box is always empty. It is empty because by definition you cannot know what is in there. However, the things that are in your magic box are visible to other people, just as the contents of other people's magic boxes are visible to you. Race calls this the magic box because in it are all those things you are good at but do not recognise as anything special or significant.

Unconscious uncompetence (the danger box)

In this quadrant go all the things that you do not know you cannot do. As with items in the magic box, once you become aware of the things you cannot do they are no longer invisible to you and so belong in the conscious uncompetence quadrant (the transit box). Again, this means that from your perspective your danger box is always empty. However, the things in your danger box are visible to other people, just as the contents of other peoples' danger boxes are visible to you. Race calls this the danger box because someone who thinks they can do something well but actually does that thing poorly has the potential to be a danger to self and others (the driver who does not recognise how bad their driving is, for example).

If we apply Race's model to the situation between Mark and Khim (see Case 11.2) we can see how it might be of benefit to their educational relationship.

You will recall that on this new placement Mark wants to be left to get on with the things he knows he can do well. He knows he can do these things well because he has already been signed off as competent by other mentors in previous placements. This means that there are plenty of things that Mark can identify as belonging in his 'target' box. So if Khim (his mentor on this new placement) asked him to complete this 'conscious competence' box it would contain a lot of information and would be backed up by the evidence of earlier mentor assessments of Mark's performance in a range of nursing competencies. In effect Mark would be making a self-assessment of his competencies.

Mark might previously have undertaken a self-assessment by using, for example, a SWOT – strengths, weaknesses, opportunities and threats – analysis. Identifying one's strengths and weaknesses is a useful way of working out which things you can do well and which things you need to improve, so in this sense it serves a similar function to the conscious side of Race's model. Yet there is a more explicit line in Race's model between being able to do some-thing (however well or poorly) and not being able to do it at all. In relation to this it is useful to think of Race's horizontal line as representing a minimum threshold of competence: in Race's model this is the 'unconscious/conscious' line but for our present purposes we will refer to this as the 'threshold line'. Thus anything Mark locates at or just above the threshold line is something he can do but only at the most basic level and is something that is likely to benefit from further development; similarly, anything that falls below the threshold line will be something that Mark cannot yet do. In assessing his competences in this way Mark can see for himself, and indicate to his mentor, those things he needs to learn how to do (or to learn how to do better) and this will allow Khim to help him to plan his placement learning.

Mark has indicated that he does have a clear idea of what he needs to learn while on this placement, which means that he will have some things ready to place into his 'conscious uncompetence' box (things that he knows he cannot yet do, but knows he needs to be able to do). He may even have identified these things as learning objectives or outcomes for the placement. This reflects Mark's strong sense of what he knows and of what he believes he can do well and it is useful for him to focus in this way. However, if he has not taken account of the unconscious side of the competence model his assessment of his learning needs will remain incomplete. Such unrecognised learning needs can lead to poor or even dangerous practice. The following example should help to illustrate the point.

Case 11.2 (continued)

Mark feels slightly aggrieved when Khim (his mentor) asks him if he knows what he is doing when he measures patients' blood pressures. He is surprised to be asked this as he was assessed as competent in this task while a first-year student on his very first placement; and he has been left to get on with doing it without the need for supervision on each subsequent placement. In terms of Race's model, Mark would assess himself as scoring high on his level of competence and high on his level of awareness. This means that *he thinks it is something that he knows he can do well*. Because of this Mark resents any implication to the contrary and thinks his mentor is wasting time even asking the question.

However, Khim is a skilled mentor and asks Mark to imagine that she is a first-year student who knows very little about blood pressure measurement. In this way Khim can begin to assess his skill as a facilitator of learning as well as his knowledge of blood pressure measurement and monitoring. Her experience has shown her that individuals rarely know how much or how little they really understand about something until they try to share what knowledge they have. As Mark begins to explain the procedure, Khim plays her part by asking seemingly innocent questions such as:

- Is it best to use the right or left arm of the patient?
- What do you do if the patient is wearing a dressing gown or thick cardigan?

Mark is able to answer Khim's initial questions with ease and begins to warm to his task. He starts to think teaching is not such a big deal and that it should not be too difficult to meet the placement outcomes for learning and teaching. However, as Khim gently increases the probing nature of her questions, Mark begins to flounder and he starts to have trouble answering some parts of her questions.

For example, when Khim asks: 'what do the numbers displayed against MAP mean?', Mark finds himself at a bit of a loss. He resorts to telling her exactly what he was told when he first learned about using the machine, that those numbers represent 'mean arterial pressure' and are not important. 'If they are not important, why are they there at all?' is Khim's immediate follow-up question, at which point Mark has to admit that he does not know. Similarly, when Khim asks him to demonstrate and explain the use of a manual sphygmomanometer, Mark finds himself on unfamiliar ground. 'I have not been asked to use one of these on a real patient before' he says. Khim then goes on to ask him if he knows when it might be appropriate to use an old-fashioned sphygmomanometer with a stethoscope and about the relationship between Korotkoff's sounds and *systolic* and *diastolic* blood pressure. Mark finds he does not really have satisfactory answers to these questions and finally concedes that his knowledge of blood pressure measurement is less complete than he had previously believed.

Khim might have asked other probing questions about the recommended length and width of the inflatable bladder held within the cuff; or about the consequences of using an inflatable bladder that is insufficiently long or insufficiently wide, but she decides to stop once Mark admitted to not knowing as much as he thought he knew. What Khim has done in this brief interlude is to offer Mark a glimpse into his unconscious uncompetences; in other words, she has demonstrated to Mark that there are *things he does not know he does not know* and further that *some of these are things he will need to know* (or at least be aware of) if he is to be a safe and effective practitioner. She has also illustrated to Mark the value of receiving feedback from others when undertaking a self-assessment so that one's unconscious competencies and uncompetences are not ignored.

This is all a bit of a revelation to Mark, who recognises that he does indeed have more to learn than he had realised. As a result of Khim's gently probing questions, Mark has come to realise that his earlier self-assessment was incomplete precisely because he had little input from other, more knowledge-able or more experienced individuals. Now that Mark has acknowledged this he can, with the help of his mentor, begin to identify a wider spread of learning needs and be in a position to take more control of his learning.

The value of the unconscious side of Race's model then lies not in filling the boxes but in acknowledging their existence. The recognition that there are things that you do not know you cannot do is in itself important because it allows you to remain open to the possibility that there are new things you need to learn even if you do not yet know what these things are. This may help you to accept that you will not always see the relevance of some of the things other people think you need to learn. In other words, when you struggle to under-stand what any particular thing you are being asked to learn has got to do with nursing, it may be that you just do not yet know or understand its relevance in relation to the safe and effective care of patients and clients.

Part 3: Exploring learning and teaching

In Part 2 of this chapter we outlined some of the things that go to make a good teacher and from this we identified the important role the teacher has in setting up an environment in which learning can take place. As Part 3 progresses we hope you will begin to recognise the limits of the teacher's part in the educa-tional process and start to acknowledge the way in which learners themselves influence the quality of each learning and teaching situation. We start here with a brief review of the things identified as making a good teacher.

Activity 11.2
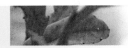

Compare the items in List 11.1 with the items in List 11.2.
Why do you think the things in one list are not merely the opposite of the things in the other?

As you might suspect, lists of the things that make a poor teacher generally identify things that are the opposite of the features that appear on lists of what makes a good teacher. Yet List 11.2 does not merely list the opposites of features in List 11.1. This suggests that there are some things that students particularly dislike in their teachers, the absence of which does not necessarily make a good teacher and vice versa. So while teacher enthusiasm is something students appreciate, a lack of enthusiasm may not of itself make a poor teacher; similarly, it may be that a modicum of open-mindedness is sufficient whereas its absence may be a significant obstacle to learning.

Thus far we have contrasted the 'good' with the 'poor' teacher. While these are words that many students use to describe their teachers, the terms have only limited descriptive value. The words good and poor can mean different things to different people, so in the remainder of this chapter we will refer to 'effective' and 'ineffective' rather than 'good' or 'poor' respectively. Thus we will now be talking about effectiveness in learning and teaching. The effective teacher, then, is the one who provides the environment in which learning is most likely to take place. This learning environment is not merely a matter of the physical environment of a classroom or a placement but includes a range of factors, some of which have been identified in the lists in List 11.1 and List 11.2 above. However, the importance of the physical environment should not be underestimated. It is, after all, difficult to concentrate on the content of a lecture when sitting in a cold classroom. Similarly, it may be hard to engage in learning when faced with a heavy workload on placement: if you are worrying that there is not time to get everything done before the end of your shift you are unlikely to give your full attention to the mentor's explanation about, for example, hyper- and hypoglycaemia.

Many factors contribute to the learning environment and other people (mentors and other staff in placement settings; other students and teachers in the classroom and so on) have an important role in determining the effectiveness of any given learning situation. Wenger's (2000) concept of 'communities of practice' is an attempt to describe this social aspect of learning as an essential and necessary feature of a learning environment if an individual is to negotiate the development of competences. Learning in practice is an important element of becoming a nurse and as such the practice environment itself impacts upon the student's capacity to learn. According to Wenger there are a set of specific dimensions necessary for a community of practice if it is to maintain the capacity to develop and support the learning of everyone within it:

- Enterprise – the level of learning energy describes the enthusiasm which a community demonstrates for maintaining learning at the centre of its action, a spirit of enquiry and a desire to find out.
- Mutuality – the depth of social capital describes the level of trust between people to ensure they feel comfortable addressing problems together: this can often take time.
- Repertoire – the degree of self-awareness describes how the concepts, language and tools of the community embody its perspective and own state of development.

(Summarised from Wenger 2000 p. 230)

Activity 11.3

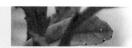

Write a short account of a recent or significant learning experience (it does not matter if this was an effective or ineffective learning experience). Have a go at seeing how far any of the three dimensions described above were present in the setting in which this learning experience took place.

We anticipate that the more these dimensions were present in the learning situation you describe, the more you learned. You might have described a placement or a classroom learning experience as these dimensions are relevant across the range of learning situations. For example, seminar groups provide the type of environment where students can learn with and from each other in a way that supports those who at any point may be struggling to learn. In the placement environment the attitudes of the qualified staff can be a significant factor in a student's capacity to learn. It seems that trust has an important part to play if effective learning is to take place. The following vignette illustrates a community of practice in which effective learning is occurring:

Case 11.3

Ann, the manager of a unit in a local hospital, understands the value of providing an environment in which learning is encouraged. She contributes sessions to students of nursing at the local university and because she has budgetary control has appointed an education facilitator to work with staff. Ann encourages all staff to reflect on their practice and discuss aspects of their reflections with others to help improve practice. The education facilitator contributes to these discussions whenever possible and organises formal study events and training sessions on topics or issues highlighted during the discussions. Over time this has helped the staff to recognise the value of learning in this way and the culture of the unit has developed as a learning community.

Individual learning style is the process of self-evaluation to understand and identify the approaches and strategies that one most commonly employs in learning.

In a learning community such as this, everyone is involved and learning takes place both formally and informally which helps individuals to build their capacity for learning.

Activity 11.4

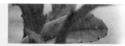

- Have another look at the items in Lists 11.1 and 11.2.
- Identify the things in List 11.1 that you think are most likely to aid effective learning.
- Identify the things in List 11.2 that you think are most likely to inhibit effective learning.
- Now swap your new lists with another student, what do you notice?

We think that the things you identify as most likely to aid and inhibit learning will not be exactly the same as the those identified by other students. This suggests that individuals learn in different ways. In fact, the idea that not everybody learns in the same way is a well-documented phenomenon referred to as a matter of **individual learning style**.

Research focus 11.1

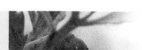

In a comprehensive review, Coffield *et al.* (2004) found that the literature on learning styles falls into three distinct areas: (1) theoretical, (2) pedagogical and (3) commercial. The review identified 71 models of learning styles. Some discuss the workings of the brain, others explore personality traits, some emphasise the importance of previous experience and environmental factors, and some emphasise the importance of understanding one's own learning biography.

The impact of theoretical frameworks on the teaching and learning process is clear. However, different disciplines have interpreted learning theory in ways specific to their own particular academic discipline: thus learning theory is understood differently within the disciplines of psychology, sociology, management, education, nursing and so on. As a consequence the impact of learning theory varies in the practice of teaching and learning across different disciplines.

The contrast between nursing and teaching is of interest. Teaching began as an academic process and has gradually moved towards an emphasis on classroom practice whereas nurse education emerged from clinical practice and has developed into an academic discipline in its own right. Despite these different antecedents the learning contexts for those learning to become teachers is broadly similar to those learning to become nurses.

Learning styles

There are many ways to categorise how different individuals learn. Common in the different descriptions of learning styles is the idea that people will not simply fit into one category of learner. Rather, most people can be categorised (or will categorise themselves) as having a preferred learning style even if they do not always make use of that style in all learning situations. This insight is important for several reasons that we will explore shortly. First though we will outline one popular and commonly used learning style; one that has its roots in the psychology of personality.

Honey and Mumford (1992) describe learners as predominately falling into one of four categories: activists, reflectors, theorists, and pragmatists:

- *Activists* like to participate and try things out for themselves. Activists tend to be keen to get involved whenever the opportunity arises.
- *Reflectors* like to think about things first. Reflectors may be content to watch others try things out before getting involved.
- *Theorists* like to use models and theories to understand things. Theorists may try to avoid being swayed by emotions or first impressions.
- *Pragmatists* like to experiment. Pragmatists prefer practical rather than abstract ideas and like to see how they work in the real world.

Most people find they can identify themselves as fitting one (or more) of these categories and you may already have recognised yourself as primarily a pragmatist, a theorist, a reflector, or an activist; or as a combination of more than one. There is no evaluative undercurrent here; this is to say that, in general terms, no one learning style is necessarily better or more effective than any other, although there are some situations in which one style is more likely to result in effective learning. For example, students who prefer an activist learning style are likely to be most comfortable getting involved in learning the practical skills of things such as cardiopulmonary resuscitation, where theorists might struggle. Nevertheless, the theorist who can adopt an activist approach when faced with learning practical skills will be an effective learner in that situation. This is an important point because it suggests that effective learners are those who can adapt their learning style to suit the requirements of learning particular topics in particular situations. Conversely, the student who is reluctant to adopt a different learning style to the one they most prefer is likely to struggle to learn in those situations that benefit most from alternative learning style approaches. The fact that individual students have preferred learning styles also has significant implications for the teacher when designing, planning and implementing programmes of learning.

This next activity is designed to help you begin to understand some of the ways in which learners influence both the learning environment and the quality of learning that takes place in any learning situation.

Activity 11.5

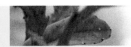

Make a list of the things you think make an effective learner. When you have completed your list, identify the five most important things on your list. Now read on and compare your list with the one we have compiled from the responses of nursing students who have undertaken this activity over the years (List 11.3).

Clearly, one of the implications of individual learning styles is that those students who are able to adapt their learning style to the meet the demands of particular learning situations are more likely to be effective learners across a wide range of learning opportunities. In addition to this, teachers think that few learners recognise the role they (the learners) play in influencing the quality of their own educational experiences. Teachers generally understand learning as an active process, whereas (teachers believe) most students think of education as more of a product; this may be in terms of being 'assessment-driven' (see explanation of this point in Part 1 of this chapter) or in terms of education being merely **instrumental** in character. If this is true then the learner who takes an active role in an educational process is more likely to benefit from a given learning and teaching situation. In other words: the more active the learner is, the more effective their learning is likely to be.

Instrumental understandings of education: some students (and some teachers) see education purely (or primarily) as a means to a particular end. So the student nurse who thinks classroom teaching is largely irrelevant to the so-called 'real world' on placement might be described as using the classroom merely as a way of achieving their desired end of becoming a registered nurse. For such a student education is the **instrument** of getting to where they want to get.

List 11.3 Common responses of nursing students to the question: what makes an effective learner?

We have found that student nurses think effective learners:

- are committed
- take a questioning approach to learning
- are enthusiastic
- pay attention
- are keen to learn
- are motivated
- have goals/objectives.

Just as with the lists for the 'what makes a good teacher' activity in Part 2 of this chapter (see List 11.1 and List 11.2) we suspect that your list will contain similar things to the list we have compiled here. This indicates that you already know a great deal about effective learning and teaching.

List 11.4 Common responses of nursing students to the question: what makes an ineffective learner?

We have also found that student nurses think that ineffective learners may:

- not listen
- be uninterested
- lack enthusiasm
- be unmotivated
- be distracted
- think they know it all.

One important point here is that there are common aspects of approaching learning that will influence the effectiveness of learning regardless of individual learning styles. The person who thinks they 'already know it all' is likely to be less receptive to new ideas than the person who knows they have things to learn. To return to Race's competence model: the student nurse or practitioner who thinks they 'know it all' is either unaware of their own uncompetences (i.e., does not know what they do not know or cannot do) or has chosen to ignore their uncompetences (i.e., knows what they do not know but is, for some reason, unwilling to do anything about it). In either case, such a person is likely to become an unsafe practitioner without recognising this as a danger to their practice and to the patients in their care.

Developing aptitudes to learning

While the characteristics and approach of the teachers will have a significant influence on the learning experience of each student, the role of the learner in creating an effective learning situation should not be underestimated. The teaching style of the teacher will often depend on the nature of the topic being taught but the fine detail of the session will reflect the teacher's own views about how people learn. This alone does not determine the learning that takes place. While the primary responsibility for setting the environment in which learning can take place may lie with the teacher, it is the learner who is ultimately responsible for their own learning. If this is true then it should be clear that each learner needs to build their learning capacity so as to make best use of the available learning resources and opportunities. In other words, what and how much a student learns will be influenced not only by what it is that is to be learned but also by the way in which the learner approaches learning. We will now explore briefly some of the aptitudes that have the potential to enhance students' learning.

Self-awareness

Successful engagement with the learning process requires you as a learner to develop an understanding of how you best learn. This will necessarily require that you engage with some form of self-evaluation in order to gain insight into your particular learning potential and to understand what conditions offer you the best chance of maximising your learning. As we mentioned earlier, Claxton (2002) encourages learners to build their learning power through engagement in self-evaluation and through exploration of a variety of approaches to learning in a range of different settings.

Claxton suggests that there are four different learning dispositions which need to be developed and extended in order to build one's learning capacity. He categorises these as follows:

- Resilience: being ready, willing and able to lock on to learning
- Resourcefulness: being ready, willing and able to learn in different ways
- Reflectiveness: being ready, willing and able to become more strategic about learning
- Reciprocity: being ready, willing and able to learn alone and with others.

(Claxton 2002 p. 4)

These dispositions can be developed as strengths in order to understand one's own approach to learning and may involve trial and error by, for example, exploring the best environment for writing essays or by trying to find the most useful person in the workplace with whom to discuss a topic. Both examples require the dispositions described above together with a level of self-confidence in one's own capacities. It may be the case that in professional practice a student nurse is not always aware of all aspects of their learning but that through

> *simply interact(ing) with the situation in a 'mindless' but observant manner, they come to master it, at an intuitive level – they do the right thing without knowing why – faster than those who keep struggling for conscious comprehension.*

(Atkinson and Claxton 2000, p. 36)

Self-awareness of the learning process is a valuable commodity, particularly in the workplace where formal learning opportunities are not always made explicit. This capacity together with an emergent awareness of learning power can enable the student to recognise informal and formal learning opportunities in the workplace and beyond.

Open-mindedness and flexibility

We have already noted that each individual has a preferred learning style and we suggested that those learners who, when the occasion requires it, are able to adopt a style of learning other than their preferred style are likely to increase their learning power. This is important in a profession such as nursing precisely because learning opportunities occur in various forms (both formal and informal) and learning to be flexible in choosing an appropriate learning style for a specific task will enhance learning which in turn will help to develop and improve practice. For some individuals becoming flexible in this way will require effort but can be assisted by cultivating open-mindedness. Open-mindedness requires a person to remain open to the possibility of being wrong and open to the possibility of a need to change behaviour: including learning behaviour. These are demanding requirements but the alternative is to be either closed-minded or credulous (Sellman 2003), and either of these will reduce the learning opportunities available to students and registered practitioners alike.

The capacity to be flexible and open-minded is consistent with the idea of self-actualisation as explored by Rogers (1989), who noted that in order to be successful an individual must experience unconditional approval to reduce anxieties about their own perceptions and abilities. This is important for nurses as learners as they build learning capacity from contact with peers, mentors, patients and others in the practice environments.

Reflection

Reflection provides individuals with an opportunity to identify what they know, what they do not know and what they need to do in order to fill in the gaps in their knowledge, understanding and skills. Reflection is a major theme in Chapter 13 of this book so here we will confine ourselves to a few brief comments. Reflection has become an important aspect of many practical occupations (including nursing and teaching) as a method by which individual practitioners can develop their practice. Schön (1987) presents three levels of reflection: knowing-in-action; reflection-in-action; and reflection-on-action.

Knowing–in-action implies that thinking is embedded in actions, that it is implicit. The student nurse in the workplace would demonstrate their knowledge through the actions in which they are engaged. This form of learning is particularly relevant to learning for professional practice. While a student or practitioner may have considerable knowledge, if they are unable to enact the knowledge (i.e., use their knowledge to inform their practice) they will struggle to be a safe and effective registered nurse. For Schon, knowing-in-action is demonstrated when, for example, a student successfully gives an injection or accurately assesses the nursing care needs of a patient.

This is distinct from *reflection-in-action* which involves a conscious standing back to think critically and to question whether merely continuing with existing knowledge-in-action is appropriate in a particular situation. Reflection-in-action may be momentary and might result in a change of knowledge-in-action and thus a more suitable action in what may be a novel situation. In this respect, reflection-in-action can enable the transfer of skills from familiar to unfamiliar contexts.

Reflection-on-action requires a retrospective review of actions taken and has a more structured purpose in assisting a practitioner or student to evaluate performance and to learn from that performance. Most nursing students will be encouraged to reflect-on-action as a way of providing evidence which may be used to build a portfolio of learning.

As such, reflection provides opportunities for students and practitioners to learn in and from practice.

Conclusion

Wherever and whenever nursing occurs, learning and teaching is almost certainly taking place. Student and registered nurses invariably learn things from and about patients and relatives while at the same time patients and relatives learn things from and about student and registered nurses. This learning might be incidental or deliberate, and it may be related or unrelated to patient care. When you observe a patient's reaction to a painful procedure you learn something about them and the receptive nurse will make use of that learning to inform future pain management strategies. At the same time the patient will learn something about you: they may learn whether or not you are compassionate and/or trustworthy; they may learn that you care about or are indifferent to their pain and this may affect the way they subsequently behave in your presence. This type of learning may be informal and incidental but as we indicated early in this chapter, when one person learns something from another then that other is in some sense acting as a teacher. When you explain anything to another person, be it how to engage in discussion

with a depressed patient, how to manage a long-term urinary catheter, how to measure and monitor blood pressure or how to give advice on healthy eating you are engaged in a form of teaching precisely because you are trying to get that other person to learn something.

Thus teaching is directly related to nursing practice in all sorts of ways and in all nursing situations and it follows that a basic knowledge and understanding of learning and teaching is an essential aspect of safe and effective nursing practice. As a student nurse, and subsequently as a registered nurse, other people (patients, relatives and carers, students, health care assistants and so on) will learn from you whether or not you intend this to happen. Hence you have a choice. You can either ignore the influence you have on what it is that others learn from you or you can take active steps to encourage particular sorts of learning in those around you.

The Nursing and Midwifery Council state that 'You must *facilitate* students and others to develop their *competence'* (2008, emphasis added) and this makes it clear that in addition to the professional requirement to continue to learn, each registered nurse has a professional obligation to facilitate learning for others. This means that as far as the regulatory body for nursing is concerned you do not have a choice. In other words, not only must you be aware of your responsibilities in relation to learning and teaching but you must also be proactive in assisting in the development of an environment that encourages the development of the learning power of each individual in the environment.

While achieving the minimum threshold level of competence consistent with safe and effective practice is necessary in order to register as a nurse, the importance of developing a positive approach and attitude towards learning for self and others remains the cornerstone of the maintenance of professional nursing practice.

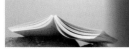

Suggested further reading

Quinn, F. M. (2007) *Principles and Practice of Nurse Education* (5th ed.), Cheltenham: Nelson Thornes.
Race, P. (2006) *The Lecturer's Toolkit* (3rd ed.), London: Routledge.

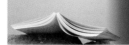

References

Alexander, R. (2004) *Towards Dialogic Teaching: Rethinking classroom talk.* Cambridge: Dialogos.
Atkinson, T. and Claxton, G. (2000) *The Intuitive Practitioner: On the value of not always knowing what one is doing.* Buckingham: Open University Press.

Chambers, M., Powell, G. and Claxton, G. (2004) *Building 101 Ways to Learning Power.* Bristol: TLO.
Claxton, G. (2002) *Building Learning Power: Helping young people to become better learners.* Bristol: TLO.
Coffield, F., Moseley. D., Hall, E. and Ecclestone, K. (2004) *Learning Styles and Pedagogy in Post-16 Learning: A systematic and critical review.* London: Learning Skills Research Centre.

Dewey, J. (1916) *Democracy and Education: An introduction to the philosophy of education.* New York: Macmillan.

Greenhalgh, T. (2006) *How to Read a Paper: The basics of evidence-based medicine.* Oxford: Blackwell.

Honey, P. and Mumford, A. (1992) *The Manual of Learning Styles.* Maidenhead: Honey & Mumford.

NMC (Nursing and Midwifery Council) (2004) *Standards of Proficiency for Pre-registration Nursing Education.* NMC: London.
NMC (2008) *The Code: Standards of conduct, performance and ethics for nurses and midwives.* NMC: London.

Race, P. (2006) *The Lecturer's Toolkit* (3rd ed.). London: Routledge.

Rogers, C. (1989) [first published 1961] *On Becoming a Person*. London: Constable.

Sacks, O. (1995) *An Anthropologist on Mars*. London: Picador.

Schön, D. A. (1987) *Educating the Reflective Practitioner: Towards a new design for teaching and learning in the professions*. San Francisco: Jossey-Bass.

Sellman, D. (2003) Open-mindedness: a virtue for professional practice. *Nursing Philosophy* **4** (1), 17–24.

Smith, F. (1998) *The Book of Learning and Forgetting*. New York: Teachers' College Press.

Tharp, R. G. and Gallimore, R. (1988) *Rousing Minds to Life*. Cambridge: Cambridge University Press.

Vygotsky, L. S. (1978) *Mind and Society: The development of higher psychological processes*. Cambridge MA: Harvard University Press.

Wenger, E. (2000) Communities of practice and social learning systems. *Organisation* **7** (2), 225–246.

Chapter 12

Management and leadership

Iain Snelling, Cathryn Havard and David Pontin

Learning outcomes

After reading and reflecting on this chapter, you should be able to:

- Explain key theories of leadership and management and their application in a health care setting;

- Outline how conceptual and theoretical knowledge can be used to develop personal effectiveness and underpin ways of working in practice;

- Discuss developing effective strategies for managing self and others within the work environment.

Related NMC Standards of Proficiency for Pre-registration Nursing Education (NMC 2004)

- Identify, collect and evaluate information to justify the effective utilisation of resources to achieve planned outcomes of nursing care.

- Use appropriate risk assessment tools to identify actual and potential risks.

- Identify environmental hazards and eliminate and/or prevent where possible.

- Communicate safety concerns to a relevant authority.

- Manage risk to provide care which best meets the needs and interests of patients, clients and the public.

- Take into account the role and competence of staff when delegating work.

- Demonstrate the ability to co-ordinate the delivery of nursing and health care.

- Demonstrate effective leadership in the establishment and maintenance of safe nursing practice.

Introduction

Increasingly, nurses are managers as well as deliverers of care and act as leaders. This doesn't mean that nurses are away at meetings all day, or spend all their time fulfilling bureaucratic functions. Management and leadership means much more than this. Being responsible and accountable for the actions of others in the health care team, which is a core function in the work of most nurses, means that you manage them.

The chapter is divided into three parts.

In Part 1, we outline management and leadership and discuss how organisations that provide health care organise themselves to deliver their services and respond to health care policy.

In Part 2, we explain how a manager running a department, ward or outpatient clinic for example might address their challenges. This will hopefully give you some scope to reflect on your experiences on placement. A range of issues will be covered briefly, but there will be some additional details of clinical governance and service improvement, which were two areas of health policy that were identified as being particularly significant in Chapter 4.

In Part 3, we explore some critical perspectives on management and leadership.

Part 1: Outlining management and leadership

Case 12.1

Sue is a final-year student on placement on a surgical ward. She is worried about the ward. She observes that the shifts are very busy and chaotic. Although she can't point to anything that is really unsafe, or that the quality of care is not good enough, it just seems that it could be better. She has mentioned this to the Ward Manager, and she sort of agreed, but said that there was no more money to improve things, and that the staff 'should do their best'. If there were specific concerns they would be addressed, but otherwise, we should get on with it. Although Sue wants to concentrate on her nursing duties on placement, she reflects on the ward team and how the care it provides might be improved.

Why should I study management and leadership?

Over many years of facilitating learning and skills development in relation to management and leadership with pre-registration nursing students, we have noticed that at an early stage people ask: '*I didn't come into nursing to become a manager . . . so why am I studying management?*'

The particular challenge here is to focus on the wider aspects of being a registered nurse. Students are asked: 'how do you think that you will *manage* in your future professional role?' In particular: 'how will you manage yourselves, manage other people, and manage the environment in which you work?' We will return to this framework later in the chapter.

We also want to know what or who inspires and challenges you – in other words, who you look to for leadership. In the following section, we look at ideas about leadership and management and how these relate to the work of newly qualified nurses. Our aim is to encourage you to think critically about your work and to identify the sorts of people skills needed to work with patients and clients, and colleagues and other carers; and how to use information and resources effectively to promote good-quality work. We propose that an understanding of leadership, management practice and underpinning theories and concepts will help you develop greater personal, professional and organisational effectiveness.

How will this help me in my work?

Following registration as a nurse, most people's first priority is finding a job and settling in to a new role. This means finding out about the practical realities and responsibilities of the job. It also includes spending time and energy getting to know colleagues, the types of patient/client issues you will be facing and usual situations that arise. In short – managing yourself, managing others and managing the environment. You will find that there is an expectation within the workplace that the required competence level will be reached within an agreed time frame, and evidence will need to be produced to support the achievement of competence. Increasingly these will be prescribed by and linked with the requirements for the job, as mapped out via the NHS Knowledge and Skills Framework in line with Agenda for Change (DH 2004a) and managed via a personal development plan.

Your progress towards achieving competence may be affected by the quality of preceptorship and leadership in your area and not all the skills and tasks may be achieved at the same point. However, there will come a time, perhaps 3 months, 6 months, or a year into the role, when you may find yourself in a situation where you not only have to manage events but function as a leader as well.

Leadership will increasingly be a key element of the role of all health care practitioners in the future. The recent important White Paper, *High Quality Care for All*, states that '[i]n the future every clinician has the opportunity to be a practitioner . . . partner, . . . and leader' (Secretary of State for Health 2008 pp. 59–60). Developing leadership roles of clinicians is a key element of the future development of the NHS.

Aren't management and leadership just different words for the same thing?

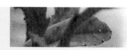

Activity 12.1

Consider the definition of management and leadership in relation to your placement experiences. Using the prompt questions below, take 5 minutes to write down as many examples as you can. Start with the most recent placement and work backwards in time.

- Who has inspired you and why?
- Who has challenged you? How were you challenged?
- Who has supported you? What did they do?

Management provides you with the ladder to reach higher: it deals with the pragmatic, logistical issues of resources, planning, monitoring and evaluating.

Leadership encourages you to reach for the stars: it reminds you of why you wanted to become a nurse in the first place by kindling your aspirations and creativity.

Look at your responses to the activity above. Who have you identified? Are they people in formal **management** or **leadership** roles in the organisation? There is a temptation to look only at people in authority roles for inspiration but you might find that you have been inspired by people who have recently qualified as a nurse or who have been nursing for a long time. They may not be nurses at all but workers in the wider health and social care team, for example a physiotherapist or a social worker. Who has challenged you? Perhaps it was a mentor who was a rigorous assessor but from whom you learned a great deal.

You may not be aware of the ways in which managers fulfil supporting roles. They are often working in the background, wrestling with targets and juggling resources. This buffering role of a manager provides shelter for clinical staff from wider internal and external forces, enabling them to focus on direct care activities. It is an essential function and often underestimated by nurses, especially if a manager is not highly visible. If you can, try to arrange to spend some time with the manager at your current placement and find out about their role and workload. It is important that you start to look outside your immediate practice area and widen your organisational horizons. Understanding the pressures and constraints of another person's role and work can be extremely helpful in promoting understanding and empathy rather than conflict and confrontation, and is consistent with the notion of shared governance.

Distinctions between management and leadership

The **authority of managers** comes from the formal roles they occupy within the organisation.

Influence is not formally linked to a role. Anyone may exert influence.

There appear to be four main distinctions in the general literature between management and leadership. We draw on Rost (1993) as a way of clarifying the difference (see Figure 12.1)

The **authority of managers** comes from the formal roles they occupy within the organisation. The organisation legitimates their power to act and requires other people to do as they are asked or told. **Influence** on the other hand is not

Management	Leadership
Authority relationship with others	Influence relationship with others
Roles classed as managers and subordinates	Roles classed as leaders and followers
Rationale is the production of goods/services for consumption and sale	Rationale is the intention to make observable changes in the work environment
The production of goods/services comes from the co-ordination of others' activities	The intention to make changes that reflects the shared purposes of colleagues or co-workers

Figure 12.1 Distinctions between management and leadership.
Source: Rost (1993).

formally linked to a role. Anyone may exert influence but they may not be able to compel someone to act. Leaders have to persuade people, either by word or deed, that they should follow their example or ideas; that is, there is a voluntary agreement to act. This is not to say that managers cannot be leaders, or vice versa. Effective managers are also leaders. Valerie Iles, for example, 'outlines a style of management . . . [called] real management . . . Real management straddles the divide drawn between management and leadership' (Iles 2005 p. 2). Whether individuals are acting as managers or leaders, or both, they do so in an organisational context, including the established structure.

Organisational structures

Health care organisations, even relatively small ones such as GP practices, are both complicated and complex. Understanding the difference between complex and complicated may help you understand the management issues you experience during your working life, and some of the ideas presented in this chapter. The differences are illustrated by Glouberman and Zimmerman (2002). Sending a rocket to the moon is an example of a *complicated* problem. There are many different aspects, and many different experts are required to find solutions to problems. Ultimately, how the rockets work will be understood in minute detail. An unexpected outcome in the smallest area may have devastating consequences. Raising a child is an example of a *complex* issue. There are no formulas for success, although evidence and experience may give some guide. Each decision may have unintended consequences, or be influenced by factors outside our control. There is no way in which even the closest studies can determine precisely what and how things will happen.

Health care organisations use rules, procedures, structures and contracts to deal with complicated issues. However, organisations are mainly made up of people working together, producing a wide range of complex issues. Ideas, concepts, models and theories give insights into how the organisation works, but they will not solve problems by creating understanding in the same way that a merely complicated problem can be solved. It might be helpful to keep this distinction in mind as you go through this chapter.

All health care organisations have a formal structure. It would be helpful if you could obtain a copy of the structure of an organisation you are working in or have worked in. You might find one on the website, or get one from the human resources (HR) department. The complicated work of the organisation will be organised very carefully so that all required tasks are completed. The structure shows how individuals in key roles work together so that everything that needs to be done is done effectively.

The organisational structure will have a number of levels. Usually it is shown from the top down, with the board of directors at the top. In explaining this we will start at the bottom, with staff who deliver the service, although the diagram will be shown in traditional form. The table in Figure 12.2 explains some different levels of management involved with delivering the service.

The levels we have identified are not a blueprint for every organisation. A very large NHS foundation trust, for example, may need to have an additional layer of management between hospital executives and individual services. Some organisations, perhaps smaller ones, prefer 'flat' structures where levels

Level	Description of role	Examples of job titles
Individual health care professional	Individuals have their own professional responsibilities, but also have management responsibilities for themselves. This will include, for example, duties to meet health and safety legislation, and a wide range of policies. All these specific tasks will be included in the job description.	Staff nurse, Physiotherapist, doctor
Team leaders	Health care professionals work in teams, which need to be co-ordinated to work effectively. An individual nurse might be a member of several different teams – a team of nurses, an interprofessional team working with a group of patients, or a project team working on a specific development. A team leader may need to allocate tasks, complete duty rosters, supervise team members, and ensure communication is effective between team members.	Senior staff nurse, team co-ordinator, shift leader
Operational manager	Operational managers will make sure that the service runs effectively, but at this level they are more likely to be concerned with making sure that teams have the facilities and support needed. The operational manager will tackle issues that affect the whole department, and will also make sure that any requirements of the organisation are completed. This is likely to include staff management issues and managing a budget.	Ward sister or charge nurse, department manager
Middle management	Middle managers will typically be responsible for a number of wards or departments. They have duties to support the running of services, for example in solving major problems, or introducing major changes. They will also have important roles in the organisation, ensuring that organisational policies are developed and that external requirements are met.	Matron, service manager, general manager
Executive director	Executive directors are concerned with the whole organisation. Formally, they are members of the Trust board which is the highest decision-making body in the organisation (see Box 12.1). Executive directors have specific responsibilities, as well as a collective overall responsibility. As well as executive directors there are non-executive directors, who are appointed on a part-time basis to ensure that the board serves its stakeholders, and a chair.	Director of nursing, medical director, director of finance, director of operations
Chief executive	The chief executive is the person at the top of the organisation. Everyone in the organisation is ultimately accountable to him or her. He or she is accountable to the chairman and the board.	

Figure 12.2 Different levels of management

of management are reduced, so that for example operational managers report directly to directors or perhaps deputy directors.

The table explains the structure for managers who have specific responsibility for delivery of services. Alongside this structure there are a range of functions that are needed to support services, for example finance, human resources and estates. Staff delivering health care services are not normally accountable to managers in these functions, although clearly they fulfil important roles. Accountability is discussed in more detail below.

The diagram in Figure 12.3 shows these levels presented in an organisational chart. You may find it interesting to compare this diagram with the organisational chart of organisations you are working in, or have worked in.

This organisational chart shows details for ward staff in orthopaedics. In this case, the general manager is accountable to the clinical director, who is

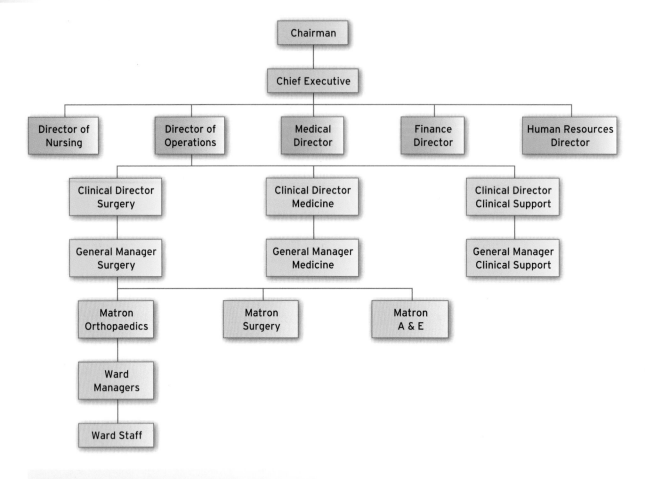

Figure 12.3 An example of an organisational chart

often a doctor. At the level of the directorate in this structure there is no nurse manager, though the general manager may have a nursing background. The clinical director is accountable to the director of operations.

These accountabilities are for line management. For professionally qualified staff, there is also 'professional accountability' for professional issues which a line manager may not be able to judge. So all medical staff, including clinical directors, are accountable to the medical director for their professional practice, and all nurses are ultimately accountable to the director of nursing.

Box 12.1 Attending a board meeting

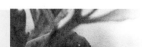

You will have experienced team management and operational management in your placements. To get a picture of how the top level of management and leadership works, you can attend a board meeting as a member of the public. At least some parts of board meetings are held in public; confidential issues are dealt with at the end of the meeting after the public has been excluded. Board papers are also available; agendas, minutes, and supporting reports. These will be available on an organisation's website or from the chief executive's office.

Part 2: Explaining management and leadership

The standards of proficiency outlined at the beginning of the chapter are particularly concerned with safety and risk, and these will be themes running through the chapter. In this section, management and leadership will be explained in more detail. This will be structured around four areas:

1. Managing self.
2. Managing and leading others.
3. Managing resources.
4. Managing the environment.

Managing self

Chapter 13 considers personal and professional development in some detail, concentrating particularly on reflective practice. In this brief section, we'll consider the implications for your development with reference to management and leadership

Activity 12.2

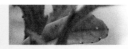

Go back to the beginning of this chapter, and have another look at the learning outcomes, and the *Standards of Proficiency for Pre-registration Nursing Education*. Reflect on your experiences relating to these standards of proficiency, and identify possible areas for development.

How did you complete this task? Chapter 13 gives some models of reflection, particularly relevant to reflecting on individual events, and how you experienced them. In the context of the learning outcomes of this chapter, it is important for you to be able to take an overview of your practice and how you may need to develop in order to improve your effectiveness in a range of management tasks. Two related issues frequently identified as development needs are improving time management and coping with stress.

Time management

You can only do so much in the time available. The answer to pressure of tasks building up is not to increase the time available, for example by staying late, arriving early, or skipping breaks. To make the most effective use of your time, you need to do two things: undertake each task as efficiently as possible, and prioritise your tasks.

For many tasks, there is a trade-off between time taken and quality. It takes longer to do something well than it does to do it badly. That may be true up to a point, but it is likely that after a while extra time devoted to a task adds very little, if any additional quality. Quality might even begin to fall after a while. Conversations or meetings might fall into this category. If you are involved in a meeting you might find that although it begins with energy and focus, after a

Classification	Important	Not important
Urgent	Do it	Delegate it
Not urgent	Plan it	Leave it

Figure 12.4 Prioritising strategies

while people become tired and think about other things they might be doing. New agenda items are not dealt with as well. Later still the meeting might become ineffective, as people leave or begin to get irritated with others' behaviour under the pressure of time.

The second issue to consider is prioritisation – doing the right things. Tasks might be categorised in two dimensions: their urgency and their importance. A common problem is that urgent tasks, even relatively unimportant ones, take precedence over important ones. The grid in Figure 12.4 suggests some strategies for prioritising tasks based on this categorisation.

There are some pitfalls in prioritising:

• Your personal priorities may not be the same as others.
• Staff priorities may not be patient priorities and vice versa.
• There may be different views within teams.
• There may not be anyone available to delegate to.

Case 12.1 (continued)

Sue observed that the ward was 'busy and chaotic'. She made a list of tasks which staff undertook routinely during their work and identified those which she thought they might be able to do more quickly without reducing the quality, and those where if they had more time, the quality would be increased. She also used the urgent/important grid. Her first example was the handover between shifts. She marked this as urgent and important, but felt that it could be done more quickly if it was better organised.

Activity 12.3

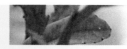

Identify other tasks from your placement experiences which you think might be managed better. Use the urgent/important grid. Managing the task better might mean spending more time, or less, or delegating it, or not doing it at all.

Prioritising tasks is not only key to managing yourself, it is also important in planning and delivering care.

Management standard	Competency	Examples of positive management behaviour	Examples of negative management behaviour
Demands	Managing workload and resources	• bringing in additional resources to handle workload • aware of team members' ability • monitoring team workload • refusing to take on additional work when team is under pressure	• delegating work unequally to team • creating unrealistic deadlines • showing lack of awareness of how much pressure team are under • asking for tasks without checking workload first

Figure 12.5 Examples of positive and negative management behaviour relating to the demands of your job.

Stress

The Health and Safety Executive (HSE 2005) defines **stress** as 'the adverse reaction people have to excessive pressure or other types of demand placed on them'. Some pressure at work is helpful – it stimulates and motivates – but after an optimum level of performance is reached, additional pressure reduces performance, and can lead to stress. According to the HSE, about 1 in 5 people find their work either very or extremely stressful. They (Mackay *et al.* 2004) identify the primary risks for stress at work as (NHS Employers 2008):

• The demands of your job.
• Your control over your work.
• The support you receive from managers and colleagues.
• Your relationships at work.
• Your role in the organisation.
• Change and how it is managed.

The management standards approach gives a framework for risk assessment and action planning on an organisation level, identifying and tackling risks in these six areas. The Health and Safety Executive and the Chartered Institute of Personnel and Development have published guidance for line managers and for HR departments (HSE 2007). They identify, in each of the six areas of the management standards, management competencies and examples of positive and negative management behaviour. An example is given in Figure 12.5.

Case 12.1 (continued)

Sue was able to observe positive and negative management behaviour on the ward relating to the demands of the job. For example the Ward Manager did check how busy the nurses on the ward were before allocating a new task (collecting a patient from theatre) but some nurses did appear to be more busy than others.

If you are feeling under stress, you should first try to understand the cause, and then discuss it with your manager. Many of the examples of positive management behaviour require partnership between managers and staff, so you should do what you can to support improvement. It is not enough for you simply to hand the problem over.

Managing and leading others

It is when thinking about the way that you relate to others that the distinction between management and leadership becomes most important. An element of the distinction relates to formal authority and accountability arrangements within the organisation. A managerial relationship is formal – each employee should be clear about who their line manager is. A leadership relationship is less formal. In this section we will consider some specific issues relevant to management and leadership:

- Delegation and accountability.
- Team working.
- Managing and leading change.

These three areas have been chosen because they are most relevant to the specific aims of this chapter. Other chapters in the book, for example, Chapter 1 on professional accountability, Chapter 4 on health policy, Chapter 5 on inter-professional working and Chapter 9 on communication, will be particularly relevant to management and leadership.

The discussion about management and leadership in Part 1 identified that both are essentially to do with people. Management and leadership are social sciences drawing on a range of other disciplines, including sociology and psychology. This section will draw on a range of theories, but first it will be useful to consider what management theory is, and how it will help you think about your role as a nurse.

Think about infection control. There is a great deal of knowledge about how infections are spread, and how health care professionals can reduce the spread of infection. The development of knowledge in this area has a number of clear implications that for practical purposes are true, for example in emphasising the importance of hand hygiene. You know what you should do (even though you may not need to know all the fine details of microbiology) and you know that if you follow the basic rules, the chances of you being responsible for the spread of infection will be reduced. In the sections below theories will be introduced about, for example, how to achieve change. The theories will have some key implications, for example in emphasising the importance of balancing roles in developing a team.

However, the theories are not scientific explanations that are either true or false. Research in management and leadership does not identify basic truths, it offers likely explanations. Even if a theory offers a clear prescription, you should think about it, and apply it to your situation, and your experience. The application to practice will not necessarily give the results you want. For many reasons your practice may be more complex than the prescription might suggest. Applying theory to practice requires critical reflection, rather than just knowing what to do.

Delegation is the process of passing on responsibility for a task to another person, in an agreed planned way.

A **competent** person is able to perform a specific task. What a person needs to know and understand and the skill required to perform a specific task are defined in a competency.

Accountability is individual responsibility for behaviour or the achievement of a specific objective. Accountability should include reference to the person or body to whom an individual is accountable.

Objectives are explicit statements of tasks to be performed or outcomes achieved.

Authority is an acknowledged right to influence or direct people. It is often related with the idea of power. Considering authority leads to questions about how the right to influence is acknowledged, and where the limits of the authority lie.

Delegation and accountability

Within any structure, the process of delegation is the key to effective provision of services. The chief executive is accountable for all the service that an organisation provides but he or she cannot be in charge of everything. So, responsibilities are **delegated** to individuals, who are **competent**, along with the **accountability** to achieve specific **objectives**, and the appropriate **authority**.

The highlighted terms are all important. Simple definitions are given in the margin. You might find it interesting to consider what you understand by these terms, as they are applied to your practice. Many have a specific professional meaning and application discussed in Chapter 1.

We have identified delegation in a broad and simple sense. There are many elements of good practice in delegation. Pearce (2006) has developed a 10-step guide for effective delegation, which is explained in Box 12.2. These steps are aimed at people who are delegating but your experience of delegation may be being the person to whom the task is delegated. It should be clear that the process that Pearce outlines is mutually supportive and developmental, not just someone getting rid of their work. The principles apply to a chief executive delegating responsibility for nursing issues to the director of nursing, or a ward sister delegating a specific task to a staff nurse, or a third-year student nurse delegating care to others in their final placement.

Professional issues and positions

The NMC *Code* states that:

- You must establish that anyone you delegate to is able to carry out your instructions.
- You must confirm that the outcome of any delegated task meets required standards.
- You must make sure that everyone you are responsible for is supervised and supported.

(NMC 2008)

Box 12.2 Ten steps to effective delegation

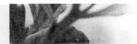

Step 1   Decide what you delegate

Step 2   Be clear what you delegate

Step 3   Decide who you delegate to

Step 4   Inform other team members

Step 5   Decide how to brief subordinates

Step 6   Decide how to guide and develop subordinates

Step 7   Assign responsibility and authority

Step 8   Monitor performance

Step 9   Give feedback

Step 10   Evaluate the experience

(Pearce 2006)

There are a number of colleagues who you could delegate to:

- Someone who has an *equivalent* qualification, role and function (that is, someone from your own peer group).
- Someone who has a *different* qualification, role and function, for example doctors and other health care professionals, health care assistants, support workers, carers and students.
- Someone who has *no formal* qualifications, for example patients and informal carers.

The Royal College of Nursing (RCN) contributed to a collaborative paper which addresses supervision, accountability and delegation. It stated that:

> *When delegating work to others, registered practitioners have a legal responsibility to have determined the knowledge and skill level required to perform the tasks within the work area. The registered practitioner retains accountability for the delegation, and the support worker is accountable for accepting the delegated task and responsibility for his/her actions in carrying out the task. This is providing that the support worker has the skills, knowledge and judgement to perform the delegation, and that the delegation of task falls within the guidelines and protocols of the workplace, and the level of supervision and feedback is appropriate.*

(RCN *et al.* 2006 p. 8)

Assessing competence is very important in making sure that delegation is safe and effective.

Activity 12.4

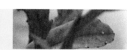

Think of anything that you know you are good at - sport, hobby or activity.

- How do you know this?
- How could other people know this?
- What evidence would confirm this?

Now apply this to yourself in a work context and link with your self-assessment of current skill level. As mentioned previously, it is important that you are competent in the tasks being delegated so if you identify that there are gaps in your knowledge/skills, you will need to make a plan to fill them. Now apply this to working with other staff. When you do not know them or their background you will need to make an evaluation and assessment of them by:

- Asking questions about their qualifications and asking for proof or evidence.
- Exploring their previous experience.
- Asking them to explain or demonstrate the elements of a skill or procedure that you wish them to undertake.
- Observing their practice.
- Evaluating standards of care.

This gets more complicated in practice, because of a range of contextual and cultural issues related to delegation including:

- High workload.
- Fast throughput.
- Variously qualified staff.
- Variable numbers of staff.
- Increasing ethnic diversity in staff and patients.
- Increasing public expectations.

Because of the complexity of health care, it is crucial that registered nurses are able to critically appraise and evaluate evidence (from a range of sources) and supervise and evaluate the performance of others and self.

Objectives

Setting objectives is particularly important. Thinking about what is to be delegated is the first step in deciding who it should be delegated to and whether they are competent and have the authority to carry it out. A popular guide for objectives is that they should be SMART:

- **Specific.** It should be possible to identify whether the objective has been achieved or not.
- **Measurable.** How the achievement is to be measured should be clear.
- **Achievable.** The objective should be achievable, which is not the same as saying it should be easy to achieve. Whether it is achieved will depend in large part on the performance of the person who has been set the objective.
- **Relevant.** To both the staff member and the organisation.
- **Time-bound.** To be achieved within a defined period.

Team working

'A **team** is a small number of people with complementary skills who are committed to a common purpose, performance goals and approach for which they hold themselves mutually accountable' (Katzenbach and Smith 1993 p. 45).

Health care emphasises **team** working, and particularly interprofessional teams providing care. The terms 'clinical team', or 'management team' are often used, and 'project teams' are often formed for specific purposes. So, developing an understanding of how teams can improve their effectiveness is an important area for management research. This is important for those who lead teams, but also for those who are team members. The first issue to consider is 'what is a team?', and 'how does it differ from a collection of individuals, or a group?'

Activity 12.5

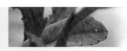

What do you think is the difference between a team and a group?

In considering this question, think of some specific examples from your professional or other experience. If you can undertake this activity in a group (or team!), discuss your ideas with others, and try to agree key points.

The margin definition is used in a publication from the NHS Institute for Innovation and Improvement and the RCN (RCN 2007) entitled *Team Effectiveness Guides*. Like other management concepts, the ideas explained in the guide do not give absolute truth, but perspectives which may help you to reflect on your own experiences.

There is a great deal of research about team working which can be described only superficially here. Four areas of theory are briefly presented, and an activity will ask you to consider how they may help you to understand better the development of teams.

The four are:

1. The team performance curve (Katzenbach and Smith 1993).
2. Stages of team development (Tuckman 1965).
3. Team roles (Belbin 1993).
4. Team working and effectiveness in health care projects (Borrill *et al.* 2002).

Based on research on private sector companies, Katzenbach and Smith (1993) developed a team performance curve which represents how team effectiveness contributes to high performance. On the curve are five key points which represent teams of differing effectiveness and performance impact (see Figure 12.6).

They explain some of the characteristics of each of the identified points (Figure 12.7).

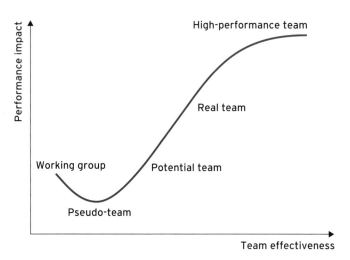

Figure 12.6 The team performance curve.
Source: Katzenbach and Smith (1993).

Case 12.1 (continued)

Sue used this model to consider where the ward team might be on the team performance curve. She thought that it might be at the 'potential team' stage. There is a need for a team with 'a common purpose, performance goals and approach'. Issues like performance goals (standards) are discussed at ward meetings, but the discussions don't often seem to lead to new ideas. Some staff say that their job is just to complete their own work, suggesting that the team has not established mutual accountability.

Working group	• No significant need that would require it to become a team • Members interact primarily to share information • Makes decisions to help each individual to perform within their area of responsibility • No common purpose or joint-work products
Pseudo-team	• There could be a need that would require it to become a team, but is not trying to achieve it
Potential team	• There is a need that requires it to become a team, and it is trying to achieve it. Requires more clarity of purpose, goals or work products • Has not established collective accountability
Real team	• Team members have complementary skills and are equally committed to a common purpose, goals and a working approach for which they hold themselves mutually accountable
High-performing team	• In addition to the features of the real team, has members who are deeply committed to one another's personal growth and success

Figure 12.7 Characteristics of identified points on the team performance curve.
Source: Katzenbach and Smith (1993).

This model helps teams to develop but it does not suggest that these are necessary stages in development. Tuckman's model (1965) suggests that during their establishment, new teams need to go through four phases before they become effective. Some teams that you are a member of may have been established for a long time before you joined them, but high turnover or a change in role may, in effect, push a team backwards in its development.

The four stages are:

1. Forming.
2. Storming.
3. Norming.
4. Performing.

The forming stage relates to that time when team members are getting to know each other and the purpose of the team. After this has been accomplished, teams develop into the storming phase, characterised by conflict. As team members get to know each other better they may be more willing to give opinions, especially about the task or purpose of the team. There may be an element of 'jockeying for position'. As these conflicts are resolved, the team will develop a way of working. This is the norming stage, where attention will be given to the group rather than the task. Finally, the team will develop to the performing stage, where it begins to work effectively.

Belbin's (1993) analysis concentrated on roles within a team. She identified that the most successful teams had nine identifiable roles. There are a number of questionnaires available which can help people to identify what their naturally preferred roles are, but it is important to remember that these are roles and not people acting helplessly in the only role they are able to fulfil. Being aware

Team roles	Description
Plant	Creative, imaginative, unorthodox, solves difficult problems.
Resource-investigator	Extrovert, enthusiastic, communicative. Explores opportunities. Develops contacts.
Co-ordinator	Mature, confident, a good chairperson. Clarifies goals, promotes decision-making, delegates well.
Shaper	Challenging, dynamic, thrives on pressure. Has the drive and courage to overcome obstacles.
Monitor evaluator	Sober, strategic and discerning. Sees all options. Judges accurately.
Teamworker	Co-operative, mild, perceptive, and diplomatic. Listens, builds, averts friction, calms the waters.
Implementer	Disciplined, reliable, conservative and efficient. Turns ideas into practical actions.
Completer	Painstaking, conscientious, anxious. Searches out errors and omissions. Delivers on time.
Specialist	Single-minded, self-starting, dedicated. Provides knowledge and skills in rare supply.

Figure 12.8 Team roles.

Source: Belbin (1993).

of the need for different roles can help team members to adapt their natural behaviour. It does not mean that every team has to have at least nine members, each able to act in their own natural preference. The roles are listed in Figure 12.8 with the descriptions given to them by Belbin (1993 p. 22).

Case 12.1 (continued)

Sue has observed that discussions at team meetings about standards didn't often lead to new ideas. One area where there was often progress was in infection control where there was a link nurse who was very passionate. Sue thought that she might be acting as a 'specialist' and that such a role might be missing for other areas where improvements could be made.

The conclusions of the 'Team working and effectiveness in health care project' were that:

- Health care teams that have clear objectives, high levels of participation, emphasis on quality, and support for innovation, provide high-quality patient care. Such teams also introduce innovations in patient care.
- Members of teams that work well together have relatively low levels of stress.
- In primary health care teams particularly, a diverse range of professional groups working together is associated with higher levels of innovation in patient care.

- The quality of meetings, communication and integration processes in health care contribute to the introduction of new and improved ways of delivering patient care.
- Clear leadership contributes to effective team processes, to high-quality patient care, and to innovation.

(Borrill *et al.* 2002)

Activity 12.6

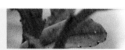

Having considered some ideas relating to teams, and illustrated them through the case study, reflect on whether any of these ideas help you to understand any team that you are part of. For example, have you been part of a new team that has experienced conflict fairly soon after its establishment? Can you think what your preferred team role is, and can you identify others' through observing their behaviours? You may find that different models are useful for different types of teams.

Research focus 12.1

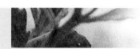

Organisations

are not inanimate objects, staffed by inconvenient things called individuals who would be much easier to deal with if they really were just human resources, a name we give them in the hope that they will be as docile as our fork-lift trucks or as programmable as our computers... Organizations of course are not objects. They are micro-societies.

(Handy 1999 p. 9)

This quotation sums up the complexity of management and leadership research that draws on many areas of social science. The evidence base is not the same as much clinical research which comes from a much more scientific background. The management researcher may try to understand a specific case in detail rather than generalise through big studies that control variables and look for statistical evidence. Applying the knowledge produced in a management research project in one setting to another context requires critical analysis of the new context, which will include critical reflection on a manager's own experiences in that context.

One study in the NHS that adopted a more scientific method (West *et al.* 2002) looked at whether the way that staff were managed in acute hospitals, particularly relating to training, teamworking and appraisal, had an effect on mortality rates. A range of numeric data in these areas were collected. A number of factors that might affect mortality were controlled, such as size, local health needs, and the number of doctors available. The statistical analysis showed that hospitals who had developed training and appraisal systems and whose staff worked in teams achieved lower mortality rates. The study acknowledged some limitations in its design, relating to the data, and concluded that more research is needed to explore the 'underlying mechanisms responsible for these associations. But, at the least, the findings suggest an important new line of enquiry into hospital care and hospital performance' (West *et al.* 2002 p. 1309).

Managing and leading change

We live in an era where change is constant. Much of this change is related to developing technologies, but social change is also rapid. The importance of service user involvement, and working in interprofessional teams, for example, are relatively recent developments. Pressures such as achieving improvements in service, and dealing with resource issues, all require change. When the difference between management and leadership was considered earlier, the definition of leadership was particularly concerned with change.

Like other areas that we have considered, there are many textbooks on change in a health care setting, and we can only touch on the subject here. In Chapter 4, the significance of change in the policy context was emphasised – the Government's commitment to increasing resources available for the NHS was based on an explicit requirement that the way that the service was delivered would change – the word reform is often used.

The NHS Modernisation Agency was established to support this process, mainly through establishing a wide range of projects to examine in detail the process through which health care was being provided. In 2005, the Modernisation Agency function became part of the NHS Institute for Innovation and Improvement, which 'supports the NHS to transform healthcare for patients and the public by rapidly developing and spreading new ways of working, new technology and world class leadership' (NHS Institute for Innovation and Improvement, 2008a). The NHS Institute for Innovation and Improvement has published a number of resources to help staff lead change. There is a series of Improvement Leaders' Guides (NHS Institute for Innovation and Improvement 2007), which are widely used in the NHS. At the time of writing (January 2009) there were 15 guides available.

The first guide, *General Improvement Skills*, starts with a quotation from Winnie the Pooh:

> *Here is Edward Bear, coming downstairs now, bump, bump, bump, on the back of his head, behind Christopher Robin. It is, as far as he knows, the only way of coming downstairs, but sometimes he feels that there really is another way, if only he could stop bumping for a moment and think of it.*
>
> (Milne, 1926)

The theories and tools described in the Improvement Leaders' Guides are presented to help clinicians think about changes that will improve services and how they can be implemented. One of the Guides is called *Managing the Human Dimensions of Change*. It presents a model which gives two approaches to improvement: the anatomical and the physiological. These are not alternatives – in order to effect an improvement each project should be an appropriate combination of both approaches. The differences are explained in Figure 12.9.

An example of a change where the approach might be mainly anatomical is the introduction of a new computer system. There may be opportunities for staff to get involved in many different ways, but there will need to be a precise plan to implement the change. On the other hand, an improvement project might address some issues in the way that drugs are dispensed on a ward – there may be problems for example with timing, or interruptions, or supervising patients taking their drugs. The answer for this problem may involve the ward staff thinking through possible changes to make an improvement, and trying them out in practice.

Anatomical approach to improvement	Physiological approach to improvement	In practice, both approaches to improvement are necessary
Change is a step by step process	Outcomes cannot be predetermined	You need to set a direction but need to be flexible
It is typically initiated top-down	Change comes typically bottom-up	Top-down support is needed for bottom-up change
Objectives are to set in advance (and set in stone)	There is no end point	Objectives need to be set and the team should be congratulated when each objective is achieved, but improvement never ends
It goes wrong because of poor planning and project control	It goes wrong because of people issues	Planning and monitoring is important but gaining the commitment of people is *vital*

Figure 12.9 Anatomical and physiological approaches to change.
Source: NHS Institute for Innovation and Improvement (2007).

Activity 12.7

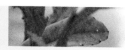

Identify three or four changes you have been involved with. For each change, draw a line across a page, with 'Anatomical' at one end, and 'Physiological' at the other. Mark a cross on the line which represents the balance between these approaches that was adopted. Give your reasons and compare your views with others.

Even formal top-down change, at the anatomical end of the continuum, will need people to change, requiring leadership more than management. Solutions to problems should not be dictated by managers; involving staff at all stages of change management processes is key to managing change successfully. Individuals who want to resist change, or sabotage it, are unlikely to give a manager an opportunity to discipline them for misconduct, for example for failing to follow a new procedure. They are much more likely to reduce the effectiveness of change simply by not engaging in the change or the reasons for it. The best way to ensure that change is successful is to reduce the effect of the factors that can hinder it, and many of these will involve staff.

Managing resources

Both you and the people you work with are resources that have to be carefully managed, but in this section finance is considered. Budget management is an important area for NHS managers. 'Keeping within my budget' is regarded as a very important objective. In recent years, although the NHS has had a large increase in the available resources overall, there have been significant difficulties in managing services within budgets. Even if a service manager considers their budget as adequate, and does not need to find ways of saving money, it remains important that a service runs efficiently. Inefficient services deny the opportunity to invest resources elsewhere. In this section, some of the key issues of financial management will be identified which will hopefully help you to develop some insight into some of the actions and decisions that your managers might make.

What is a budget?

A budget is a plan. Although a budget is often thought of in terms of an amount of money that is available to spend, it should also be linked to other key aspects of performance, particularly activity, since it is activity that determines costs. Budgets are determined through the planning process. The planning process for the following year starts early. Organisations predict key targets they need to achieve, such as meeting waiting times or improving infection control, assumed activity levels and other priority improvements. Priorities are determined through external influences, particularly the requirements of commissioners to meet DH guidelines, but also internal processes that identify strengths and weaknesses of currently provided services. Usually a planning process will seek bids from departments or directorates for additional investment to meet specific objectives – for example if a department is experiencing an increase in demand, it might put forward a bid for additional staff.

Financial management and control

How do managers spend the money they have available to deliver the services they are responsible for? An organisation will have strict processes for controlling how money is spent, to make sure that it is spent wisely and to prevent its mangers spending too much. In effect this would mean spending money that the organisation does not have. A key issue for financial control are levels of authorisation; who does the organisation allow to spend its money? Usually this will be a person who holds the budget. That person is responsible for ensuring that the budget is not overspent, and used for the purposes for which it is intended, and as a general rule, it should be that person who authorises expenditure.

Value for money

If a service reduces its costs by buying the same things (staff and non-staff) for less money, it becomes more **economic**.

If a service produces the same amount of work with fewer resources (staff and non-staff) it becomes more **efficient or productive**.

Value for money is a term which you will come across from time to time; another related term is cost-effectiveness. Producing as much benefit as possible from the money available (money which, it should not be forgotten, comes from all of us in tax) is an important objective of management. How can you judge whether you can improve the cost-effectiveness of your service? The model below describes the NHS Production Pathway (Wanless *et al.* 2007 p. 11). It shows how cost-effectiveness measures how money produces benefits. This is broken down into three separate stages:

- The money 'buys resources'. For the NHS these are mainly staff, but also equipment and supplies. Cost-effectiveness can be improved here by reducing the cost of these resources, becoming more **economic**.
- The resources are used to produce activities, which might for example be nursing interventions, or district nurse visits. Cost-effectiveness might be improved here by producing the same output with fewer resources (or more output with the same resources) which might mean for example fewer staff, becoming more **efficient or productive**.

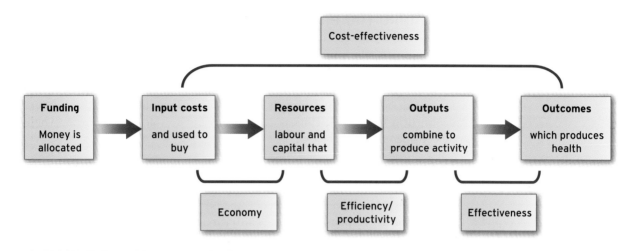

Figure 12.10 The NHS production pathway.

Source: Wanless *et al.* (2007).

If a service gets better at achieving its goals, it becomes more **effective**.

- The outputs of the process are not goals in themselves. Goals are expressed in terms of outcomes, which in general are described as 'health' but might also include other desirable outcomes such as 'independence' or 'safety'. Cost-effectiveness might be improved here by producing the same outcome with fewer activities, becoming more **effective**.

The model is shown in Figure 12.10.

The important thing is that cost-effectiveness is maximised. Attempts to improve one part of the model may not increase cost-effectiveness overall.

Case 12.1 (continued)

Sue thought about this model when a ward meeting was discussing how the ward could make savings, and someone had suggested that they could save on food because a lot was wasted. If the right portions were given to all patients which resulted in less food being sent from the kitchen, there would be an increase in efficiency. However, the purpose of food is to maintain and enhance nutritional status, and a lot of wasted food may suggest that this was not being achieved. Perhaps increasing the quality of the food (and its cost), and helping patients to eat their food if they were having difficulty, would lead to more food being eaten, and better achievement of the goal. In that case, the process would become less economic and less efficient. It would become more effective. It would be difficult to know if the whole process had become more or less cost-effective.

Activity 12.8

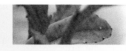

Think of an outcome you produce, and how you might be able to increase cost-effectiveness by being more economical, efficient, or effective.

Managing the environment

In this section, the environment in which you work will be discussed. It is called 'Managing the environment' but it might be called 'Managing *in* the environment' – it depends if the particular aspect of the environment can be influenced, or if it just needs to be responded to. Two important themes were identified in Chapter 4; clinical governance and service improvement. These are considered in turn below.

Clinical governance

Clinical governance is 'a framework through which NHS organisations are accountable for continuously improving quality of their services and safeguarding high standards of care by creating an environment in which excellence in clinical care will flourish' (DH 1998 p. 33).

Clinical governance was introduced to the NHS in 1997. Previously there had been no formal responsibility for health services to deliver high-quality care. The only formal duty they had (for which the chief executive was accountable) was for the use of resources. Clinical governance introduced a statutory duty for the quality of care.

Clinical governance creates a set of systematic ways in which it should become increasingly difficult for an organisation to give poor-quality service. As clinical governance was being developed over a number of years, some reports addressing scandals gave the issue importance and urgency. The most important of these were the poor outcomes achieved in paediatric heart surgery at the Bristol Royal Infirmary between 1984 and 1995 (Kennedy 2001), and Dr Harold Shipman's murder of 215 of his patients between 1975 and 1998 (Smith 2002). In Bristol, although individual doctors were disciplined by the GMC, it was the failings of the system that were identified as the main cause of the problem. In Shipman's case, although the deaths were the result of Shipman's action, the system he worked within allowed him to continue. He was only caught when he forged a patient's will. Clinical governance attempts to create *systems* of care which reduce the likelihood of poor quality.

In 1998, a consultation paper, *A First Class Service* (DH 1998) was published which gave more details about clinical governance. It was defined as 'a framework through which NHS organisations are accountable for continuously improving quality of their services and safeguarding high standards of care by creating an environment in which excellence in clinical care will flourish' (DH 1998 p. 33). The Commission for Health Improvement (CHI) was set up to support the development of clinical governance. It established a more detailed framework for clinical governance, which would be used to inspect Trusts. CHI identified seven components of clinical governance (CHI 2001):

- Consultation and patient involvement.
- Clinical audit.
- Clinical risk management.
- Research and effectiveness.
- Staffing and staff management.
- Education, training and continuing professional development.
- Use of information.

Since CHI set out these areas of inspection, and since a bad CHI Clinical Governance Review could have severe consequences for organisations (and particularly their senior managers), these seven areas became accepted as the definition of clinical governance. Trusts were inspected every four years by CHI and as well as inspecting various aspects of care, CHI spoke with patients, staff and other stakeholders. Their reports, which included a score against each of these seven areas, were published and the Trust was required to produce and publish an action plan to address issues that were raised.

In 2005, the system of specific Clinical Governance Reviews was replaced by the Annual Health Check. National standards are now published (DH 2004b) and every year Trusts have to assess their compliance against them. The standards and the processes of checking compliance are discussed in general in Chapter 4.

Safety

A number of the national standards are concerned with safety and the management of risk. The safety of health care was given priority in 2000 with the publication of a consultation document, *An Organisation with a Memory* (DH 2000). The government responded by establishing the National Patient Safety Agency to support learning from adverse incidents and near misses. As well as the system for reporting and analysing incidents, it was also acknowledged that factors such as a reporting culture, education and development, and managing change were crucial. Progress has recently been reviewed (DH 2006a). Although progress has been made, the report claims that patient safety does not always have the same priority from Trusts as activity or financial targets, and that the reporting systems are not yet fully effective. A range of proposals have been made to improve progress. One of the recommendations was a national patient safety campaign, which is now being managed by the NHS Institute of Innovation and Improvement.

There are four core standards in the patient safety domain of the NHS national standards (see Figure 12.11). The process for assessing whether a health care organisation is meeting the standards is that they undertake a self-assessment using additional criteria produced by the Healthcare Commission (2007) (Care Quality Commission from April 2009). These criteria give some guidance for each standard about how the organisation can judge whether it is meeting the standard or not. Often these criteria refer to other standards and guidelines.

These standards identify a number of specific areas for concern; infection control, child protection, NICE guidelines, medical devices, decontamination and medicines management. The Care Quality Commission's criteria for assessing whether a Trust is meeting each standard refers to a range of other guidelines and organisations, including:

- The National Patient Safety Agency (NPSA). The NPSA has a National Reporting and Learning System which Trusts have a duty to support.
- The NHS Litigation Authority. The NHSLA (2008) has published standards for risk management. There are five standards, relating to:
  1. Governance.
  2. Competent and capable workforce.
  3. Safe environment.
  4. Clinical care.
  5. Learning from experience.

Core standard C1	Health care organisations protect patients through systems that: a. identify and learn from all patient safety incidents and other reportable incidents, and make improvements in practice based on local and national experience and information derived from the analysis of incidents. b. ensure that patient safety notices, alerts and other communications concerning patient safety, which require action, are acted upon within required timescales.
Core standard C2	Health care organisations protect children by following national child protection guidelines within their own activities and in their dealings with other organisations.
Core standard C3	Health care organisations protect patients by following National Institute for Health and Clinical Excellence (NICE) interventional procedures guidelines.
Core standard C4	Health care organisations keep patients, staff and visitors safe by having systems to ensure that: a. the risk of health care-acquired infection to patients is reduced, with particular emphasis on high standards of hygiene and cleanliness, achieving year on year reductions in methicillin-resistant *Staphylococcus aureus* (MRSA) b. all risks associated with the acquisition and use of medical devices are minimised c. all reusable medical devices are properly decontaminated prior to use and that the risks associated with decontamination facilities and processes are well managed d. medicines are handled safely and securely e. the prevention, segregation, handling, transport and disposal of waste is properly managed so as to minimise the risks to the health and safety of staff, patients, the public and the safety of the environment

Figure 12.11 Core standards in the patient safety domain.
Source: DH (2004b).

- A guide (*Working Together to Safeguard Children*) produced by the Government for inter-agency working to promote child protection (HM Government 2006).
- The Health Act 2006 Code of Practice for the Prevention and Control of Health Care Associated Infections (DH 2006b).
- DH guidance for the management of controlled drugs (DH 2006c).

This list is really only a demonstration of the volume of guidelines, standards and criteria that exist. All of these documents are in the public domain, and you can look them up if you need to.

Activity 12.9

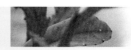

Find the NPSA's risk management standards on its website. Which criteria are most relevant to your work? Identify any detailed guidance or requirements relevant to you.

Although there is a whole range of specific measures and guidance, the importance of good management is fundamental to creating a culture where safety is a top priority. Organisational culture was identified in *An Organisation with a Memory* as of vital importance. It . . .

> is central to every stage of the learning process – from ensuring that incidents are identified and reported through to embedding the necessary changes deeply into practice. There is evidence that 'safety cultures', where open reporting and balanced analysis are encouraged in principle and by example, can have a positive and quantifiable impact on the performance of organisations. 'Blame cultures' on the other hand can encourage people to cover up errors for fear of retribution and act against the identification of the true causes of failure, because they focus heavily on individual actions and largely ignore the role of underlying systems. The culture of the NHS still errs too much towards the latter.
>
> (DH 2000 p. ix)

All staff have roles in developing and maintaining a safety culture, which might mean for example making sure that concerns are properly reported, often using an incident reporting form.

General principles of risk management

A **hazard** is a situation that may cause harm.

A **risk** is a specific incident that may occur to cause harm.

Hazards, both natural and man-made, are all around us all the time and health care is a particularly risky business. We cannot avoid them entirely so they have to be managed. When we have the expertise for doing this we become comfortable, even with the most hazardous situations, but we should never become complacent. First it is important to differentiate between **hazards** and **risks**, and some general examples are given in Figure 12.12.

Hazard	Risk
Wet floor	Slips and falls
Electrical equipment	Electrocution; burns
Hot water/baths/drinks	Scalds
Body fluids	Infection; cross-infection
Invasive procedures e.g. catheterisation; biopsy	Infection; trauma
	Peri- and postoperative complications
Surgical interventions	Adverse reactions
Blood transfusion	Injury; infection; cross-infection;
Sharps/needles	inadvertent inoculation
Medicines	Errors; adverse drug reactions
Violent/abusive patients or visitors	Damage or trauma to staff
Major incidents/terrorism	Damage to property

Figure 12.12 Examples of hazards and risks.

Hazards are always present – you cannot just avoid them so hazard awareness is imperative and reporting of actual and potential hazards essential. What is needed is a strategy to manage and minimise risk and this starts with making an effective assessment.

Activity 12.10

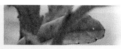

Think back to your last placement and identify any specific hazards present and how these were assessed and managed.

- What assessment tools were used and how was this documented?
- Did you observe any incidents or accidents?
- How were these managed and what did you learn from this?

Assessing and managing risk

Risk assessment is a systematic and effective method of identifying risks and determining the most cost-effective means to minimise or remove them (NPSA 2008).

Although managing risks is important in the provision of safe care, it is possible that an organisation can go too far. Managing risks has a cost, as well as implications for the actions of staff. In order to strike the right balance organisations will use systematic **risk assessment** processes.

Risks are assessed against two dimensions:

1. Impact. If the risk that has been identified actually happens, how serious would it be?
2. Likelihood. What are the chances of the risk happening?

These dimensions can be shown as a matrix (see Figure 12.13).

	Low likelihood	High likelihood
High impact		
Low impact		

Figure 12.13 Risk assessment matrix.

Assessing risk in this way will help managers to decide what to do about a risk. If a risk is very unlikely to happen, and even if it did the impact would be low, it might be decided that no action should be taken. If a risk is likely to happen, and if it did the impact would be very serious, the organisation may put great effort, and significant resources, into reducing the chances that it will happen, and reducing its impact if it does.

Activity 12.11

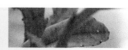

Identify risks from your experience (in your personal and professional life) and use the matrix in Figure 12.13 to assess them.

	Impact	Likelihood
1	Negligible	Rare
2	Minor	Unlikely
3	Moderate	Possible
4	Major	Likely
5	Catastrophic	Almost certain

Figure 12.14 The NPSA risk matrix.

Source: NPSA (2008).

While it is easy to determine priorities between low likelihood/low impact and high likelihood/high impact, the other two quadrants in the matrix are more difficult. What is more important: a risk which is unlikely to happen but with high impact, or one which is likely to happen but with low impact? While it may be relatively simple to understand the likelihood of an event, different sorts of impacts have to be considered. How do you compare, for example, the importance of possible injury to a patient with financial loss or adverse publicity? It might be useful to revisit the risks you have identified. Are most of the risks you have identified mainly about patient safety? How would you compare other risks, which might lead to financial loss?

A systematic process for assessing and prioritising risk is required. If the impact and likelihood are given a numeric score against criteria to make sure that the scoring is consistent, then multiplying the scores together will give a single risk score. This will allow comparisons to be made, and help organisations decide where to put the most effort and resources to manage risk.

The NPSA has published a risk matrix to help managers assess and manage risk. For impact and likelihood they have developed a five-point scale, with 1 being low, and 5 high – the general descriptors are shown in Figure 12.14. The NPSA also give descriptors which help to assess consistently the impacts of risks against different domains. Eight domains are identified, and for each domain there are examples of descriptors in each of the five impact scores ranging from negligible to catastrophic.

Activity 12.12

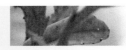

The table in Figure 12.15 gives the eight domains in the NPSA risk matrix, and some examples of descriptors in each domain. Go through the table comparing the impact of these risks, and note what impact (from Figure 12.14) score you think each descriptor might have. The answers are given at the end of the chapter.

Service improvement

For many NHS staff, an interest in management may start through an understanding that something about the service they provide should be improved. In Chapter 4, the context for the recent emphasis on modernisation was explained. In 2000, the NHS Plan was published (Secretary of State for Health 2000),

Domain	Example of a descriptor	Impact score?
Impact on the safety of patients, staff or public (physical/psychological harm)	E1. Increase in length of hospital stay by more than 15 days	
Quality/complaints/audit	E2. Treatment or service has significantly reduced effectiveness	
Human resources/organisational development/staffing/competence	E3. Very low staff morale	
Statutory duty/inspections	E4. Reduced performance rating if unresolved	
Adverse publicity/reputation	E5. Potential for public concern	
Business objectives/projects	E6. 5–10% over project budget	
Finance including claims	E7. Claim(s) between £100,000 and £1 million	
Service/business interruption Impact on environment	E8. Loss/interruption of more than one week	

Figure 12.15 The eight domains of the NPSA risk matrix.
Source: NPSA (2008).

which delivered significant additional resources for the NHS, but also called for the service to be 'redesigned around the needs of the patient'. The NHS Institute for Innovation and Improvement was introduced above when we were discussing managing and leading change. It was the successor organisation to the NHS Modernisation Agency which was set up in 2001 to support change in the NHS. The Institute has established projects in a number of areas to improve care, and has a wide range of services available. In 2008/9 the Institute has six priority areas (NHS Institute for Innovation and Improvement 2008b):

1. Safer care
2. Delivering value and quality
3. Commissioning for health improvement
4. iLinks (which is about improving the accessibility of their support materials)
5. Building capacity for a self-improving NHS, which is about improving learning and leadership
6. National Innovation Centre.

It would be impossible to summarise the work of the Institute, and the NHS Modernisation Agency before it, in a few pages. You may find it useful to browse their website at http://www.institute.nhs.uk. You have to register on the site but this is easy and free. The section on Safer Care will be particularly useful. The *Improvement Leaders' Guides* (NHS Institute for Innovation and Improvement 2007) are important publications.

Improvement Leaders' Guides

The *Improvement Leaders' Guides* were discussed earlier in the section about change. They are 15 booklets which support staff in making improvements to their service. They are aimed at all staff, because one of the key principles of service improvement is that it is everybody's business. It is not just a management responsibility, and a number of the tools and techniques introduced in these guides are about making a series of small changes to services, in a continuous drive for improvement – the physiological change in the model introduced earlier. One project in the Institute is to include improvement techniques into pre-registration curricula, so that newly qualified nurses and other staff are equipped with some of the tools of improvement, and have the motivation to take responsibility for improving services. The *Improvement Leaders' Guides* suggest that the 'discipline' of improvement has 'four equally important and interrelated parts':

1. *Involving users, carers, staff and public.* If services are to become more responsive to the needs and preferences of patients and carers, staff involved in improvement need to develop techniques for understanding what these needs and preferences are. This applies to individual patients as well as groups of patients, and prospective patients.

2. *Process and systems thinking.* Health care is provided through complex systems, many of which have evolved over many years. An often used quotation is that 'every system is perfectly designed to achieve the results that it gets' (Institute for Healthcare Improvement 2008). So if the system that you work in achieves outcomes like long waits, or high rates of infection, as opposed to short waits or low rates of infection, it is as if someone had designed the way that care is provided in order to achieve these outcomes. So in order to improve services it is often necessary first to understand the system that produces the results that it gets.

3. *Personal and organisation development.* All health care is provided by teams who work in organisations. This part of improvement discipline helps leaders to build cultures within teams and organisations that support improvements, and recognise differences between individuals helping to mobilise engagement.

4. *Making it a habit: initiating, spreading, and sustaining.* Improvement should not just be a specific initiative to address a specific issue. It should be a constant search to provide better services, and achieve better outcomes. That requires improvement activities being part of everyday work.

The *Improvement Leaders' Guides* address all these areas. They are available to be downloaded on the NHS Institute website, and you will also be able to order a boxed set by ringing a number that is printed on the back cover, or you can order online.

A **process map** is a diagram that shows all the tasks required to complete a process for a patient's care and treatment, in the sequence that they are completed.

Described in the *Improvement Leaders' Guides*, **process mapping** is a key technique to help teams identify suggestions for change. This helps teams develop a detailed understanding of the process that produces the outcome that is the subject of the improvement. When a team develops a process map, it is important that it records what actually happens, not what should happen, or what the most important person in the room thinks happens. The idea behind process mapping is that the system that has developed to complete a task may have evolved over many years, and is unlikely to be understood in detail by any person with a responsibility for improving the outcome of the system. Process mapping creates this understanding, and when it has been achieved, the process can be changed to improve its performance.

The model for improvement (Langley *et al.* 1996) is widely used, and is shown in Figure 12.16.

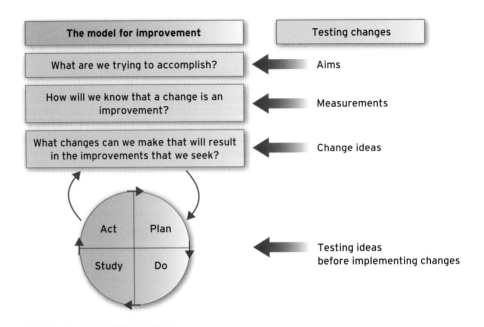

Figure 12.16 The model for improvement.

Source: Langley *et al.* (1996).

NHS Scotland (2006) Diagnostic Collaborative Programme. There are many different versions available. http//www.scotland.gov.uk/Resource/Doc/96540/0023357.pdf

Case 12.1 (continued)

Several patients from Sue's ward had complained that when they were taken to X-ray, they were kept waiting for a long time in a cold corridor. A small team from the ward, the X-ray department, and the porters got together and completed a process map so that they could fully understand what the process was. The process involved requests being taken from the wards and being checked in the X-ray department before being put in a tray for the porters. There were several delays in the process which led to problems – for example the porter often found that the patient was not available, and some patients had to be taken immediately because the X-rays were needed. Because of these delays the porters tried to maintain a queue in the department so that there was always someone waiting. This led to patients waiting for a long time, before and after their X-ray. The process map identified all the stages and delays, and helped the team suggest areas for improvement.

A **PDSA** (Plan, Do, Study, Act) cycle is a rapid way of trying and evaluating a small change in a work process to see if the change leads to an improvement.

Change ideas are tested, in the model for improvement, through Plan, Do, Study, Act (**PDSA**) cycles. In Case 12.1 above, the team may have suggested that the wards try to write on the form a time by when the X-ray is required to help prioritisation, or times when the patient might be unavailable. It might be agreed that the X-ray department could call for more portering help if there was more than one patient waiting. These changes could be tried in PDSA cycles. PDSA cycles are rapid change cycles, so that a momentum for improvement is established in a team. It is a method that is particularly useful in achieving 'physiological' change, which was described earlier. If the change achieves an improvement, it can be made permanent. If it does not, then it can be amended or another suggestion tried.

Activity 12.13

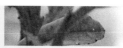

Download the guide entitled *Process mapping, analysis and redesign.* In a team identify a process that might be improved, and produce a process map. Identify changes that might be considered for PDSA cycles. Use the search facility at http://www.institute.nhs.uk

PDSA cycles will help to develop a culture where everyone has a responsibility for changing the service, and where changes can be tried out. If a change does not result in an improvement, effective learning can still be achieved. However, there are some changes that could be made, where a failure would not be acceptable, particularly relating to patient safety. Introducing a new treatment or procedure, for example, is likely to have a clear procedure within a Trust's governance framework. So, although there are efforts being made to empower clinicians who deliver services to make changes, these changes have to be made within the context of the organisation and its governance arrangements.

Complaints

Complaints provide valuable feedback from which organisations and individuals should learn, not only about safety issues, but about the whole range of the patient's experience. The natural reaction to a complaint may be to be defensive, but they offer, as well as an opportunity to address issues a complainant may have, an opportunity for improving services. In 2007 the DH produced proposals for consultation (DH 2007a) to make complaints procedures more flexible and locally driven. Procedures included provisions for independent review by the Healthcare Commission (now Care Quality Commission), and final referral to the Health Service Ombudsman, were not easily understood (DH 2007a). The new arrangements, which will be developed through the experience of early adopters from 2009, will be more consistent with the principles of developing locally responsive organisations, with a strong regulatory framework, which was explored in Chapter 4. Previously, local resolution was managed by the organisation, with a formal response being sent by the chief executive. In the new system, local services will be invited to respond and develop service improvements as a result. Organisations will get involved if the complaint is too complex to be dealt with locally, and the right of referral to the Ombudsman will remain. Local clinical leadership will become more important in developing learning from incidents, including complaints.

Part 3: Exploring management and leadership

To conclude this chapter on management and leadership we discuss a number of issues which provide some critical perspectives. First, we will consider some views about whether the NHS has too many managers, which seems to be a popular view among many members of the public and health professionals. We will also briefly consider some more substantive critiques:

- The relationship between managers and health care professionals.
- Evidence-based management.
- Unexamined assumptions which support established interests.

In 2007, the NHS Confederation, which represents NHS organisations, published a report entitled *Management in the NHS: The facts* (NHS Confederation 2007). This addressed key issues such as why the NHS needs managers, and what they do, noting that they 'often find themselves criticised and derided for being faceless bureaucrats or pointless pen-pushers' (NHS Confederation 2007 p. 2). The NHS Confederation pointed out that 'the traditional image of NHS managers – perpetuated by TV programmes such as *Casualty* and *Holby City* – is of men in sharp grey suits, who are not really interested in patients' (NHS Confederation 2007 p. 6). The reality is that 59 per cent of managers and senior managers in the NHS are female, and over 50 per cent have a clinical background. Only 2.7 per cent of the NHS workforce are managers, compared with 15 per cent of the UK workforce as a whole. Management costs were around 4 per cent of total NHS expenditure in 2005, and this has fallen from 5 per cent in 2000. In addition, as we have discussed in this chapter and others, the NHS is going through major changes which have to be managed.

Evidence such as this might give an objective view, but figures on this scale are difficult to relate to in practice. There are some difficulties in defining exactly what a manager is – would you, for example, count a Ward Sister or Charge Nurse as a 'manager'? The views of many of NHS staff may be formed more by their experience of management, rather than statistical evidence.

There has been a considerable amount of practical interest in the relationship between managers and health professionals. For example, the Audit Commission published a report in December 2007 called *A Prescription for Partnership* (Audit Commission 2007) which highlighted the importance of clinical engagement in financial management. This is just one report in a long line.

One reason that tensions remain between the medical profession and managers is the changing way that health care is delivered, with greater emphasis on uniformity in clinical processes, with care and treatment being increasingly 'systematised' (as opposed to being based on individual decisions of clinicians), and increased efficiency becoming more important (Degeling *et al.* 2003). Degeling *et al.* (2003) offer some international evidence on attitudes to various aspects of modernisation. Figure 12.17 shows how medical clinicians and managers, nurse clinicians and managers, and general managers view key issues in health service reform.

From the chapters in this book, particularly this one and the one on health policy, hopefully you will recognise the four key elements of modernisation in the table. Interestingly, nurse managers is the only group supporting all four elements, and the paper goes on to argue that managers and doctors should

Elements of health services modernisation	Medical Clinicians	Medical Managers	General Managers	Nurse Managers	Nurse Clinicians
Recognise connections between clinical decisions and resources	Oppose	Support	Equivocal	Support	Oppose
Transparent accountability	Oppose	Support	Support	Support	Oppose
Systematisation	Oppose	Oppose	Support	Support	Equivocal
Multidisciplinary team	Oppose	Oppose	Equivocal	Support	Support

Figure 12.17 Attitudes on modernisation.

Source: Degeling *et al.* (2003).

engage more directly with nursing and allied health colleagues. This paper suggests that nurses as managers and clinicians have a particular perspective, outside the much-discussed divide between management and medicine.

The rise in the evidence-based health care movement has provided the inspiration for calls for managers to use similar processes of using evidence in their decision-making. The recent report of the High-level Group on Clinical Effectiveness (DH 2007b) identified the importance of using and developing an evidence base on how to implement evidence-based practice. There are clear differences in evidence-based clinical practice and evidence-based management, particularly in the availability of evidence. Difficulties in applying evidence to management practice are widely acknowledged and relate to issues which include differing cultures, the strength (or lack) of the research base, and the nature of decision-making. A lack of a body of knowledge in health care management has led to a view that to attempt to apply the principles of evidence-based clinical practice to management is simply misconceived. Instead a call has been made to examine the 'craft' of management, which draws on the work of Schon (1983) on the 'reflective practitioner' to create a more critical and 'evidence aware' approach (Hewison 2004). The debate about evidence-based management raises some questions about the status of the 'profession' of management, how its practitioners should be educated, and how they should relate to health care professionals who have an increasing reliance on an explicit evidence-base.

There has been considerable growth in research about management in the health service in recent years. Learmonth (2005) reviewed the literature relating to a number of key issues, and concludes that much management research 'takes commonsense managerial imperatives as simply a natural part of the way that the world is, assumptions used to construct particular worlds' (Learmonth 2005 p. 110). In other words, there is insufficient examination in much management research of basic assumptions; they give 'a version of the world [that], whilst appearing neutral, tacitly supports elite interests' (Learmonth 2005 p. 93). These assumptions might include the inevitability of legitimate power in organisations, or the importance of management techniques.

An example of this is given in McDonald (2004), in a study of an initiative in a PCT to 'empower' staff, which is a theme of recent service improvement initiatives, as discussed earlier. She suggests that the 'empowerment' of staff may be seen as a different way of exercising control, through moulding identities acceptable to the organisation, to value staff who are 'loyal, positive, and embrace change' (McDonald 2004 p. 946).

This serves to reinforce a point made in the chapter. Management is not a science which gives you the right answers in a specific context. Understanding management and leadership require sustained critical reflection on your experience, with the help of a range of models, theories, and concepts. As this last section has attempted to show, there are some fundamental debates about the status of management, its role in the NHS and its relationship with the health care professions.

Conclusion

In this chapter, we have asked you to think about management and leadership not only as part of your working environment, but also as important activities that you will undertake from the very beginning of your career. Theories and concepts in management and leadership do not contain truths which can tell you, for example, what management behaviour will make a team successful, or what is the 'correct' way to assess risk. But they do give you ideas which you can use to help reflect on your experiences to develop your understanding of your work environment, and how you develop your own role and behaviour.

The importance of clinical professionals being leaders has recently been emphasised in a major review of the NHS (Secretary of State for Health 2008). Further improvements in the NHS, particularly in the quality and safety of services, will not happen unless staff at all levels are prepared to take on responsibility not only for their own professional actions, but also as leaders. In your career you may also wish to follow a management route. In either case, we hope that this chapter has given you some useful ideas to consider.

Answers to impact scores

Example E1, 4; E2, 3; E3, 4; E4, 2; E5, 1; E6, 3; E7, 4; E8, 4.

Suggested further reading

NHS Institute of Innovation and Improvement. *Improvement Leaders Guides* http://www.institute.nhs.uk - these guides are free to download once you have registered on the site, and are highly recommended.

Barr, J. and Dowding, L. (2008) *Leadership in Health Care*, London: Sage.

Iles, V. (2005) *Really Managing Health Care* (2nd ed.), Maidenhead: Open University Press.

Moullin, M. (2002) *Delivering Excellence in Health and Social Care*, Buckingham: Open University Press.

References

Audit Commission (2007) *A Prescription for Partnership*. London: Audit Commission.

Belbin, R. M. (1993) *Team Roles at Work*. Oxford: Butterworth-Heinemann.

Borrill, C., West, M., Dawson, J., *et al.* (2002) *Team Working and Effectiveness in Health Care Project. Findings from the Health Care Team Effectiveness Project.* Birmingham: Aston Centre for Health Service Organisation Research.

CHI (Commission for Health Improvement) (2001) *A Guide to Clinical Governance Reviews in NHS Acute Trusts*. London: CHI.

Davies, H. T. O. and Harrison, S. (2003) Trends in doctor-manager relationships. *British Medical Journal* **326**, 646–649.

Degeling, P., Maxwell, S., Kennedy, J. and Coyle, B. (2003) Medicine, management, and modernisation: a 'danse macabre'? *British Medical Journal* **326**, 649–652.

DH (Department of Health) (1998) *A First Class Service. Quality in the new NHS.* London: DH (http://www.dh.gov.uk).

DH (2000) *An Organisation with a Memory*. London: DH (http://www.dh.gov.uk).

DH (2004a) *The NHS Knowledge and Skills Framework (NHS KSF) and the Development Review Process*. London: DH (http://www.dh.gov.uk).

DH (2004b) *National Standards, Local Action. Health and Social Care Standards and Planning Framework. 2004/5–2007/8*. London: DH (http://www.dh.gov.uk)

DH (2006a) *Safety First. A report for patients, clinicians, and health care managers.* London: DH (http://www.dh.gov.uk).

DH (2006b) *The Health Act 2006 Code of Practice for the Prevention and Control of Health Care Associated Infections*. London: DH (http://www.dh.gov.uk).

DH (2006c) *Safer Management of Controlled Drugs: Guidance on strengthened governance arrangement*. London: DH (http://www.dh.gov.uk).

DH (2007a) *Making Experiences Count. A new approach to responding to complaints.* London: DH (http://www.dh.gov.uk).

DH (2007b) *Report of the High-level Group on Clinical Effectiveness. Chaired by Professor Sir John Tooke*. London: DH (http://www.dh.gov.uk).

Glouberman, S. and Zimmerman, B. J. (2002) *Complicated and Complex Systems: What would successful reform of Medicare look like?* Discussion paper 8, Commission on the Future of Health Care in Canada. (http://www.change-ability.ca/Health_Care_Commission_DP8.pdf) Last accessed 6 January 2009.

Handy, C. (1999) *Understanding Organizations* (4th ed.). Harmondsworth: Penguin.

HM Government (2006) *Working Together to Safeguard Children*. London: The Stationery Office.

HSE (Health and Safety Executive) (2005) *Tackling Stress: The management standards approach*. London: HSE (http://www.hse.gov.uk).

HSE (2007) *Line Management Behaviour and Stress at Work – Guidance for line managers*. London: HSE (http://www.hse.gov.uk).

Healthcare Commission (2007) *Criteria for Assessing Core Standards in 2007/8. Acute trusts*. London: Healthcare Commission (http://www.healthcarecommission.org.uk).

Hewison, A. (2004) Evidence-based management in the NHS: Is it possible? *Journal of Health Organisation and Management* **18** (5), 336–348.

Iles, V. (2005) *Really Managing Health Care* (2nd ed.). Maidenhead: Open University Press.

Institute for Healthcare Improvement (2008) *Improvement Tip: Want a new level of performance? Get a new system*. London: Institute for Healthcare Improvement (http://www.ihi.org/IHI/Topics/Improvement/ImprovementMethods/Improvement Stories/ImprovementTipWantaNewLevelofPerformanceGetaNewSystem.htm). Last accessed 29 December 2008.

Katzenbach, J. R. and Smith, D. K. (1993) *The Wisdom of Teams: Creating the high-performance organisation*. Boston: Harvard Business School Press.

Kennedy, I. (2001) *Learning from Bristol: The Report of the Public Inquiry into Children's Heart Surgery at the Bristol Royal Infirmary 1984–1995*. CM 5207 London: The Stationery Office.

Langley, G., Nolan, K., Nolan, T., Norman, C. and Provost, L. (1996) *The Improvement Guide: A practical approach to enhancing organisational performance*. New York: Jossey-Bass.

Learmonth, M. (2005) Making health services management research critical: A review and a suggestion. *Sociology of Health and Illness* **25** (1), 93–119.

Mackay, C. J., Cousins, R., Kelly, P. J., Lee, S. and McCaig, R. H. (2004) Management standards and work-related stress in the UK: policy background and science. *Work and Stress* **18** (2), 91–112.

McDonald, R. (2004) Individual identity and organisational control: empowerment and modernisation in a Primary Care Trust. *Sociology of Health and Illness* **26** (7), 925–950.

Milne, A. A. (1926) *Winnie-the-Pooh*, London: Methuen and Co.

NPSA (National Patient Safety Agency) (2008) *A Risk Matrix for Risk Managers*. London: NPSA (http://www.npsa.nhs.uk).

NHS Confederation (2007) *Management in the NHS: The facts*. London: NHS Confederation.

NHS Employers (2008) *Staff: Are you stressed*? London: NHS Employers (http://www.nhsemployers.org/practice/practice-4010.cfm) Accessed 29 July 2008.

NHS Institute for Innovation and Improvement (2007) *Improvement Leaders' Guides*. London: NHS Institute for Innovation and Improvement (http://www.institute.nhs.uk)

NHS Institute for Innovation and Improvement (2008a) (http://www.institute.nhs.uk/organisation/about_nhsi/about_the_nhs_institute.html) Accessed 24 April 2008.

NHS Institute for Innovation and Improvement (2008b) *Business Plan 2008/9*. London: NHS Institute for Innovation and Improvement (http://www.institute.nhs.uk).

NHS Litigation Authority (2008) *NHSLA Risk Management Standards for Acute Trusts*. London: NHS Litigation Authority (http://www.nhsla.com).

NMC (Nursing and Midwifery Council) (2004) *Standards of Proficiency for Pre-registration Nursing Education*. London: NMC (http://www.nmc-uk.org).

NMC (2008) *The Code. Standards of conduct, performance and ethics for nurses and midwives*. London: NMC (http://www.nmc-uk.org).

Pearce, C. (2006) Ten steps to effective delegation. *Nursing Management* **13** (8), 9.

Rost, J. (1993) Leadership development in the new millennium. *Journal of Leadership and Organizational Studies* **1** (1), 91–110.

Royal College of Nursing (2007) *Team Effectiveness Guides*. London: RCN (http://www.rcn.org.uk).

Royal College of Nursing, Royal College of Speech and Language Therapists, The British Dietetic Association, and The Chartered Society of Physiotherapy (2006) *Supervision, Accountability and Delegation of Activities to Support Workers*. London: RCN (http://www.rcn.org.uk).

Schon, D. (1983) *The Reflective Practitioner*. New York: Basic Books.

Secretary of State for Health (2000) *The NHS Plan*. Cm 4818-I. London: The Stationery Office.

Secretary of State for Health (2008) *High Quality Care for All. NHS Next Steps Review Final Report*. Cm 7432. London: The Stationery Office.

Smith, J. (2002) *The Shipman Enquiry. First Report*. London: The Stationery Office.

Tuckman, B. (1965) Developmental sequence in small groups. *Psychological Bulletin* **63** (6), 384–399.

Wanless, D., Appleby, J., Harrison, A. and Patel, D. (2007) *Our Future Health Secured? A review of NHS funding and performance*. London: King's Fund.

West, M. A., Borrill, C., Dawson, J. *et al.* (2002) The link between the management of employees and patient mortality in acute hospitals. *International Journal of Human Resource Management*, **13** (8), 1299–1310.

Chapter 13

Personal and professional development

Clare Hopkinson

Learning outcomes

After reading and reflecting on this chapter, you should be able to:

- Outline the nature of reflection, critical reflection and reflexivity;
- Identify a range of methods for reflecting effectively;
- Explain different ways of knowing in nursing;
- Begin to develop a professional portfolio and private personal diary;
- Recognise the importance of continuing professional development;
- Raise questions about your own practice;
- Recognise the emotional impact of caring for others.

Related NMC Standards of Proficiency for Pre-registration Nursing Education (NMC 2004)

- Use professional standards of practice to self-assess performance.

- Identify one's own professional development needs by engaging in activities such as reflection in, and on, practice and lifelong learning.

- Develop a personal development plan which takes into account personal, professional and organisational needs.

- Share experience with colleagues and patients and clients in order to identify the additional knowledge and skills needed to manage unfamiliar or professionally challenging situations.

- Take action to meet any identified knowledge and skills deficit likely to affect the delivery of care within the current sphere of practice.

- Contribute to the learning experiences and development of others by facilitating the mutual sharing of knowledge and experience.

Introduction

Personal and professional development is an important part of becoming and remaining a registered nurse. The need to continue to develop arises from the recognition of the changing nature of what is known and from the need to improve one's skills in order to ensure the delivery of safe and effective care. In this Chapter I hope to convince you of the value of reflection as a means of being systematic and thoughtful in developing your personal and professional skills.

The chapter is divided into three parts.

In Part 1, I offer some insights into the value for nursing practice (and thus, if only indirectly, for patient care) of the relationship between reflection on the one hand and personal and professional development on the other.

In Part 2, I begin to outline the nature of reflection. I offer some definitions while noting that universal agreement about the nature of reflection is not forthcoming. This is unsurprising given that reflection can take a variety of forms and be undertaken in different ways. In this Part, I also offer a brief description about a number of different models of reflections.

In Part 3, I begin to explore the implications for nursing practice of different ways of knowing and how these can help you think about ways in which you might develop your practice. I conclude the chapter with some ideas that may help you to reflect, together with some practical suggestions about keeping and maintaining a reflective portfolio.

Part 1: Outlining personal and professional development

Case 13.1

Julia is a third-year student nurse who has been involved in a drug administration error. She has been asked by her mentor (Tariq) to write a reflective piece about the incident. Tariq knows that Julia is not a natural reflector so he has asked her to structure her writing using Johns' model of reflection. For her part Julia is reluctant to put pen to paper, as she knows she will be required to endure a three-way discussion (with her university tutor and her mentor, Tariq) and thinks that this meeting should be the end of it. She finds it difficult to understand why Tariq thinks she should spend time writing about the incident when she already knows what happened and what now needs to be done. In short, she thinks it a bit of a waste of time, and further she thinks Johns' model demands too much detail. However, Julia also knows that Tariq will be responsible for assessing her competencies and she does not want to mess up her chances of getting a good report or reference. She realises that she will need to spend some of her precious spare time tonight before going out writing her reflection in order to have it ready for Tariq in the morning.

As a student nurse you should find it easy to complete the sentence: 'my course would be so much better if only . . .' This is because most students will have at least one idea of how their programme could be improved. Similarly many students will be able to identify easily what a particular lecturer or mentor needs to do in order to be better at their job. We all engage in the kinds of conversations in which the shortcomings of systems, organisations or other people are identified and where simple solutions for making things better are suggested. Unfortunately, the same cannot always be said in relation to ourselves: indeed, we rarely engage in conversations that identify our own shortcomings, let alone provide solutions for improving our performance as nurses. If nothing else, reflection provides an opportunity to review the effects and consequences of our behaviour and actions. Tariq has asked Julia to use a structured form of reflection in an attempt to enable her to identify her role in the incident and to help her begin to understand how the incident might have been avoided altogether. From this Tariq hopes Julia will consent to construct a plan of action to assist her personal and professional development.

To develop is to improve. Development occurs when things can be said to have improved. Development is intimately bound with thinking; thinking about the way things are now and thinking about the way things might be improved: and to engage in thinking about things in this way is to engage in reflection. Thus reflection is an essential feature of development, and as suggested above, most of us engage with this type of activity on an everyday basis. We might not normally call this 'reflection' but when we think about how things are and how they might be improved we are reflecting on what is and what might be.

Personal development is personal improvement, while professional development involves improving experiences of health and nursing care for patients. So in a professional sense, engaging with reflection (i.e., thinking about how things are and thinking about how they might be improved for patients) must be accompanied by action (i.e., actually doing something in an attempt to make things better for patients). Thus reflection is an integral part of personal and professional development.

In this chapter the focus is on reflection as a method of pursuing personal and professional development in order to help you to learn from and about your practice as a nurse. I hope that reading this chapter will encourage you to have a go at reflection and find for yourself its value in your development as a professional nurse. In this way you can learn to become a reflective practitioner and begin to use your personal and professional experience as a means for continuing development (Ash 1992).

Poem 13.1 — A manual handling incident by Clare Hopkinson (14 April 2005)

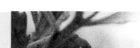

Let's move this patient
From the trolley to the bed
How are we going to do this?
The health care assistant said

All hands to the deck are needed
We could really do with six
Better still, use the slide sheet
Cos we've definitely judged the risk

But the slide sheet can't be found
It's not readily at hand
Oh let's move her anyway then
But be careful how you stand

Fill in the incident form, later
That'll do the trick
But how safe is it to whistle blow?
Cos mud will often stick

Hurry up, time to go home now
The stupid form can wait
We're really fed up of staying behind
So today we won't be late

You need lots of incident forms anyway
Before managers will ever act
What's the point of even trying
There's no money and that's a fact

Staff shortages and cutting corners
Are now part of the working day
Leaving the workforce feeling, what?
Unwilling to have their say?

Activity 13.1

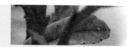

Consider the feelings evoked by Poem 13.1.

- What questions does it raise?
- What are the assumptions in it?
- What are the tensions and possible contradictions in the poem?
- How does this relate to your own experiences of moving patients?
- Could a poem like this help to change practice for the better?
- What do you imagine might be some of the difficulties in attempting to change practice?
- How effective is the poetry for helping to reflect on practice?

Reflective practice
involves noticing, imagining, challenging, inquiring, reframing, acting and developing different ways of knowing the world in order to become a more effective practitioner.

I wrote Poem 13.1 following a difficult experience when returning to nursing after a gap of 10 years. In writing the poem I hoped to capture the reality that practice does not always follow the theory propagated in college (but I am sure you already know this!). I offer this poem not because it is particularly well crafted but because it shows the value of asking questions of nursing practice. It illustrates one possible way of inquiring into some of the difficulties of practising effectively when working with others. At a personal level I was struck by the power of the group dynamics to silence my objections to moving the patient without a slide sheet and by the general lack of will to feedback to the organisation issues that were affecting practice. In sharing my personal story perhaps you can recognise similar problems in your own practice. **Reflective practice** can be a powerful process in learning from such less than perfect and difficult (although not uncommon) situations. In this way, reflective practice can challenge, and help to change for the better, attitudes and behaviours and this in turn can hopefully lead to improvements in the quality of nursing care as experienced by patients and clients.

The language used in relation to reflection can be difficult to understand, so one purpose of this chapter is to help you understand some of the terminology. Nursing is predominately an oral profession: it seems easier to talk about nursing than to write about it. In this chapter I suggest there is value in writing but also that there are varied and creative ways to reflect. For example, through using poetry to write about my experiences of practice I was encouraged to reflect and question my caregiving. I suggest also that having a safe, critically reflexive friend (Taylor 2006) who will both support and challenge your development as you talk about your stories of practice can be invaluable. This person must not merely agree with you or take your side but help you to explore your experiences in ways that allow you to see those experiences differently, to challenge your assumptions of practice, and to encourage you to develop further changing your practice for the better. Another feature of the oral tradition of nursing is that many (if not all) nurses find it difficult to articulate the 'taken for granted' aspects of nursing knowledge (i.e., the embodied knowledge that guides actions) because this tacit and intuitive knowledge is difficult to express.

The overall aim of this chapter is to present a realistic picture of the process of reflection and to show that at times reflecting is not an easy process. It takes curiosity, courage, tenacity, commitment, resilience, assertiveness, empathy, a sense of humour and an openness to learn from everyday experiences. For me, reflection is like a mystery tour: I think I know where I am going so I tend to jump to conclusions about where I will end up. However, if I do this, I rush to the end too soon and miss both the positive and negative experiences of the journey. In allowing the journey to unfold, the sense of adventure and anticipation of not knowing quite where one will end up allows the learning and the development to take place in sometimes surprising ways. Sometimes this is pleasant, sometimes unpleasant, but either can stimulate strong emotion. I have found that a significant proportion of my most important learning has been from the unpleasant experiences.

Arguably, the predominant view of reflection in the nursing literature is that it is primarily a solitary pursuit. My preference is to understand reflection as three interlinked processes: that is, first-, second- and third-person inquiry (Marshall 1999, 2004, Torbert 2001). The language of first-person, second-person and third-person inquiry is rather cumbersome therefore I prefer to call these respectively: personal reflection (where the nurse reflects on her own); relational reflection (where the nurse reflects as part of a group or in a one-to-one relationship with another person); and organisational reflection (where the nurse contributes to the way the organisation learns and changes its practices as a consequence of reflective activities).

Despite being in her third year and close to qualification (and registration) and despite being required to incorporate reflection in various assignments throughout her course, Julia has managed to avoid the level of reflection that Tariq is expecting. She thinks she will need only a few minutes to get something written down, just as she has done for those reflective assignments she has completed during her course. She will then be free to enjoy her evening with friends. Sadly for Julia (although she does not know it yet), Tariq will be unimpressed by her half-hearted attempt at reflection and ultimately Julia will find herself slightly embarrassed by her efforts. This chapter follows Julia as she comes to realise that not only is becoming a nurse a more serious business than she has previously taken it to be but also that there may be some value in this thing called reflection after all.

Part 2: Explaining personal and professional development

Case 13.1 (continued)

Tariq is a staff nurse and a mentor to Julia (our third-year student nurse). One of the things Tariq has found so surprising since becoming a staff nurse is the way that so many nurses just keep on doing the same old thing day after day despite being full of complaints about the way things are and full of statements about how much better things would be if only . . .

Tariq knows how busy and pressurised nursing work can be and he is beginning to suspect that the majority of nurses are just too tired and too overwhelmed by the sheer volume of demands on their time to do anything about their complaints or with their ideas for improvement. He hears lots of nurses complaining about the way things are but he sees few nurses doing anything to change their situations. Because he has only been qualified a relatively short time and because he feels many of the nurses in his practice area have fallen into the 'this is the way we do it here' trap, he feels he should put his efforts into encouraging students. Thus when the drug administration error occurs he seizes the opportunity to engage Julia with ideas about personal and professional development.

Personal and professional development requires a willingness to acknowledge in oneself a need to continue to learn. Many of the skills and attitudes required for effective learning are explored in Chapter 11, so the focus in this chapter is less on the building blocks of learning and teaching and more on the nature of reflection as a process with which to enable personal and professional development. Reflection is a way of identifying what and how things might be improved. Therefore capturing that learning in a form that can be included in a portfolio is one way of demonstrating your personal development as well as your contribution to the development of professional practice. Such developments need not be large scale for consistent with the idea of improving the lot of patients, is the idea that it may be in the little things that the patient experience is enhanced.

Personal and professional development also requires a willingness to move on from merely complaining about a current unsatisfactory state of affairs; it requires taking action in an attempt to make things better. Nevertheless, arguably, the act of complaining does at least demonstrate a minimum form of reflection (i.e., thinking that things could be better than they are) but without some form of action, complaining tends to become an end in itself and leads to stagnation rather than development. Thus development requires reflection plus action: the term reflective practice captures this requirement for action and is therefore often used as the preferred term in practice-based professional occupations such as nursing.

There are several terms common in the literature including 'reflection', 'critical reflection', 'reflective practice' and 'reflexivity'. These terms are sometimes used interchangeably although each has been the subject of a particular definition by different authors, nevertheless it is generally accepted that reflection without some form of development is a sterile activity. Indeed, the vast majority of the literature on reflection focuses on the personal reflective stories of individuals' experiences as a way of creating, modifying, developing and thus improving practice (e.g., Bolton 2005, Burns and Bulman 2000, Ghaye 2005, Ghaye and

Lillyman 2000, 2006, Johns 2006, Johns and Freshwater 1998, Kim 1999, Moon 2004, Taylor 2006).

Kember *et al.* (2001) suggest that formal definitions of reflection are hard to find because reflection is variously understood as ranging from casual ways of thinking about practice at one extreme to highly structured processes based on the philosophical underpinnings of, for example, Dewey, Habermas, and Gadamer (Johns 2000, Kember *et al.* 2001, Taylor 2006) or Bourdieu (Grenfell and James 1998) at the other. According to the *Oxford English Dictionary*, reflection is 'to throw back, reconsider, go back in thought, serious thought or consideration' (OED 2006 p. 1208).

This OED definition offers only a simplistic view that corresponds with the 'casual thinking about practice' end of the continuum. The value of this form of reflection tends to remain in the intellectual rather than practical domain and, in common with many other definitions, suggests reflection as a solitary pursuit. Given that nursing is a practical and (more often than not) collective activity, the developmental value of isolated individual reflection may be limited.

Reflective learning is the process of internally examining and exploring an issue of concern, triggered by an experience which creates and clarifies meaning in terms of self, and which results in a changed conceptual perspective.

(Boyd and Fales 1983, p. 100)

A process of consciously examining what has occurred in terms of thoughts, feelings and actions against underlying beliefs, assumptions and knowledge as well as against the backdrop (i.e., the context or the stage) in which specific practice has occurred.

(Kim 1999, p. 1209)

The definitions offered by Boyd and Fales (1983) and by Kim (1999) recognise reflection as a process for improving practice through increased self-understanding and inquiry into the context and structures that support practice. Kim's notion of 'consciously examining' practice (and this includes examining the context in which care is delivered) implies a depth missing from the OED definition. Reflexivity is a third common term, that Johns (2000) described thus: 'looking back and seeing self as a changed person is the essential feature of reflexivity. It is not an endpoint but is always open to and anticipatory of future experiences' (p. 61).

Reflection has been criticised on, the grounds of timing (affecting recall), interference from stress and emotions, particularly anxiety (Ixer 1999, Mackintosh 1998, Newell 1992) and lack of universal definition (Mackintosh 1998). This last assumes that a single definition is necessary for understanding a complex phenomenon and that there is only one way of knowing. However, one purpose of reflective practice is to transform and widen one's perspective (Mezirow 1981, Taylor 2006) as well as to appreciate and accommodate alternative perspectives. This makes it unsurprising that numerous definitions exist.

Using the experience illustrated in Poem 13.1, I would want to explore at least:

- The reason(s) for slide sheets being unavailable in the unit.
- The cost of getting slide sheets.
- Why staff are reluctant to use the slide sheets and fill in the risk assessment forms.
- Who would it be necessary to tell to effect a change in practice.

Critical reflection involves reflecting at a deeper level because it is linked to making changes or with transforming perspectives (Mezirow 1981). In being reflexive I would be asking myself both 'why had I not been my usual assertive self?' and 'what was it that stopped me from completing an adverse incident form?' I might ask myself specific questions such as:

- Did my need to be liked and accepted by the team get in the way of my responsibilities to the patient?
- Could I have exerted a positive influence on those other members of the team who consider form-filling a waste of time?
- Have I learned anything about my own assertiveness in the face of opposition?
- Is there knowledge that would support me to act differently next time I find myself in a similar situation?

This focus on asking questions, on analysis, on evaluation and on possible solutions is central to critical reflection, but more than this, critical reflection also implies an emotional and political awareness of the need to effect change. It requires an understanding of responsibility, authority and influence. This understanding is important if nurses are to make use of their influence to effect change for the better. A commitment to development then is a commitment to not only acknowledge that one has some influence over the way things are but also to demonstrate leadership in one's role regardless of the level of that role. In other words, a commitment to personal professional development is a commitment to act so as to make a positive difference to practice.

Of course, effecting change is easier said than done. In part this is because we often lack sufficient insight into our own shortcomings (Dunning 2005), and it can be difficult to receive useful and honest feedback about those shortcomings; just as it can be challenging to alert others to their shortcomings. Add to this the unequal power relationship between individual practitioner and institution (hospital system, primary health care trust, etc.) then the challenge of effecting change can seem overwhelming.

Activity 13.2

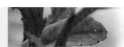

Think of a story from practice that you recently shared with a friend.

- With whom would you share this story?
- What kinds of stories would you not want to share with a consultant? A ward manager? Your mentor? Your personal tutor?
- Why would you tell some people but not others?
- What sort of power relationships might silence your stories?
- Is your reluctance based on fear or anxiety of what might happen to you?
- Is it possible that this fear/anxiety might be more imagined than real?
- To what extent can you realistically influence practice in the area where you work?
- What would stop you trying?
- What would encourage you to give honest feedback to those with whom you work?
- Consider how you might limit your learning by not sharing some stories from practice.

Reflection-in-action is reflection that occurs at the same time as an action or experience; sometimes described as thinking on one's feet, or having an intuitive grasp of a situation.

Reflection-on-action is a retrospective activity; an intentional and purposeful looking back at occurrences.

The literature is further complicated by the various ways in which reflection is categorised. I have already noted that reflection may be a personal, relational or organisational process, and commonly a distinction is made between **reflection-in-action** and **reflection-on-action**. In addition, different levels are indicated (suggesting a developmental process from non-reflection, through reflection to critical reflection); and a bewildering array of reflective models can be found (e.g., Boud *et al.* 1985, Gibbs 1988, Holm and Stephenson 1994, Johns 1995, 2006, Taylor 2006).

Personal reflection

> I observe myself and so I come to know others. Lao-Tze

Personal reflection (or first-person inquiry) refers to self-study or self-reflective inquiry (Marshall 1999, 2004, Torbert 2001). The purpose of personal reflection is to understand one's behaviours, communications, intentions, attitudes, values, beliefs, emotions and thoughts in the attempt to develop more effective working relationships and practices. Personal reflection allows an individual the opportunity to identify strengths and weaknesses (e.g., contradictions, distortions, defended behaviours, blind spots) as well as values, hopes, intentions, dreams and achievements. It helps in processing emotional aspects of nursing work by removing obstructive negative feelings and by encouraging a reframing to positive feelings thereby facilitating learning (Boud *et al.* 1985).

Relational reflection

Relational reflection (or second-person inquiry) involves other people either in a one-to-one relationship or as part of a group process and can be formal or informal. Torbert (2001) describes second-person inquiry as 'speaking-and-listening-with-others' (p. 253). I take second-person inquiry to be relational because Torbert argues it occurs in dialogue with others and involves 'public testing of our interpretations' (p. 255). Relational reflection often takes place in groups in educational settings or as a formal clinical supervision process. It may have value in enabling nursing teams to engage with the primary purposes of their practice in particular settings but this has yet to be fully realised and researched. Relational reflection might be encountered in, for example, action learning sets, nursing handovers, work-based learning days, multidisciplinary (or nursing) team meetings, over coffee or in corridor conversations. Relational reflection requires the use of appropriate communication skills (see Chapter 9); especially the ability to challenge effectively and supportively while avoiding demonising or blaming specific individuals, so that poor or unsatisfactory practice can be questioned and confronted.

Organisational reflection

> Do you continually curtail your effort till there be nothing of it left? . . . By
> non-action there is nothing which cannot be effected. Lao-Tze

Organisational reflection (or third-person inquiry) takes place at the organisational level where the 'research/practice, focuses primarily on the exercise of mutual power to co-construct the future' (Torbert 2001, p. 257). Put more simply, where collaborative efforts of nurses lead to the development of new and effective ways of working, this can influence working practices across and throughout the organisation. Learning from a story of practice can lead to organisational learning and wider practice changes. This level of reflection and development can be difficult, but it is not impossible to achieve. Indeed, it may be that the developmental potential of personal and/or relational reflection is restricted unless accompanied by some sense of organisational reflection that leads to change in organisational working. This means reflective practice becomes embedded within the organisation (Gould and Baldwin 2004) and is not just a deconstruction of practice. For example, this can be achieved through risk assessments and specific practice developments.

Reflection-on-action and reflection-in-action

Schon (1983), one of the most influential writers on reflection, suggests that practice is messy and complex. He suggests the context of practice needs to be explored and understood as a source of knowledge and learning in its own right. He used the term 'theories in use' to describe knowledge situated in practice, which, with Arygis (Arygis and Schon 1978), he found to be different from the theories that practitioners claim to use as a basis for practice (espoused theories).

In Poem 13.1 the use of a slide sheet is the espoused theory while the 'theory in use' is moving the patient using six people. In other words, we do not always do what we say we do or know we 'should' do. For Schon, practical knowledge arises from what people do and not from what they say they do; and this may be (at least in part) because of the failure of theory to translate into action (i.e., the theory practice gap, or the need for classroom theory to be adapted before it can be used in practice), or because practice has not been understood sufficiently in its specific context. Schon also noted that professionals often find it difficult to articulate their 'theories in use'. It is possible that nurses are drawn to Schon's ideas because it emphasises values, the 'difficult to articulate' aspects of nursing work so often devalued by the emphasis on scientific knowledge (Mantzoukas and Jasper 2004).

While difficult to verify, reflection-in-action enables nurses to ask themselves whether or not what they are doing is effective, and to try out alternative actions in the midst of the action. This on-the-spot experimentation is something that many nurses claim to do all the time, yet we have all come across nurses who adopt an uncritical and largely uniformed *we-have-always-done-it-this-way* approach to practice. Reflection-in-action allows us to know why we are doing what we are doing, when we are doing it.

On a personal level I experienced this when incontinent following hip replacement surgery. I refused catheterisation unlike the lady opposite in a similar predicament who, having a catheter *in situ* until having her bowels open (4 days in her case), developed a urinary tract infection that delayed her mobilisation programme and her discharge from hospital. When asked about the evidence for the practice of waiting for a bowel movement before catheter removal, the response from the nurses was on the lines of 'we do it this way because sister insists upon it'. This story illustrates a singular failure to develop practice precisely because of a reluctance to engage with reflection at either the personal or relational level. It also highlights the power one individual can exert on inhibiting professional development amongst a group of staff.

Activity 13.3

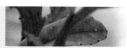

Write a description of your next placement at the end of your first day there. Try to include as much specific detail as possible. The following questions might help in this task.

- What did it look like?
- What did it smell like?
- What kinds of noises did you become aware of?
- How were you welcomed?
- What were you feeling like?
- What nursing did you carry out?
- How well would you judge your nursing ability?
- What helped or hindered your learning that day?
- How do you feel about it now you are looking back on that day?
- How might that day set the tone for your learning experience?

The detail you note on the first day in placement will not be so easy to identify subsequently. If you repeat this exercise a month later you will find it difficult to give such a detailed account. This is because many things you notice now will become routine and 'taken for granted'. This means that you will have become part of the culture of that practice environment and consequently will find it harder to identify the need for change and development.

Models of reflection

There are a growing number of models and frameworks for reflection. Some include a series of prompt questions designed to help develop reflective skills (e.g., Cook 1999, Driscoll 2000, Gibbs 1988, Holm and Stephenson 1994, Johns 1995, Thomas 2004). These models are particularly helpful for nurses who find reflection difficult. Other models provide a framework for analysing and re-evaluating experiences as a way of encouraging the nurse to generate their own practice questions (e.g., Atkins and Murphy 1993, Boud *et al.* 1985, Goodman 1984, Kim 1999, Mezirow 1981, 1990, Taylor 2000). These models are suitable for nurses who prefer a less structured approach. In addition, there are several models developed from specific respective research studies (e.g., Benner 1984, Johns 1997, Kim 1999, Taylor 2000). A brief overview of some models of reflection is given below, however you should note that there are many other models available.

Boud, Keogh and Walker (1985)

Boud, Keogh and Walker's approach is more of a process than a model. This can be a bit daunting for a novice reflector, as it requires a self-generated set of questions and making links between existing and new knowledge. It is designed to enable reflection on new experiences in a cyclical manner and to enable a reframing of negative feelings, although this may be difficult without the help of a critical friend. The process is staged under the following headings.

1. Experience:
   - behaviour, ideas and feelings.
2. The reflective process:
   - returning to the experience;
   - utilising positive feelings and attitudes;
   - removing negative feelings by reframing and processing them;
   - re-evaluating the experience.
3. Outcomes/actions:
   - new understandings and appreciations;
   - new knowledge and perspectives;
   - change in behaviour, attitudes or skills;
   - readiness to put knowledge into practice.

Gibbs' reflective model (1988)

The simple cyclical structure of Gibbs' model makes it easy to use and popular among nurses, indeed it is the model Julia has previously used for assignment purposes. It is useful as it emphasises the link between reflection and action (and this can assist in setting a personal development plan). However, it neither encourages consideration of other people in (or affected by) the event nor does it require examination of motives, values, knowledge, or congruence between thoughts and actions. While action-based and thus relevant for professional development it may not encourage deeper reflection of self and thus may be limited in terms of *personal* development (see Figure 13.1).

Johns' fifteenth model of structured reflection (2006)

Johns frequently updates his reflective model and is now on his fifteenth version, which still incorporates Carper's (1978) ways of knowing. This model offers a level of detail that may be particularly helpful for those who struggle with reflection. It makes direct links between past experiences and values on the one hand and experience on the other. The development of empathy is encouraged by asking nurses to imagine the consequences of their actions as well as the feelings of other people associated with the event. It also helps to identify the knowledge base (or ways of knowing) being utilised in the situation and encourages gaps in knowledge to be identified. It is for these reasons that Tariq has asked Julia to use this model to structure her reflection on the drug administration error.

In his fifteenth version Johns asks the nurse 'to bring the mind home'. By this he means become grounded or setting aside thoughts of the past or future in order to focus on the present. Clearly, this is difficult to do as the past influences the present. However, by focusing on your body and clearing your mind of the chattering thoughts that are often present it is possible to become

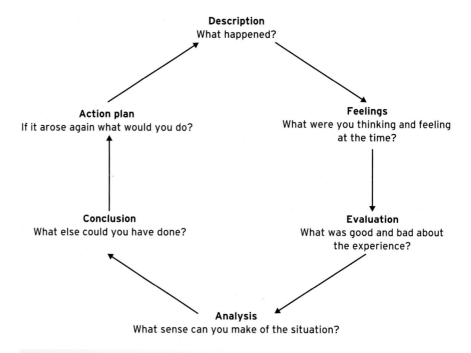

Figure 13.1 Gibbs' reflective model (1988).

more attentive and contemplative. Johns' model is based on focusing on a description of an experience that seems significant in some way and responding to a set of reflective cue questions.

Aesthetics:
- What particular issues seem significant to pay attention to?
- How were others feeling and why did they feel this way?
- What was I trying to achieve and did I respond effectively?
- What were the consequences of my actions on the patient, others and myself?

Personal:
- How was I feeling and why did I feel that way?
- What factors influence the way I was/am feeling, thinking and responding to this situation?
- How does this experience connect with previous experiences? (also reflexivity)
- What factors might constrain me from responding in new ways?
- How do I NOW feel about this experience?

Ethics:
- To what extent did I act for the best and in tune with my beliefs?

Empirics:
- What knowledge did or should have informed me?

Reflexivity:
- Given the situation again, how might I respond differently?
- What would be the consequences of responding in new ways for the patient, others and myself?

- Am I able to support myself better as a consequence?
- What insights have I gained?
- Am I more able to realise desirable practice?
- What have I learnt through reflecting?

The house that Johns built

Ali Moss (a nurse and post-registration student) saw Johns' model as a house in which to wander; with each room having something different to offer. Using this idea in a group reflection, we enlarged the image by including an attic, foundations, garden and garden shed. A specific experience opens the door to reflection allowing exploration of the different rooms of personal knowing, aesthetics, empirics, ethics and reflexivity. The foundations might contain hidden experiences that shape the way of seeing the house. A series of questions suggest themselves which might include:

- What is kept out of sight in the attic or the garden shed?
- Who else gets invited into the house?
- Is it an open house or a private sanctuary?
- Do we tidy the house in advance of a viewing (an assignment, or portfolio piece)?

Holm and Stephenson's student's perspective, reflective model (1994)

This model was developed by two students who claim that it can also be used to structure or act as a checklist for many written assignments. It takes the following form.

After describing the event ask yourself:
- What was my role in the situation?
- Did I feel comfortable or uncomfortable? Why?
- What actions did I take?
- Was it appropriate?
- How could I have improved the situation for myself, the patient, my mentor?
- What can I change in future?
- Do I feel as if I have learnt anything new about myself?
- Did I expect anything different to happen? What and why?
- Has it changed my way of thinking in any way?
- What knowledge from theory and research can I apply to this situation?
- What broader issues, for example, ethical, political, social, arise from this situation?
- What do I think about these broader issues?

Taylor's model of reflection (2000, 2006)

Taylor based her model on the work of the German philosopher Jurgan Habermas. She identified three types of reflection (technical, practical and emancipatory) which she proposed as connected rather than discrete categories.

It is important to consider these categories as ways of creating a tidy framework on which to hang certain broad principles. There is no form of reflection which is better than another, each has its own value for different purposes.

(Taylor 2000, p. 149)

Technical reflection focuses on the nature and effects of work practices and how they may be changed through technical reflection. It examines empirical knowledge, that is, knowledge obtained from the senses, scientific knowledge and evidence-based practice. This type of reflection allows for prediction when subsequently meeting a similar experience.

Practical reflection relates to the communicative aspects of nursing work and to interpersonal relationships. It is based on lived personal experience, being subjective and examining the inner self. Practical reflection also examines intersubjectivity, that is, how the nurse relates to others in the social world or her dialogue with others.

Emancipatory reflection requires a more critical view of practice and is linked to transformative action. It involves freedom, choice and empowerment. It challenges power, political aspects of care, and inhibiting cultural and social effects. The nurse is required to be influential and to raise awareness of issues that are often taken for granted practices or assumptions.

The benefits of reflective practice

Reflective practice enables nurses to review what they do and the effect they have on other people (patients, relatives, other staff and so on). Reflective practice is ideally suited to exploring the complexities of practice and practice contexts. It can offer a route to critical examination of effective as well as poor, habitual and routine practice (Kim 1999): it is not merely about dramatic events or critical incidents. It offers scope for exploring emotional and ethical dilemmas faced by nurses and a way of encouraging professional and personal development in support of therapeutic relationships with patients, their family and loved ones (Hopkinson 1998). Reflective practice also encourages an articulation of the knowledge gained in and from practice as well as the knowledge that supports practice. It emphasises the process of learning, not just an outcome to be translated into nursing action. It generates a questioning approach to practice that helps to prevent nurses from becoming complacent about their work.

Research focus 13.1

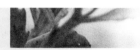

There are a large number of papers relating to reflective practice that support its worth (e.g., Atkins and Murphy 1993, Burton 2000, Clarke 1986, Clarke *et al.* 1996, Cook 1999, Freshwater 2004, James and Clarke 1994, Platzer *et al.* 2000, Rich and Parker 1995, Rolfe 1997), but surprisingly few empirical research studies on reflection-on-action in nursing. Some qualitative studies have made use of journals and interviews (e.g., Duke and Appleton 2000, Durgahee 1996, Glaze 2001, 2002, Hallet 1997, Smith 1998, Teekman 2000, Wong *et al.* 1995). Two studies examine perceptions of reflective practice, one by adopting a qualitative design (Burnard 1995), and the other a small sample size quantitative questionnaire approach (Cadman *et al.* 2003).

There are even fewer research studies carried out in a clinical setting (Mantzoukas and Jasper 2004, Powell 1989). What remains under-explored is what enables or inhibits interaction with reflection as a learning process. Powell (1989) uses a non-participant observation strategy in a small-scale study to inquire into the complex concept of reflection-in-action. Mantzoukas and Jasper (2004) use an interpretive ethnographic approach with unstructured observation, semi-structured interviews and content analysis on written structured reflective writing to examine the organisational culture and reflective practices. They found reflection was belittled in the ward setting and that the hierarchical structures and power struggles between the different staff inhibited reflective processes. Where nurses were able to reflect, they did so in their personal time.

There are a growing number of studies using retrospective reflection away from the bedside (e.g., Glaze 2001, 2002, Gustafsson and Fagerberg 2004, Johns 1997, Kember *et al.* 2001, Kim 1999). Focusing entirely on personal reflection, Johns (1997, 2000) uses a qualitative design to interview practitioners following the introduction of clinical supervision in a primary care nursing unit. He suggests that practitioners could become reflective practitioners by being more available to patients, responding to the person, and knowing and managing the self within caring relationships.

When Tariq reads Julia's reflection he is not surprised by what he reads. In her writing she provides a full description of the events leading up to the error in drug administration and this part of her reflection is comprehensive. However, the remainder of Julia's reflection is brief and non-committal. She is vague about what she was trying to achieve, why she responded in the way she did, and the consequences for the patient, herself and others (the aesthetics). She mentions that she feels 'a bit guilty' but says nothing about her internal state at the time (the personal); she is particularly vague about the relationship between her actions and her beliefs (the ethics) and about the knowledge she might have used to inform what she did (the empirics), although she does mention the NMC guidance on the administration of medicines. She writes nothing about how this incident relates to previous experience and suggests how she might do things better next time only in abstract terms. She offers no responses to the reminder of the prompts under the reflexivity heading.

Tariq tries not to show his disappointment as he asks Julia if she found the exercise useful and how she went about writing it down. Julia eventually confesses to spending very little time on it and admits that her responses to the cue questions are perfunctory at best. During the discussion with Tariq she does begin to demonstrate greater insight into the issues raised by the error and reluctantly acknowledges that she has learned something about herself in the process. She agrees to revise her reflection in the light of their discussion and to try to give more thoughtful responses to the cue questions. They agree to meet again in a couple of days to review her revised reflective account.

Part 3: Exploring personal and professional development

Development is underpinned by knowledge: before you can know what needs to change it is necessary to know how things are. Whether or not there is such a discrete thing as nursing knowledge is the subject of a vigorous debate that will not be entertained here. However, because reflection (as a means to development) requires coming to know something that was previously unknown or at least unacknowledged it cannot be ignored altogether. Many nurses subscribe to the idea that practical knowledge differs from theoretical knowledge, or as Polanyi (1967) describes it: 'knowing how' and 'knowing that' respectively. Reflective practice can be seen as an attempt to bring these two forms of knowledge together so that a nurse may learn in and from practice in the pursuit of development. In this sense, practice can generate knowledge as much as, if not more than, knowledge can inform practice. Some understand this relationship as helping to minimise the so-called 'the theory–practice gap' (e.g., Atkins and Murphy 1993, Cooney 1999, Durgahee 1996, Hallett 1997, Heath 1998).

The important point here about this distinction between practical knowledge ('know how'/tacit knowledge) on the one hand and theoretical knowledge ('know that'/propositional knowledge) on the other is that while the latter is relatively easy to articulate, the former is not. Propositional knowledge is the kind of knowledge you use when you answer an examination question about, for example, how to catheterise a patient. Tacit knowledge is the type of knowledge demonstrated when you successfully perform a catheterisation.

When composing her reflection on the drug administration error Julia found it easy to write a description of events because it was based on 'know that' type of knowledge. However, she struggled to respond to the cue questions in Johns' model and this can be explained in part by the idea that she needed to draw from different forms of knowledge. One of the things she admitted to Tariq (her mentor) was that she did not really understand the categories of aesthetic, personal, ethical and empirical knowing. She had always assumed knowledge to be uncontroversial; at school she always turned up for lessons and now at university she attends all scheduled classes, pays attention and does her best to learn and use that learning in her assignments. She does work hard on her assignments but often struggles to know what is required and rarely gets marks above 50 per cent. The idea that there may be different forms of knowledge is new to her and she has agreed to read something about different ways of knowing before revising her reflective piece about the drug administration error. She is not really looking forward to this because she thinks it is going to be difficult.

What knowledge informs nursing practice?

Real knowledge is to know the extent of one's ignorance. Confucius

Activity 13.4

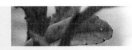

Spend 10 minutes writing an account of what you do on a typical day working as a nurse. Imagine you are writing this for a friend who knows nothing about nursing. When you have finished writing, think about the following questions:

- Does what you have written capture the essence of nursing?
- From reading what you have written, would your friend have a clear grasp of what being a nurse involves?

If you have done Activity 13.4, then you will have been doing some reflection, but the main purpose of the exercise is to illustrate how difficult it is to articulate the nature of nursing. Like Julia's description of events, the chances are that your description of a typical working day focuses on particular tasks (e.g., washing patients, giving out medications, doing the observations, and so on) because these things are relatively easy to describe: they also tend to fall into the category of 'knowing that'. The other parts of nursing (e.g., the caring, the responding to human suffering, the allaying of fears, the explaining of what is going on) are much more difficult to write down and yet for most nurses, these 'difficult to articulate' things are what make nursing the special occupation that it is. Reflection is one way in which the knowledge that underpins these difficult to articulate aspects of nursing can be expressed.

The implication here should be clear. A large part of what nurses do remains obscure because the emphasis on easily describable knowledge focuses attention on tasks, client group, or speciality: hence the standard categorisations of, for example, mental health nursing, care of the older person, emergency care and so on. Nursing is more than this: it is a complex social practice requiring a wide and varied knowledge base to support the choices made in caring for the well-being of others. Two different approaches to ways of knowing are explored briefly below.

Ways of knowing 1 (women's ways of knowing)

Research focus 13.2

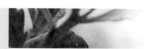

Combining Gilligan's (1982) 'ethics of care' and Perry's (1970) study of the evolving knowledge of male students, Belenky and colleagues (1986) describe five different perspectives they call 'women's ways of knowing'. They claim that the self-concepts of women are interwoven with their ways of knowing. They further suggest women struggle to claim the power of their own minds because of the stereotypical view of women as emotional and intuitive as opposed to the purported logic and rationality of men. Belenky *et al.* argue that while gender-related, the five identified characteristics (silence, received knowledge, subjective knowledge, procedural knowledge and constructed knowledge) are not gender-specific and may be found in some men. They claim that, unlike male-dominated ways of knowing, women's ways of knowing do not exist as a hierarchy.

Belenky and colleagues (1986) identify five characteristics (silence, received knowledge, subjective knowledge, procedural knowledge and constructed knowledge) that they claim typify women's ways of knowing. They note a lack of any hierarchy in this scheme, which may be important as it leaves the way clear for nurses to draw upon whichever knowledge base best fits a particular practice situation. These different ways of knowing link directly to the reflective process and suggest reasons why some nurses favour a structured rather than a free-form expressive approach to reflection. Additionally, it may be that different levels of structured reflective models are appropriate for different types of experiences.

Silence

The first perspective identified by Belenky and colleagues is silence. The silent women, while few in number in the study, were among the youngest and most socially, economically and educationally deprived. They have no voice and see words as weapons to be used against them. The silent women describe themselves as 'deaf and dumb' in terms of their abilities and find it almost impossible to describe any aspects of themselves as individuals. They use the word dumb to reflect both their feelings of stupidity and their lack of conversation with others. They see themselves as passive in relation to external and powerful authority figures. These women tend to have little sense of their own worth and become uncomfortable when asked to reflect on anything they do because reflection will unlock their silence. Silent women will only begin to reflect when encouraged within a highly supportive environment.

Received knowledge: listening to the voices of others

She never did and never could put words together, out of her own head. George Eliot, *Middlemarch*

The women in this category learn by listening to others and perceive listening as a way of knowing. They tend to polarise ideas as right or wrong, true or false, good or bad, black or white and so on. They tend to assume only one answer will be correct for a given question and consequently see alternative answers as just plain wrong. Belenky and colleagues note:

while received knowers can be very open to take in what others have to offer they have little confidence in their own ability to speak. Believing the truth comes from others, they still their own voices to hear the voices of others.

(1986 p. 37)

Received knowers have little confidence in their ability to speak out; they tend to perceive authority figures as the source of knowledge. Learning tends to be understood as the regurgitation of facts and they struggle with the idea of being original because they have not learned to trust or value their own opinions; as a result they find coursework challenging when it requires independent creative thought. Belenky and colleagues suggest this type of learner may be successful in courses 'that do not demand a reflective relativistic stance' (p. 42). Received knowers tend to consider the judgements, ideas and opinions of others as more important than their own. They often channel increasing awareness of self into empowering and caring for others through listening and responding, which in certain circumstances may lead to a valuing of their own judgements, ideas and opinions. While reluctant reflectors, structured models of reflection may assist received knowers to begin at the descriptive level of reflection. Given the appropriate form of encouragement (role models who will encourage the received knower to value their own judgements, ideas and opinions) the received knower may begin to listen to their own inner voice.

Subjective knowledge: the inner voice and the quest for self

Women in this category see truth and knowledge as personal and private; being subjectively known through intuition. They rely on gut instinct and may refuse to accept answers from other people. They tend to mistrust learning from books but value learning from direct experience or personal involvement, and from their feelings or senses. They prefer to work things out for themselves and because they do not possess a solid sense of self find it difficult to talk about themselves or to ask for help. Nevertheless, they retain a basic commitment and responsiveness to others' needs. Belenky *et al.* suggest this growing reliance on intuitive processes is an important step in the process of women becoming assertive, self-protecting and self-determining; and thus moving towards reflective and critical thought. However, the subjective knower is reticent about sharing personal thoughts in public although they may share them with friends. This makes them reluctant reflectors (despite valuing experience) although structured reflective models may help them to connect with both their own feelings and the feelings of others. According to Bolton (2005), trying to imagine the perspectives of others can assist subjective knowers to develop reflective skills and this, in turn, can lead to recognising the value of alternative sources of knowledge from which to base decisions and actions. This can help the subjective knower to move beyond entrenched positions common among this group.

Procedural knowledge: separate and connected knowing

Procedural knowers highlight the way separation and attachment influence how men and women think through and approach experience (Hartog 2005). Women operating from procedural knowledge invest in learning and tend to operate from either separate or connected knowing. Gilligan (1982) refers to 'separate knowing' as the sense of being apart from others. She claims men develop their sense of morality from separateness with its emphasis on objectivity, evaluation and justice while women's moral sensitivity arises from a connected, relational and caring ethic. This connected knowing values relations with others, caring, empathy, subjectivity, acceptance and appreciation of others' points of view.

Connected knowers value reflection and find identifying the affective (feeling) component of experience easier than recognising the underpinning knowledge. Hence a structured reflective model will encourage them to identify the gaps in their knowledge base and encourage a deeper level of reflection. Connected knowers tend to value conversations with critical friends (Taylor 2006) who will challenge and support their reflections. They may be willing to keep a diary or learning journal.

Separate knowers have difficulty with the ideology of reflection because it challenges the objectivity of separateness. Nurses operating from this perspective prefer a structured reflective model although they tend to have difficulty identifying their feelings and would tend to write themselves out of events. They prefer to focus their analysis on others' experiences because this allows them to be more objective. However, a comprehensive reflective model that encourages consideration of self as well as others, such as Johns' (1995, 2006) model, can help seperate knowers to move towards deeper reflection.

Constructed knowledge: integrating the voices

Belenky and colleagues describe constructed knowers as articulate and reflective individuals aware of their own thoughts, judgements, desires and moods. They draw knowledge from reason, intuition and others' expertise. They view knowledge as contextually bound and they notice and care about the lives of other people. They want to make a difference through their actions and are committed to action. Constructed knowers are consummate critical reflectors and probably do not need the security of structured models of reflection as they have an embodied reflexivity that allows them to ask appropriate and probing questions of their practice.

Activity 13.5

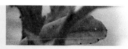

Review the five characteristic ways of women's knowing offered by Belenky *et al.* and consider the following questions:

- Do you recognise in yourself one of these ways of knowing?
- Can you identify each of these ways of knowing amongst others with whom you work in practice?
- If you and your mentor have different ways of knowing, how might this impact on your development as a nurse?

Ways of knowing 2 (Carper)

Carper's (1978) claim of four fundamental patterns of knowing (empirical, aesthetic, ethical and personal) has been influential in nursing. For Carper, each pattern of knowing is of equal value and each has a contribution to make to practice, dependant on the particularities of a given set of circumstances. Carper's claims form the basis for Johns' reflective model (1995, 2006).

Empirical knowing is gained from the senses and is based on observation, systematic investigation and testing embedded in the positivist or quantitative paradigm (Berragan 1998). It can be regarded as the science of nursing.

Aesthetic knowing refers to the action of nursing as it involves perception, understanding and empathy. It is described as the art of nursing in which the value of everyday experience is acknowledged. It is associated with the interpretive, qualitative paradigm and phenomenology (Masterson 1996). Berragan (1998) links aesthetics to intuitive actions.

Ethical knowing relates to moral issues and value judgements, and enables nurses to engage with difficult philosophical questions about good in relation to health and nursing practice.

Personal knowing recognises that each nurse brings a unique contribution to practice precisely because of a personal history of experience and emotional responses to situations. Carper describes personal knowing as knowing oneself. Personal knowing is a central concept for reflective practice.

Having read this short review of some different ways of knowing you might be getting a sense of where Julia might be located against these different categories. It may not come as a surprise to you to find that Julia is part subjective knower and part separate knower. If you return to these sections you will see that subjective knowers *find it difficult to talk about themselves or to ask for help* but *retain a basic commitment and responsiveness to others' needs* and are *reticent about sharing personal thoughts in public.* Separate knowers *tend to have difficulty identifying their feelings and tend to write themselves out of an event.* If we were able to point these things out to Julia we can be pretty sure that she would recognise herself in this depiction. It certainly fits with Tariq's impression of Julia and this explains why he was so keen for her to use Johns' model of reflection.

Activity 13.6

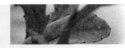

Re-read your written account of your typical working day (Activity 13.4).
Try to add some more detail to your description of what it is you do every day, paying particular attention to those 'difficult to articulate' aspects of everyday nursing.

- Make a list of the different types of knowledge needed to complete all the things you describe as the work of nurses.
- Add some brief notes against each type of knowledge you identify explaining where (and when) you obtained that particular type of knowledge (i.e., where and when did you learn to do that particular activity).

Hopefully, this activity will have helped you to realise that nursing practice draws on a wide and varied knowledge base. This recognition is important for effective personal and professional development. As suggested earlier, in order to know what needs to be improved (or developed) it is necessary to know what is already known; and this applies to all the different types of knowing that contribute to the knowledge base of nursing. Reflection thus contributes to development by enabling nurses to acknowledge their existing knowledge base and to identify what further knowledge they need in order to be effective in the role of registered nurse.

Of course, knowledge (or more precisely, what is known) changes over time. So nurses will need to review and add to their knowledge if their practice is to remain informed by what is currently known. However, this is complicated by three related factors: (i) what is currently known is often contested; (ii) some types of knowledge receive greater legitimacy than others and; (iii) the type of knowledge valued in the university is not always the same as that valued by practice-based staff.

In order to become a registered nurse, it is necessary to learn both in a practical and an academic setting, integrating rather than separating and then applying all forms of knowledge. As a registered nurse you will need some way of working out which type of knowledge provides the best guide for action in any specific situation. Reflection is one means of achieving this.

Inevitably conflicts of ideas, contradictions and tensions will arise between practitioners who value different aspects of nursing knowledge. This should be regarded as an opportunity for development as practitioners engage in critical discussion (in the form of relational reflection) of 'the what' and 'the how' of best practice. Unfortunately, many nurses seem to become locked into polarised views of practice in which simplistic right or wrong assumptions abound. Reflection as an ongoing process of continuing professional development can assist in more subtle and nuanced thinking about nursing work and this can ultimately benefit patient care.

Activity 13.7

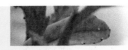

Spend 10 minutes writing about a significant event in your life. Try not to take your hand off the page. Don't worry about sentence construction, punctuation or paragraphs, just let the words flow.

- What did the exercise feel like?
- Is there anything that surprises you as you read over what you have written?

Keeping a reflective diary

How can I know what I think till I see what I say? E. M. Forster

A deeper understanding of ourselves can be achieved through writing. Written reflection is a common theme in the literature as a way of reflecting on action but it is strewn with confusing language. There are learning logs, journals, portfolios, structured accounts, reflective models, reflective reviews and personal diaries. Some reflective writing is public (e.g., a portfolio for an assignment) while other writing is private (e.g., a diary). Through writing, nurses can be encouraged to reflect on critical incidents from practice (I prefer the term 'stories of experience'). These stories are usually prompted by some emotional or ethical discomfort (e.g. Bolton 2005, Burns and Bulman 2000, Crathern 1998, Ghaye and Lillyman 2006, Glaze 2002, Gould and Baldwin 2004, Johns 2006, Moon 2004, Taylor 2006). Stories can focus on positive or negative experiences and allow you the chance to view events from a distance, considering:

- What happened, paying attention to the context and detail of the story.
- What you did and why you did it.
- What you felt about the experience and how this may connect with past experiences.
- What you have learned about yourself, others, your practice.
- What were the gaps in your knowledge, attitudes and skills.
- What could be done differently.
- How your practice has changed now you have read or considered a different way of working.

The stories help you to identify areas of knowledge and skills for development and help you to explore the context in which you practise. As Figure 13.2 illustrates, and as the previous discussion on models identified, there are many questions that you can ask yourself to develop your learning from a story of practice. This can form part of your informal diary writing or more formal writing for a public portfolio document. As you get more practised at writing you will develop your own ability to ask questions in order to develop your practice insight.

However, writing does not come easily to everyone and some individuals may need regular practice if patterns are to emerge or if deeper learning from experience is to take place. When you first start, it can be useful to share your writing with others: a tutor or a friend, perhaps, who can help you to question your practice. Depending on your preferred way of knowing you may find it more or less challenging. Do not be put off writing just because it is difficult. Try experimenting with different ways of writing, either with different models or just putting your thoughts down in no particular order, just as they come (free-fall writing) and your ability to analyse your experiences will begin to develop. Getting in the habit of writing regularly may also help in your coursework.

My preference is to use an A5-size notebook and write two or three times each week. Like many people, I find it easier to write about negative (rather than positive) experiences. However, this tends to remind me of my weaknesses rather than my strengths and this can undermine my self-esteem. Sometimes I go weeks without writing; other times I write in short bursts of 10 minutes most days.

Writing two or three times a week allows me to process the emotional component of work and re-reading old diaries provides me with insights into my patterns of thinking and behaviour, allowing me to make changes. Several of my diary entries involve pre-planning and these sometimes become 'to do' lists (these help me to clarify my need to act). I have evolved my own method of

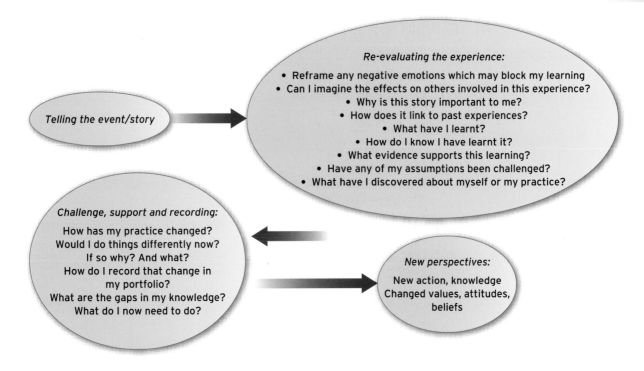

Re-evaluating the experience:

- Reframe any negative emotions which may block my learning
- Can I imagine the effects on others involved in this experience?
- Why is this story important to me?
- How does it link to past experiences?
- What have I learnt?
- How do I know I have learnt it?
- What evidence supports this learning?
- Have any of my assumptions been challenged?
- What have I discovered about myself or my practice?

Telling the event/story

Challenge, support and recording:

How has my practice changed?
Would I do things differently now?
If so why? And what?
How do I record that change in my portfolio?
What are the gaps in my knowledge?
What do I now need to do?

New perspectives:

New action, knowledge
Changed values, attitudes, beliefs

Figure 13.2 The reflective process.

keeping a diary which often is just free-fall writing. When I do structure my writing I tend to use the following:

- *I notice* – this tells the story of what happened.
- *I feel* – this notices how I felt and how I feel after writing.
- *I imagine* – this involves me thinking about others involved in my experience. If I am critical of others what is this saying about myself? What might be some of the consequences of this for myself and others?
- *I want* – this often turns into a 'to do' list of actions as it is not always easy to decide what I want. Sometimes I decide what I do not want first!
- *What have I learned or achieved?* – even if the experience has been difficult this helps to reframe it and allows me to let go of the emotional component.

Research focus 13.3

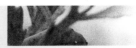

Several research studies have analysed nurses' use of diaries/journals during programmes of learning (Richardson and Maltby 1995, Wong *et al.* 1995) and some have analysed assignments (Duke and Appleton 2000, Jasper 1999, Maclellan 2004, Mountford and Rogers 1996, Watson 2002). As Taylor (2000) notes, few nurses sustain diaries/journals beyond the end of a course and she suggests there is 'relatively little guidance in how to do reflection in a practical and sustained way'.

Jasper (1999), Smith (1998) and Durgahee (1996) found nurses valued learning about themselves through writing diaries/journals and found emotions from work were released through the process of writing. However, Jasper (1999) notes the voyage of self-discovery can be threatening, danger-ous and even risky. She advocates developing techniques for 'damage limitation' by, for example, keeping a balance between a focus on strengths and achievements on the one hand and a focus on weaknesses on the other.

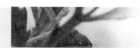

Poem 13.2   **Reflecting through diary writing by Clare Hopkinson (19 May 2004)**

To be or not to be that is the question?
Asked by greater minds than me
Still, a sense of what I am and why
Of what I also want to be

Dasein, of this time and shaping time too
Of multiple me's that conflict and grow
Which ones do I dismiss, discount, distrust?
Which ones do I willingly want to show?

I write this diary with no idea of shape or form
Poems arrive effortlessly on the page
Time and context often forgotten somehow
Twixt metaphors of sadness and rage

To do or not to do that is the question?
When life is so full why do I need you?
Too tired to think I often write
Yet re-visioning the prism, find gems anew

Do I pretend to you my friend?
Perhaps there is a flinching eye towards the day
When all these secrets held so tightly
Will break free of the page to have their say

Activity 13.8

- **What issues do you think are raised in this poem?**
- **What are the contradictions in it?**

Poem 13.2 illustrates some of the difficulties I have encountered in keeping a personal diary for professional development as well as some of my reluctance to reflect. It raises questions such as:

- For whose benefit am I reflecting?
- If I know others will read my reflections will this have an effect on what I write?
- If I am expected to show my reflections as part of my portfolio, how do I know what is safe to show and what I should keep personal?

Guidelines for starting a reflective diary

Keeping a diary can be time-consuming but I have found it to be a creative and valuable process. You should choose a format that works for you and something that can be carried around easily will allow you to make entries wherever and whenever the need arises. You may find the following considerations helpful.

1. Try a loose-leaf folder (A4). Some people prefer keeping an A5 notebook, others prefer to make entries directly onto a computer.
2. Writing on one side of the paper or half of the page allows you space to add to your reflections later on (using a second colour for later additions can be useful).
3. Try using different models of reflection until you find your preferred structure. You might find it useful to see what happens when you explore the same incident using different models.
4. Try to write soon after an incident and try not to censor the experiences or forget important contextual information.
5. Let your thoughts flow – do not worry about punctuation, spelling etc. Doodles and dreams can also be a useful key to your subconscious thoughts.
6. Keep a balance between negative and positive experiences. Writing about successful incidents can help you acknowledge your strengths, develop your self-awareness and unravel your tacit knowledge.
7. Once you get into the habit of reflective writing have a go at free-fall writing – this can be particularly helpful in developing self-awareness and understanding your responses to events.
8. Try to write at least two or three times a week. You may find this requires a bit of effort at first but you should soon find some value in the exercise. Just set aside 10 minutes and see what happens.
9. Experiment with other forms of reflection such as doodling, pictures, painting, or poetry.
10. After you have read an article or book, try jotting down your thoughts about these readings and their impact on your practice.
11. Think of your diary as a friend (rather than an enemy) and make it work for you, not anybody else!
12. Think about converting some of your informal writings into formal portfolio entries.

(Adapted from Bolton 2001 and Boud *et al.* 1985)

Julia has now spent quite a lot of time trying to write longer and more thoughtful responses to the cue questions in her reflection on the drug incident. Reading what she has written Julia is surprised by what she has begun to reveal about herself. She finds this fascinating as she has never really thought about how her behaviour affects other people. Now that she has this insight she is keen to discover more about herself so that she can modify her own behaviour to reduce any negative impact she has on other people, be they patients, relatives, or other staff. She might benefit from using the Johari window.

Guidelines for maintaining a reflective portfolio

All nurses, midwives and health visitors on the professional register have been required for some time to keep and maintain a profile or portfolio to maintain their registration (Hull *et al.* 2005). A portfolio is intended to be a vehicle for encouraging personal and professional development (Alsop 1995) and your portfolio can provide evidence of your learning which may or may not be related to specific learning outcomes. What you keep in your portfolio really is up to you but as a rule of thumb it might usefully contain your curriculum vitae (CV), evidence of qualifications, evidence of specific study and training and how this applies to your job, and a public section on your learning and reflections.

Portfolio evidence can be anything that contributes to demonstrating your learning and development and might include, for example:

- Verification of achievement of specific competencies.
- Your job description.
- Learning contracts.
- Stories from your practice.
- Reflective accounts of events.
- Learning from your days in college.
- Evidence of how your own behaviour has changed during a course.
- The impact of reading and learning about new subjects and how this has changed your practice.
- Accounts of what you have learned from visiting specific agencies or departments.
- Summaries of your learning from each placement or job.

This list is neither exhaustive nor definitive. You should try to use the portfolio in the way that is useful to you while allowing you to demonstrate your development. Of course, it will be up to you to decide if there are entries that you do not wish to make public and you might keep these in a separate removable section.

Understanding self through using the Johari window

One way of starting a diary is to begin by using a tool such as the Johari window, named after the first names of its inventors (Jo Luft and Harry Ingram). This model helps to describe the process of human interaction and has been used as a way of developing self-understanding. The four-panelled 'window' divides the self into four quadrants: the open, blind, hidden and unknown areas. Luft (1955) argued it is possible to learn about yourself either as you disclose more of yourself to others or as you receive feedback about yourself from others (Figure 13.3).

The open area is that part known to ourselves and to others. It contains the information we share with others and is not private.

The blind area is the part of ourselves known to others but not ourselves. It contains our blind spots that we can only become aware of when others tell us.

The hidden area is the part that holds our private information. We know what is in here but generally keep it hidden; although we may allow selected others access to some parts of it.

	Known to self	Not known to self
Known to others	Open area	Blind area
Not known to others	Hidden area	Unknown area

Figure 13.3 The Johari window.
Source: Luft (1955).

The unknown area is the part that holds information unknown to ourselves or others. It relates to unconscious processes and can be revealed in dreams, art, writing or, in my case, through writing poetry.

Activity 13.9

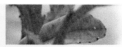

Divide a large sheet of paper into four quadrants. Number them as: 1 the open area; 2 the blind area; 3 the hidden area; 4 the unknown area. Make notes in each quadrant using the following guidance.

1. The open area:
   • Things about myself that I have no difficulty telling others.
   • Things about myself that I have some difficulty telling others.
2. The blind area:
   How do the following people see you?
   • Your best friend.
   • One of your patients/clients.
   • A specific person who dislikes you.
   • A colleague on your course.
   • Someone you have worked with recently.
3. The hidden area:
   • Write some notes about the sorts of things about yourself that you would not disclose to others.
4. The unknown area:
   This is obviously a difficult part of yourself to write about but try to 'switch off' your logical thinking brain and consider what you are really like underneath the layers of self you present to both yourself and others.
   • What might you find surprising?
   • What would surprise others?
   • Try keeping a dream diary for a week and see if this tells you anything about what is going on in your life at present.
   When you have finished each section, reflect on what you have written and consider:
   • What would happen if you allowed more people to know more about you?
   • How could you find out more about what others think about you?
   • What surprises did you find by doing this exercise?
   • To what extent do you self-disclose to others?

Creativity and models of reflection

There is a suggestion that models of reflection might stifle creativity. This is a moot point, for it is true that one of the difficulties of using a reflective model is that they are often divorced from the context of care and can lead to formulaic responses. Thus it is possible for reflection to become one more ritual in a ritualistic practice. This would be a shame, because one of the purposes of reflection is to enable a move away from the ritual and routinisation of nursing practice. It is also possible that a nurse may forget what else was happening at the time of the experience and depending on her level of self-esteem, either use the process to berate herself for her shortcomings, or use the model to justify rather than challenge her practice (Hopkinson and Clarke 2002). In this case there would be no evidence of learning or changed perspectives and hence a failure of the purposes of reflection. Sometimes a nurse can become overly descriptive in an attempt to fit answers to the specific questions within a model and in so doing lose sight of the analytical process and the purpose of learning from reflecting (Hopkinson and Clarke 2002). However, in beginning to develop a reflective approach to caregiving, models can be invaluable in getting the nurse to go deeper and look at practice from different angles. Frequently, the nurse will absorb the questioning reflective approach before moving on to develop her own reflective method which she refers to during (as well as after) caregiving as she becomes more experienced in reflecting (Hopkinson and Clarke 2002).

Creative ways of reflecting

One of the advantages of written reflection is that the nurse can trace her progress and development over time. Yet it is not the only way to reflect. Seekers (2003) linked different ways of reflecting to Gardner's theory of multiple intelligences, suggesting that everyone has a particular preferred way of reflecting (see Figure 13.4). However, in order to gain from the process of

Multiple intelligence	Narrative description	Recommended methods for recording reflections
Verbal/ linguistic	Preference for using language and reading, writing and speaking to process thoughts	Journals, diaries, written stories, poetry
Logical/ mathematical	Preference for using numbers, maths and logic to find and understand the patterns of everyday life. Often think in conceptual abstract relationships and linkages	Mind-maps, flow charts, pie charts, formulae, tables
Visual/spatial	Preference for shapes, images, patterns, designs and textures	Paint a picture, collage, sculpting, representational construction, photos, artefacts, dreams, images and metaphor
Bodily/ kinaesthetic	Preference for learning by doing and movement. Feeling knowledge through the senses is important	Taking a walk, walking the dog, dancing, gardening, cooking, driving, swimming
Musical/ rhythmic	Preference for sound and vibration as a means of gaining understanding	Music which evokes the way you felt/thought/acted. Repetitive sound can aid reflection, e.g. the roar of the sea
Naturalist	Preference for being outdoors, engaging with ecosystems, plants, animals in order to gain understanding. The elements are important aspects of everyday existence	Go on retreat, camping, walk in the rain, lie on the beach, horse riding, stroking and talking to animals

Figure 13.4 Creative ways of reflecting.
Source: Adapted from Seekers (2003).

reflection and particularly from reviewing patterns and development over a longer time frame, there does need to be some form of record-keeping. For example, if you only reflect while walking the dog and do not commit anything to paper, those reflections will become more difficult to access as time passes which can prevent you from identifying patterns in your reflections and reduce your ability to learn about yourself and your practice.

Conclusion

By the time Julia had presented her revised account of the drug incident using Johns' model to Tariq she had become convinced of the value of reflection. Julia was quite surprised to find that in taking reflection seriously, she was able to identify both her strengths and her weaknesses. She has realised that her previous attempts to reflect had all been half-hearted and only done because they were required for assignments or other things unrelated (or so she previously thought) to nursing work. Her motivation to continue to learn about herself and the effect her actions had on others (especially patients) had been gently encouraged by the support from her mentor, Tariq. He had remained non-judgemental throughout, allowing her to arrive at her own conclusions and her own plans for development. Her acceptance of the value of reflective practice as a way of continuing to develop both personally and professionally means that she is likely to recognise the importance of continuing to improve her skills in order to make a positive difference to the patients in her care. In effect, Julia can now relate to and understand the NMC *Standards of Proficiency for Pre-registration Nursing Education* (NMC 2004) listed at the beginning of this chapter and reproduced again below:

- Use professional standards of practice to self-assess performance.
- Identify one's own professional development needs by engaging in activities such as reflection in, and on, practice and lifelong learning.
- Develop a personal development plan which takes into account personal, professional and organisational needs.
- Share experience with colleagues and patients and clients in order to identify the additional knowledge and skills needed to manage unfamiliar or professionally challenging situations.
- Take action to meet any identified knowledge and skills deficit likely to affect the delivery of care within the current sphere of practice.
- Contribute to the learning experiences and development of others by facilitating the mutual sharing of knowledge and experience.

Julia now cannot wait to become a registered nurse and start to inspire the next generation of student nurses to become more reflective as a way of improving the experiences of patients within her sphere of influence.

Suggested further reading

Ghaye, T. (2005) *Developing the Reflective Team*, Oxford: Blackwell.

Ghaye, T. and Lillyman, S. (2000) *Reflection: Principles and practice for healthcare professionals*, Dinton, Wilts: Quay Books Mark Allen.

Hull, C., Redfern, L. and Shuttleworth, A. (2005) *Profiles and Portfolios: A guide for health and social care* (2nd ed.), London: Palgrave.

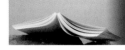

References

Alsop, A. (1995) The professional portfolio – purpose, process and practice. Part 1: portfolios and professional practice. *British Journal of Occupational Therapy* **58** (7), 299–302.

Argyris, C. and Schon, D. A. (1978) *Organisational Learning: A theory of action perspective*. Wokingham: Addison-Wesley.

Ash, E. (1992) The personal–professional interface in learning: towards reflective education. *Journal of Interprofessional Care* **6** (3), 261–271.

Atkins, S. and Murphy, K. (1993) Reflection: a review of the literature. *Journal of Advanced Nursing* **18** (8), 1188–1192.

Belenky, M. F., Clinchy, B. M., Goldberger, N. R. and Tarule, J. M. (1986) *Women's Ways of Knowing: The development of self, voice and mind*. New York: Basic Books.

Benner, P. (1984) *From Novice to Expert: Excellence and power in clinical nursing practice*. Menlo Park, CA: Addison-Wesley.

Berragan, L. (1998) Nursing practice draws upon several different ways of knowing. *Journal of Clinical Nursing* **7** (3), 209–217.

Bolton, G. (2001) *Reflective Practice: Writing and professional development*. London: Paul Chapman, Sage.

Bolton, G. (2005) *Reflective Practice: Writing and professional development* (2nd ed.). London: Paul Chapman, Sage.

Boud, D., Keogh, R. and Walker, D. (1985) *Reflection: Turning experience into learning*. London: Kogan Page.

Boyd, E. M. and Fales, A. W. (1983) Reflective learning: key to learning from experience. *Journal of Humanistic Psychology* **23** (2), 99–117.

Burnard, P. (1995) Nurse educators' perceptions of reflection and reflective practice: a report of a descriptive survey. *Journal of Advanced Nursing* **21** (6), 1167–1174.

Burns, S. and Bulman, C. (2000) *Reflective Practice in Nursing: The growth of the professional practitioner* (2nd ed.). Oxford: Blackwell Science.

Burton, A. (2000) Reflection: nursing practice and education panacea? *Journal of Advanced Nursing* **31** (5), 1009–1017.

Cadman, K., Clack, E., Lethbridge, Z. *et al.* (2003) Reflection: a casualty of modularisation? Enquiry-based reflection research group. *Nurse Education Today* **23** (1), 11–18.

Carper, B. (1978) Fundamental patterns of knowing in nursing. *Advances in Nursing Science* **1** (1), 13–23.

Clarke, B., James, C. and Kelly, J. (1996) Reflective practice: reviewing the issues and refocusing the debate. *International Journal of Nursing Studies* **33** (2), 181–189.

Clarke, M. (1986) Action and reflection: practice and theory in nursing. *Journal of Advanced Nursing* **11** (1), 3–11.

Cook, B. (1999) Reflect on the past and plan your future. *Practice Nurse* **17** (2), 98–100.

Cooney, A. (1999) Reflection demystified: answering some common questions. *British Journal of Nursing* **8** (22), 1530–1534.

Crathern, L. (1998) Steps to reflective growth. An ABC approach. *Journal of Neonatal Nursing* **4** (6), 1–4.

Driscoll, J. (2000) *Practising Clinical Supervision: A reflective approach*. Edinburgh: Balliere Tindall.

Duke, S. and Appleton, J. (2000) The use of reflection in a palliative care programme: a quantitative study of the development of reflective skills over an academic year. *Journal of Advanced Nursing* **32** (6), 1557–1568.

Dunning, D. (2005) *Self Insight: Roadblocks and detours on the path to knowing thyself*. New York: Psychology Press.

CHAPTER 13 PERSONAL AND PROFESSIONAL DEVELOPMENT   **415**

Durgahee, T. (1996) Promoting reflection in post-graduate nursing: a theoretical model. *Nurse Education Today* **16** (6), 419–426.

Freshwater, D. (2004) Analysing interpretation and reinterpreting analysis: exploring the logic of critical reflection. *Nursing Philosophy* **5** (1), 4–11.

Ghaye, T. (2005) *Developing the Reflective Team*. Oxford: Blackwell.

Ghaye, T. and Lillyman, S. (2000) *Reflection: Principles and practice for healthcare professionals*. Dinton, Wilts: Quay Books Mark Allen.

Ghaye, T. and Lillymann, S. (2006) *Learning Journals and Critical Incidents: Reflective practice for healthcare professionals* (2nd ed.). Salisbury: Quay Publications.

Gibbs, G. (1988) *Learning by Doing: A guide to teaching and learning methods*. Oxford: Oxford Polytechnic Further Education Unit.

Gilligan, C. (1982) *In a Different Voice: Psychological theory and women's development*. Cambridge, MA: Harvard University Press.

Glaze, J. E. (2001) Reflection as a transforming process: student advanced nurse practitioners' experience of developing reflective skills as part of an MSc programme. *Journal of Advanced Nursing* **34** (5), 639–647.

Glaze, J. E. (2002) Stages in coming to terms with reflection. *Journal of Advanced Nursing* **37** (3), 265–272.

Goodman, J. (1984) Reflection and teacher education: a case study and theoretical analysis. *Interchange* **15** (3), 9–26.

Gould, N. and Baldwin, M. (2004) *Social Work, Critical Reflection and the Learning Organisation*. Aldershot: Ashgate.

Grenfell, M. and James, D. (1998) *Bourdieu and Education: Arts of practical theory*. London: Falmer Press.

Gustafsson, C. and Fagerberg, I. (2004) Reflection, the way to professional development? *Journal of Clinical Nursing* **13** (3), 271–280.

Hallett, C. E. (1997) Learning through reflection in the community: the relevance of Schon's theories of coaching to nurse education. *International Journal of Nursing Studies* **34** (2), 103–110.

Hartog, M. (2005) *A Self-study of a Higher Education Tutor: How can I improve my practice?* Bath University: unpublished PhD thesis CARPP.

Heath, H. (1998) Reflection and patterns of knowing in nursing. *Journal of Advanced Nursing* **27** (5), 1054–1059.

Holm, D. and Stephenson, S. (1994) Reflection a student's perspective. In *Reflective Practice in Nursing: The growth of the professional practitioner*. Palmer, A., Burns, S. and Bulman, C. (eds). Oxford: Blackwell Science, pp. 53–62.

Hopkinson, C. (1998) *The Experience of Providing Emotional Support to Patients and Relatives By Qualified Hospital Nurses*. University of Manchester, unpublished Masters Thesis.

Hopkinson, C. and Clarke, B. (2002) Reflection in practice; the level of critical thinking. Presentation at The International Reflective Practice Conference Netherlands 6–8 June.

Hull, C., Redfern, L. and Shuttleworth, A. (2005) *Profiles and Portfolios: A guide for health and social care* (2nd ed.). London: Palgrave.

Ixer, G. (1999) There's no such thing as reflection. *British Journal of Social Work* **29** (4), 513–527.

James, C. and Clarke, B. (1994) Reflective practice in nursing: issues and implications for nurse education. *Nurse Education Today* **14** (2), 82–90.

Jasper, M. (1999) Nurses' perceptions of the value of written reflection. *Nurse Education Today* **19** (6), 452–463.

Johns, C. (1995) Promoting learning through reflection with Carper's fundamental ways of knowing in nursing. *Journal of Advanced Nursing* **22** (2), 226–234.

Johns, C. (1997) *Becoming a Reflective Practitioner*. Open University, Milton Keynes: unpublished PhD thesis.

Johns, C. (2000) *Becoming a Reflective Practitioner: A reflective and holistic approach to clinical nursing, practice development and clinical supervision*. Oxford: Blackwell Science.

Johns, C. (2006) *Engaging Reflection in Practice: A narrative approach*. Oxford: Blackwell.

Johns, C. and Freshwater, D. (1998) *Transforming Nursing through Reflective Practice*. Oxford: Blackwell Science.

Kember, D., Wong, F. K. Y. and Young, E. (2001) The nature of reflection. In *Reflective Teaching and Learning in the Health Professions*, Kember, D. (ed.). Oxford: Blackwell Science, pp. 3–28.

Kim, S. H. (1999) Critical reflective inquiry for knowledge development in nursing practice. *Journal of Advanced Nursing* **29** (5), 1205–1212.

Luft, J. (1955) *Of Human Interaction*. California: National Press Books.

Mackintosh, C. (1998) Reflection: a flawed strategy for the nursing profession. *Nurse Education Today* **18** (7), 553–557.

Maclellan, E. (2004) How reflective is the academic essay? *Studies in Higher Education* **29** (1), 75–89.

Mantzoukas, S. and Jasper, M. A. (2004) Reflective practice and daily ward reality: a covert power game. *Journal of Clinical Nursing* **13** (8), 925–933.

Marshall, J. (1999) Living life as inquiry. *Systematic Practice and Action Research* **12** (2), 155–171.

Marshall, J. (2004) Living systemic thinking: exploring quality in first person action research. *Action Research* **2** (3), 305–325.

Masterson, A. (1996) *Clarifying Theory for Practice: Study guide*. London: Distance Learning Royal College of Nursing.

Mezirow, J. (1981) A critical theory of adult learning and education. *Adult Education* **32** (1), 3–24.

Mezirow, J. (1990) *Fostering Critical Reflection in Adulthood: A guide to transformative and emancipatory learning*. San Francisco California: Jossey-Bass.

Moon, J. (2004) *A Handbook of Reflective and Experiential Learning: Theory and practice*. London: Routledge Falmer.

Mountford, B. and Rogers, L. (1996) Using individual and group learning in and on assessment as a tool for effective learning. *Journal of Advanced Nursing* **24** (6), 1127–1134.

Newell, R. (1992) Anxiety, accuracy and reflection: the limits of professional development. *Journal of Advanced Nursing* **17** (11), 1326–1333.

NMC (Nursing and Midwifery Council) (2004) *Standards of Proficiency for Pre-registration Nursing Education*. London: NMC.

OED (2006) *Concise Oxford English Dictionary* (11th ed.). Oxford: Oxford University Press.

Perry, W. G. (1970) *Forms of Intellectual and Ethical Development in the College Years*. New York: Holt, Rinehart & Winston.

Platzer, H., Blake, D. and Ashford, D. (2000) Barriers to learning from reflection: a study of the use of groupwork with post-registration nurses. *Journal of Advanced Nursing* **31** (5), 1001–1008.

Polanyi, N. (1967) *The Tacit Dimension*. New York: Doubleday.

Powell, J. (1989) The reflective practitioner in nursing. *Journal of Advanced Nursing* **14** (11), 824–832.

Rich, A. and Parker, D. L. (1995) Reflection and critical incident analysis: ethical and moral implications of their use within nursing and midwifery education. *Journal of Advanced Nursing* **22** (6), 1050–1057.

Richardson, G. and Maltby, H. (1995) Reflection-on-practice: enhancing student learning. *Journal of Advanced Nursing* **22** (2), 235–242.

Rolfe, G. (1997) Beyond expertise: theory, practice, and the reflexive practitioner. *Journal of Clinical Nursing* **6** (2), 93–97.

Schon, D. (1983) *The Reflective Practitioner*. New York: Basic Books.

Seekers, D. (2003) A journey into reflective space . . . with apologies to Star Trek. *Action Learning and Action Research Journal* **8** (1), 50–58.

Smith, A. (1998) Learning about reflection. *Journal of Advanced Nursing* **24** (4), 891–898.

Taylor, B. (2000) *Reflective Practice: A guide for nurses and midwives*. Buckingham: Open University Press.

Taylor, B. (2006) *Reflective Practice: A guide for nurses and midwives* (2nd ed.). Buckingham: Open University Press.

Teekman, B. (2000) Exploring reflective thinking in nursing practice. *Journal of Advanced Nursing* **31** (5), 1125–1135.

Thomas, J. (2004) Using critical incident analysis to promote critical reflection and holistic assessment. In *Social Work, Critical Reflection and The Learning Organisation*, Gould, N. and Baldwin, M. (eds). Aldershot: Ashgate, pp. 101–116.

Torbert, W. R. (2001) The practice of action inquiry. In *The Handbook of Action Research*, Reason, P. and Bradbury, H. (eds). London: Sage, pp. 250–260

Watson, S. (2002) The use of reflection as an assessment of practice. Can you mark learning contracts? *Nurse Education in Practice* **2** (3), 150–159.

Wong, F. K. Y., Kember, D., Chung, L. Y. F. and Yan, L. (1995) Assessing the level of student reflection from reflective journals. *Journal of Advanced Nursing* **22** (1), 48–57.

Chapter 14

Medicines management

Claire Fullbrook-Scanlon

Learning outcomes

After reading and reflecting on this chapter, you should be able to:

- Identify the organisations involved in medicines management;
- Discuss the NMC Standards for medicines management;
- Describe current legislation relating to controlled drugs;
- Discuss non-medical prescribing;
- Discuss the management of medication errors.

Related NMC Standards of Proficiency for Pre-registration Nursing Education (NMC 2004)

- Practise in accordance with the NMC Code Standards of conduct, performance and ethics for nurses and midwives.

- Consult with other health care professionals when individual or group needs fall outside the scope of nursing practice.

- Identify unsafe practice and respond appropriately to ensure a safe outcome.

- Demonstrate knowledge of legislation and health and social policy relevant to nursing practice.

- Demonstrate the safe application of the skills required to meet the needs of patients and clients within the current sphere of practice.

- Ensure that practice does not compromise the nurse's duty of care to individuals or the safety of the public.

- Apply relevant principles to ensure the safe administration of therapeutic substances.

- Communicate safety concerns to a relevant authority.

- Take into account the role and competence of staff when delegating work.

- Maintain one's own accountability and responsibility when delegating aspects of care to others.

- Literacy – interpret and present information in a comprehensible manner.

- Numeracy – accurately interpret numerical data and their significance for the safe delivery of care.

Introduction

Medicines management is an important and growing area of practice, evolving as the demands of modern health care result in the practice of nursing changing to meet patients' needs. Newly qualified nurses are required to know a considerable amount about the medicines that they administer and manage, and at the other end of the spectrum, some experienced nurses are now able to prescribe from a full range of medicinal products.

The chapter is divided into three parts.

In Part 1, the student's role in medicines management is outlined, and some key terms and organisations involved in medicines management are introduced.

In Part 2, the standards for medicines management are explained in more detail and discussed in relation to some case studies.

In Part 3, non medical prescribing and the avoidance and management of medication errors is explored in more depth.

Part 1: Outlining medicines management

Case 14.1

Josephine is a third-year student who has just started a placement on a rehabilitation ward. During the ward drug round she notices that her mentor doesn't check the name band of all the patients, especially those who have been on the ward for some time, and she doesn't ask the patients to confirm their identity, she just hands the patients a pot with their medicines, and asks the patients to take them. Sometimes the patients say that they will take the tablets later and put the pot on the locker, where occasionally they remain until the next drug round. Josephine asks why this is done and her mentor replies that the ward is very busy, and there isn't enough time to do things 'by the book'. If that was done the drug round would take all morning. Josephine accepts that the ward is busy, and that managing the medication of 30 patients is a great responsibility as well as a time-consuming one. There haven't been any incidents yet, but surely it's only a matter of time?

Medicines and medicines management

According to the Department of Health (DH) (2004a) there are almost two-and-a-half million medicines prescribed to patients in hospital and the community every day. Safe medicines management is integral to the duties of all registered nurses, and as the profession has developed, the responsibilities of the nurse in this area have increased. Not so many years ago, nurses obediently followed doctors' prescriptions and were expected to do no more. Now nurses must have detailed knowledge of the medicines they administer, and make independent judgements about medicines management for those in their care. This shift is recognised in the professional language. Where once we discussed the nurse's role in *administering* medicines, now the emphasis is on medicines *management*, encompassing administration and much more. Many nurses have completed independent prescribing courses and are now able to prescribe from a full range of medicines. This is the domain of experienced nurses, but from the first day of their registration all nurses are required to practise according to *The Code* (NMC 2008a), and be guided by other NMC guidance and publications, requiring a considerable amount of knowledge as well as the exercise of professional accountability.

There is a bewildering array of products available which claim health-giving properties. They may be obviously medicines, or food additives, cosmetics, vitamins or herbs. The Medicines and Healthcare Products Regulatory Agency (MHRA 2007) publishes *A Guide to what is a Medicinal Product* which runs to 52 tightly typed pages. This document uses the definition of 2001/83/EC directive to define a medicinal product as:

> *Any substance or combination of substances presented as having properties for treating or preventing disease in human beings; any substance or combination of substances which may be used in or administered to human beings either with a view to restoring, correcting or modifying physiological functions by exerting a pharmacological, immunological or metabolic action, or to making a medical diagnosis.*
>
> (MHRA 2007, p. 11)

The *Standards for Medicines Management* (NMC 2008b) uses a similar definition from an earlier directive. In this and other documents several words are used interchangeably. The standards define 'medicinal products' and then use the words 'medication' and 'medicine'. In this chapter I prefer the term 'medicines' but have used other terms in direct quotations. Occasionally the word 'drug' is used where it is preferred in general usage, for example in 'drug chart' or 'drug trolley'.

Medicines management has been described as:

> *the process of managing the way in which medicines are chosen, bought, delivered, prescribed, administered and reviewed, including appropriate safe, agreed withdrawal, in order to make the most of the contribution medicines can make to improving care and treatment.*
>
> (DH 2008, p. 1)

Nurses are generally not involved in the process of choosing, buying and delivering of medicines and so these aspects of medicines management will not be discussed in this chapter. However, some nurses are able to prescribe and this role will be examined and explained in Part 3. Nurses are expected to administer safely prescribed medicines and will undoubtedly be involved in reviewing medicines as part of the multidisciplinary team. In some specialties, nurses will also be involved in safe, agreed withdrawal of medications.

Medicines management is the process of managing the way in which medicines are chosen, bought, delivered, prescribed, administered and reviewed, including appropriate safe, agreed withdrawal, in order to make the most of the contribution medicines can make to improving care and treatment.

Activity 14.1

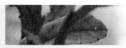

This chapter discusses the NMC standards in some detail. Before you go any further ask yourself these questions.

- Have you heard of the standards?
- Have you read them?
- Have you got a paper copy?
- Were you able to access a copy on your last placement?
- Do you know what is in the standards in relation to student nurses?
- Do you know what is in them in relation to what knowledge is required to administer medicines?

Nursing and Midwifery Council *Standards for Medicines Management*

For nurses the most important publication concerning medicines management is the NMC's *Standards for Medicines Management* (NMC 2008b). This document comprehensively sets out what is expected of registrants. It must be considered required reading and is available free to download via the NMC website. There is also a free CDRom which can be ordered from the website. If you are using this document online, links to other resources embedded within the text can be used. There are some excellent and free resources available and NMC endorsement validates their use.

There are 26 standards organised in 10 sections, and 8 further annexes which contain useful further information and guidance. Like *The Code*, the standards are written in clear language often using the imperative 'must', though there are also standards which tell a nurse what she 'may' do. In the standards, a short section of guidance follows each standard elaborating on it and here the language is more discursive – the word '*should*' replaces the word '*must*'. However, the summary of the standards states that 'it is essential that you read the full guidance and you must follow the advice' (NMC 2008b, p. 3). The document is clear that these are *minimum* standards, providing the benchmark by which practice is measured.

In Part 2 of this chapter the standards will be discussed in turn, except for the only one which specifically refers to students, Standard 18, which along with its accompanying guidance is set out in full in Box 14.1. When the term 'standards' is used in this chapter, it refers to the NMC *Standards for Medicines Management*.

Box 14.1   Standard 18

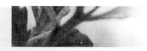

Students must never administer/supply medicinal products without direct supervision.

Guidance

In order to achieve the outcomes and standards required for registration, students must be given opportunities to participate in the administration of medication but this must always be under direct supervision. Where this is done, both the student and registrant must sign the patient's/woman's medication chart or document in the notes. The registrant is responsible for delegating to a student and where it is considered the student is not yet ready to undertake administration in whatever form this should be delayed until such time that the student is ready. Equally a student may decline to undertake a task if they do not feel confident enough to do so. The relationship between the registrant and the student is a partnership and the registrant should support the student in gaining competence in order to prepare for registration. As students progress through their training their supervision may become increasingly indirect to reflect their competence level.

(NMC 2008b, p. 31)

Throughout their programme, students need to gain experience of the duties that they will be required to undertake as registrants, and as administration of medicines is integral to the nurse's role, students need continual guidance so that they are fit for practise upon registration. *The Code* is clear that registered nurses have a duty to help students to develop their competence (NMC 2008a). Students gain experience and become competent by observing and undertaking tasks in the clinical area. When a student nurse accompanies her mentor on a medicine round it is the mentor who remains accountable for ensuring that the medicines are dispensed correctly. As the student becomes more proficient in their role the amount of delegation can be increased but students must be supervised until they become registered. A difficulty for both the mentor and the student is understanding what, exactly, is meant by the term 'direct supervision'.

The guidance accompanying Standard 18 from the NMC appears to contradict itself regarding the question of direct or indirect supervision. The standard clearly states that a student nurse must *never* administer or supply a medicinal product without *direct* supervision, and this apparently unambiguous statement is reiterated in the first line of the guidance which follows. However, later in the guidance it is suggested that as student nurses become more experienced, 'indirect' supervision may be sufficient. It seems clear that the level of supervision for a student on their first ward does not need to be the same when they are on their final ward. The level of supervision required is a matter for the accountable registered nurse to decide upon, based on a growing knowledge of each individual student's capabilities, though the student must decline tasks they do not feel competent to undertake.

Case 14.2

Mona is a third-year student on a busy surgical ward. Mr Bellchambers is two days post-surgery and requests analgesia. Mona is able to read and interpret the Medication Administration Record correctly and the patient is prescribed 1 gram of Paracetamol orally. Mona approaches the mentor who gives her the keys to the drug trolley and asks her to dispense the medication. Mona hesitates, unsure of whether she should do as she has been asked.

A number of complex issues are presented in this simple scenario. Does Mona know what the standards say about student nurses? Does she feel competent to give the tablets? Is she aware of what she needs to know about the patient, the medicine and how it must be administered? What does local policy say about student nurses having custody of the keys, for however short a period? The guidance says that supervision can become more 'indirect' as the student progresses through their training, and Mona is near the end of her programme. The mentor seems to be taking a very slack view of supervision. She has not checked the chart, asked about Mr Bellchambers' pain, checked the medicine or watched it being administered, and could be held to account for these omissions. Perhaps Mona feels capable of doing what is asked, but her mentor might find it difficult to defend supervision such as this.

Activity 14.2

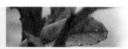

What do you think the difference between 'direct supervision' and 'indirect supervision' is? The NMC does not give any further detail, so there is not a right answer, but thinking about this might help to guide discussions with mentors in practice.

This chapter does not cover aspects of pharmacology. There are several good textbooks which cover this ground, some of which are recommended at the end of the chapter. However, in order to make the standards clear, some terms relating to medicines need to be understood. Medicines fall into a number of categories, and different legal instruments govern the prescription and supply of each category (Downie *et al.* 2008). The categories are shown in Figure 14.1.

Type	Stands for	Explanation	Example
CD	Controlled drug	Addictive drugs which produce dependence. Special controls under the Misuse of Drugs Act 1971.	Diamorphine (heroin)
POM	Prescription-only medicine	Medicines which can only be obtained with a prescription from a doctor, dentist, or independent or supplementary prescriber.	Most antibiotics
P	Pharmacy	Medicine that can only be purchased from a registered pharmacy under the control of a pharmacist. A prescription is not necessary.	Simvastatin, movicol sachets, canestan cream.
GSL	General sales list	Medicines that can be bought from any shop (some can only be bought from a pharmacy but direct supervision from the pharmacist is not required).	Paracetamol, ibuprofen. Paracetamol is limited to a maximum of 32 tablets per sale from a non-pharmaceutical sale due to the risk of permanent liver damage in overdosage.

Figure 14.1 Types of medicines.
Source: Downie *et al.* (2008).

Since loperamide was reclassified from POM to P at the request of the manufacturer in 1983, over 80 medicines have been reclassified, and there have been additions to the list nearly every year since then (Royal Pharmaceutical Society of Great Britain 2008). These medicines can be prescribed, but they do not have to be. Many prescriptions even for medication on the General Sales List (GSL) are issued, allowing the prescriber to be aware of the full range of medications taken, as well as being cheaper for many patients.

Organisations involved in medicines management

In addition to the NMC there are a number of important organisations involved in medicines management and regulation, and these are excellent sources of information and guidance. Perhaps the most important for students is the NHS Trust or other organisation where they are placed, and their policies of medicines management. Though there are national frameworks and guidance, these are not all implemented in the same way. Not all NHS Trusts use the same prescription charts, for example. Being aware of and being guided by local policy is central to safe medicines management. Many NHS Trusts have an electronic version of their policy available via their website, and if this is the case you should consider downloading it and saving it for reference. An Internet search reveals many examples.

Other resources are available from other organisations each of which has a different role in the production, prescribing and administration of medicines. Before medicines are available to the public they have had to go through a licensing procedure. In the UK all medicines and medical devices are regulated and licensed by the Medicines and Healthcare Products Regulatory Agency (MHRA). The MHRA is the government agency responsible for ensuring that medicines are acceptably safe. The MHRA only considers safety and does not take financial considerations into account when granting licences. Their website also contains information about drug safety.

The National Institute for Health and Clinical Excellence (NICE) is the organisation responsible for providing national guidance in relation to promoting good health and in the prevention and treatment of ill health (NICE 2007). In terms of medicines management, NICE is concerned with the costs and benefits relating to medicines being available to NHS patients. For example a new cancer drug would be licensed by the MHRA as safe for use. However, new cancer drugs are notoriously expensive and NICE will undertake a cost appraisal and make recommendations as to whether the drug can be used on the NHS and under what circumstances (see Chapter 2). Patients who have been denied drug treatment on the NHS are often discussed in the local and national media.

The National Patient Safety Agency (NPSA) is an arm of the NHS, responsible for promoting patient safety. The NPSA works with other health care agencies and organisations in identifying risks and helping to promote and develop good practice, including publishing national safety alerts. In relation to medicines management the NPSA has analysed medication incidents reported to the agency and identified areas of risk regarding safety in medications. Some of these findings will be discussed in Part 3.

The National Prescribing Centre (NPC) was formed in 1996 by the Department of Health. The aim of the NPC is to 'promote and support high quality, cost-effective prescribing and medicines management across the NHS, to help

Initials	Title	Role	Website
NMC	Nursing and Midwifery Council	Sets standards for practice for nurses and midwives	http://www.nmc-uk.org
MHRA	Medicines and Healthcare Products Regulatory Agency	Ensures the safety of medicines	http://www.mhra.gov.uk
NICE	National Institute for Health and Clinical Excellence	Produces guidance about which medicines should be used	http://www.nice.org.uk
NPSA	National Patient Safety Authority	Responsible for identifying risk and promoting good practice	http://www.npsa.nhs.uk
NPC	National Prescribing Centre	Support quality and cost-effectiveness in prescribing practice	http://www.npc.co.uk
UKMI	United Kingdom Medicines Information	Produces evidence-based information and advice	http://www.ukmi.nhs.uk
RCN	Royal College of Nursing	Produces some guidelines for practice	http://www.rcn.org.uk

Figure 14.2 Some organisations involved in medicines regulation and information.

improve patient care and service delivery' (NPC 2008). The NPC is primarily concerned with information about medicines and their use, education and development, and disseminating good practice. It also provides support to non-medical prescribers, MeRec publications, and new medicine schemes.

UK Medicines Information (UKMI) is an NHS pharmacy-based service. Its aim is to support the safe, effective and efficient use of medicines by the provision of evidence-based information and advice on their therapeutic use. UKMI provides resources through the National electronic Library for Medicines (NeLM), which is the largest medicines information portal for health care professionals in the NHS.

The Royal College of Nursing (RCN) also produces a number of influential guidelines. Figure 14.2 summarises the organisations and their roles.

Part 2: Explaining medicines management

This part of the chapter is based on the *Standards for Medicines Management* (NMC 2008b). Apart from Standard 18 which was introduced in Part 1, each standard is quoted in at least as much detail as in the summary document and discussed further. This chapter serves as a general discussion about medicines management. It cannot replace full reading of the standards, guidance and annexes and local policies. Sections directly quoted from the standards are indented. A summary of the standards is given in Figure 14.3.

Section	Section title	Standard number	Subject
1	Methods of supplying and/or administration of medicines	1	Method of supplying and/or administration of medicines
		2	Method of supplying and/or administration of medicines
		3	Transcribing
2	Dispensing	4	Dispensing
		5	Dispensing
3	Storage and transportation	6	Storage and transportation
		7	Transportation of medication
4	Standards for practice of administration of medicines	8	Standards for practice of administration of medicines
		9	Standards for practice of administration of medicines
		10	Self-administration – children and young people environments
		11	Administering medication from a remote prescription
		12	Text messaging
		13	Titration
		14	Preparing medication in advance
		15	Medication acquired over the Internet
		16	Aids to support compliance
5	Delegation	17	Delegation
		18	Student nurses and student midwives
		19	Unregistered practitioners
		20	Intravenous medication
6	Disposal	21	Disposal of medicinal products
7	Unlicensed medicines	22	Unlicensed medicines
8	Complementary and alternative therapies	23	Complementary and alternative therapies
9	Management of adverse events	24	Management of adverse events (errors or incidents) in the administration of medicines
		25	Reporting adverse reactions
10	Controlled drugs	26	Controlled drugs
Annexe 1	Legislation		
Annexe 2	Guidance on labelling/over-labelling of medicines		
Annexe 3	Suitability of patient's own medicinal products for use		
Annexe 4	Exclusion criteria for self-administration of medicines		
Annexe 5	Administering medicinal products in research clinical trials		
Annexe 6	Information and advice		
Annexe 7	Glossary		
Annexe 8	Contributors		

Figure 14.3 NMC *Standards for Medicines Management.*

Standard 1

Registrants must only supply and administer medicinal products in accordance with one or more of the following processes:

- *Patient-specific directions (PSD)*
- *Patient medicines administration chart (may be called a medicines administration record [MAR])*
- *Patient group direction (PGD)*
- *Medicines Act Exemption (where they apply to nurses)*
- *Standing order*
- *Homely remedy protocol*
- *Prescription forms*

(NMC 2008b, p. 11)

A **patient-specific direction** is a written instruction from a qualified and registered prescriber.

A **Patient-specific direction** (PSD) is the formal name for a written prescription. The prescription is written for a named person. It may be in the form of an instruction, for example in patients' notes, or in a hospital setting on a patient's medicines administration chart. The prescription may have been written by a doctor or a dentist. In addition nurses, pharmacists and some allied health professionals who have qualified as independent or supplementary prescribers may legally prescribe medications on patient specific directions (see Part 3).

A **patient medicines administration chart** refers to the patient's own drug chart.

Patient medicines administration chart (MAR) refers to the patient's own 'drug chart', commonly used in secondary care. Strictly speaking, it is not a prescription but a direction to administer medicine.

Patient group directions (PGDs) are written instructions allowing the supply and administration of prescription-only medications in pre-identified clinical situations without the need for individual prescription. They must be operated only by named individuals.

Patient group directions (PGDs) are written instructions allowing the supply and administration of prescription-only medications in pre-identified clinical situations without the need for individual prescription. Patients are not pre-identified prior to the treatment, the direction applying to patient groups, rather than specific patients. An example of a PGD in primary care is flu vaccinations, and in secondary care PGDs are used, for example, in emergency departments. According to the Healthcare Commission (2007) 99 per cent of Trusts use PGDs in their emergency departments. Some GP surgeries operate flu vaccine clinics where the patient will not see the GP but the practice nurse, who can administer vaccination under the direction. It is important to realise that a PGD does not simply allow anyone in that area to administer the medication; the PGD is written for specific indications, and can be operated only by named individuals. Further details on PGDs can be obtained at the NHS PGD website. See Box 14.2 for details about what PGDs should contain.

Medications Act exemption. Generally under medicines legislation drugs which are pharmacy-only (P) or prescription-only medication (POM) can only be supplied or sold by a registered pharmacy. However, in certain exemptions some health care professionals are able to sell, supply and administer some medicines directly to their patients or clients. Examples of such health care professionals are occupational health nurses or podiatrists.

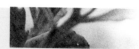

Box 14.2 Patient group directions

Each PGD should contain the following:

1. The clinical area of practice to which the PGD relates.
2. The date the PGD is valid from and when the PGD expires.
3. A description of the medicine to which the PGD applies.
4. The health care professionals who are able to supply and administer the PGD, e.g., nurses and/or specific therapists.
5. The name and signature of the author of the PGD should be written on the PGD.
6. There should be the signature of the senior doctor and senior pharmacist.
7. The clinical condition or clinical situation to which the PGD relates to.
8. Any patients who are to be excluded from the PGD.
9. Any circumstances in which the health professional must seek advice from a medical practitioner prior to administration.
10. The details of the dosage/s, together with the maximum dosage, the quantity of drugs to be given, the formulation and strength of the drug to be given, which route it is to be taken e.g., orally, intravenously, intramuscular, sublingual, topical or rectally, and the maximum or minimum period over which the medicine should be administered.
11. There should be details of any follow-up actions and special circumstances.
12. A record should be kept for audit purposes.
13. There should be a list of signatures of health care professionals who are able to use the PGD.

Standing orders. These have in the past been used by maternity services and occupational health departments under local guidelines, to supplement legislation pertaining to medicinal products that midwives or occupational health nurses may supply and/or administer (NMC 2008b). Local guidelines are not required under any legislation and indeed 'standing orders' do not exist in current medicines legislation.

Homely remedy protocol. This refers to medications that are not prescription-only (POM) pharmacy-only (P) but to medicines from the General Sales List (GSL), for example, paracetamol. Homely remedy protocols are usually used in care settings such as nursing or residential homes. If a registered nurse supplies a homely remedy she should ensure that there is written guidance as to the conditions in which she is able to administer the product and that she is competent.

Prescription forms. These are generally used in GP surgeries, hospital outpatients, dental surgeries and by nurse independent prescribers. They are numbered serially and contain anti-forgery and anti-counterfeiting features to reduce the incidence of illegal usage. There is a range of different prescription forms and they are classified as secure stationery, meaning that they have to be kept locked away when not in use.

Standard 2

Registrants (1ˢᵗ and 2ⁿᵈ level) must check any direction to administer a medicinal product. As a registrant you are accountable for your actions and omissions. In administering any medication, or assisting or overseeing any self-administration of medication, you must exercise your professional judgement and apply your knowledge and skill in the given situation. As a registrant, before you administer a medicinal product you must always check that the prescription or other direction to administer is:

- *Not for a substance to which the patient is known to be allergic or otherwise unable to tolerate*
- *Based, whenever possible, on the patient's informed consent and awareness of the purpose of the treatment*
- *Clearly written, typed or computer-generated and indelible*
- *Specifies the substance to be administered, using its generic or brand name where appropriate and its stated form together with the strength, dosage, timing, frequency of administration, start and finish dates and route of administration.*
- *Is signed and dated by the authorised prescriber*
- *In the case of Controlled Drugs, specifies the dosage and the number of dosage units or total course; and is signed by the prescriber using relevant documentation as introduced, e.g. Patient Drug Record Cards.*

And that you have:

- *Clearly identified the patient for whom the medication is intended*
- *Recorded the weight of the patient on the prescription sheet for all children, and where the dosage of medication is related to weight or surface area (e.g. cytotoxics) or where clinical condition dictates recorded the patient's weight.*

(NMC 2008b p. 17)

This is the minimum required of prescriptions and begins to tell the nurse what must be done in administering medicines. There is some overlap between Standard 2 and Standard 8, in emphasising that the patient must be correctly identified. This is the only standard which has no accompanying guidance.

Activity 14.3

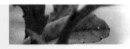

Look at the section of the drug chart shown in Figure 14.4. How many errors can you spot? (Answers are given near the end of the chapter, in Figure 14.7)

Standard 3

As a registrant you may transcribe medication from one 'direction to supply or administer' to another form of 'direction to supply or administer'.

(NMC 2008b p. 18)

REGULAR DRUGS (2)

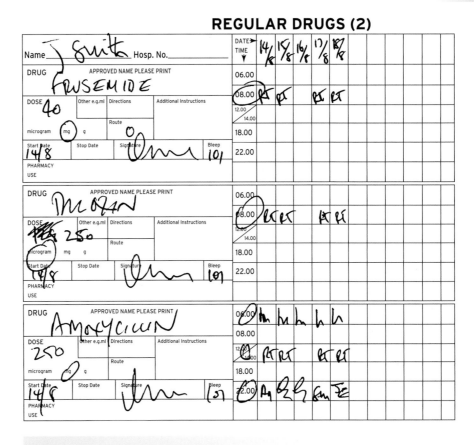

Figure 14.4 A drug chart with errors.

Transcribing medication is when a written instruction for a medicine is copied from one place to another.

Transcribing medication is when written prescriptions are copied from one place to another, for example, a direction from a patient's hospital medicines administration record to a new hospital medicines administration record. A nurse transcribing the directions is accountable for the transcription or any omissions in the transcribing process. Any transcribed medications must be signed off by a registered prescriber. It is suggested that this should be undertaken only in 'exceptional circumstances', (NMC 2008b p. 18), though many nurses will be familiar with circumstances where the space in a medicines administration record has all been used and the responsible prescriber has not yet completed a new chart to replace it. Local policy is very important here. The NMC standards allow transcription, but some local policies may not. Though the NMC regards transcription as acceptable, nurses are under no obligation to undertake it, and there is the potential that writing new records in this way becomes part of normal practice.

Standard 4
Registrants may in exceptional circumstances label from stock and supply a clinically appropriate medicine to a patient, against a written prescription (not PGD), for self-administration or administration by another professional, and to advise on its safe and effective use.

(NMC 2008b p. 20)

The NMC (2008b) defines dispensing as 'to label from stock and supply a clinically appropriate medicine to a patient/client/carer, usually against a written prescription, for self-administration or administration by another professional and to advise on safe and effective use' (p. 20). This is different from merely administering a medicine. For example, dispensing a course of antibiotics may involve putting tablets in a box or bottle, and labelling with the patient's name, the dosage and other directions, a process normally undertaken by a pharmacist. Nurses may be called to undertake such activities in dispensing doctors' surgeries. This would be seen as an extension to a nurse's usual professional practice and therefore should be covered by a standard operating procedure. Whilst there is no legal barrier to this practice, the patient can expect to have the dispensing carried out to the same standard that would be given from a dispensing pharmacist (NMC 2008b).

Standard 5
Registrants may use patients' own medicines in accordance with the guidance in this booklet Standards for Medicines Management.

(NMC 2008b p. 21)

In a practice welcomed by the NMC, many patients bring their own medicines into hospital, and of course nurses visiting patients in the community normally use patients' own medicines. These may be previously prescribed and current medicines or they may be over the counter purchases including homely remedies, herbal or complementary therapies. It is potentially dangerous if a patient self-medicates unknown to health care professionals, and nurses are responsible for ensuring that they have seen the medications and have checked their suitability for use. Additional guidance on labelling can be found in Annexes 3 and 4. The registrant must check that the medicinal products are suitable for use by ensuring:

- correct packaging and labelling
- dispensing date
- instructions for use
- dose
- the medicinal product matches what is on the label
- the patient information leaflet is enclosed
- correct patient name/ownership.

(NMC 2008b p. 66)

Discussion with the patient is very important. The nurse must explain to the patient the rationale for using or not using them. It must be acknowledged that these medications, including CDs, remain the property of the patient. They must not be removed from the patient unless they have permission and must not be used for other patients (NMC 2008b). In accordance with *The Code* for nurses and midwives (NMC 2008a), clear and accurate records of the discussions with patients must be kept especially if a patient refuses consent to use their own medication, disposal of their own medications that are no longer required or unsuitable for use or if a patient refuses to allow their medications to be sent home with a relative or carer. Patients' own medications must be stored appropriately and safely if they are to be used or kept while the patient is in a secondary care environment. Additional guidance can be found in Annexe 3.

Standard 6

Registrants must ensure all medicinal products are stored in accordance with the patient information leaflet, summary of product characteristics document found in dispensed UK licensed medication, and in accordance with any instruction on the label.

(NMC 2008b p. 24)

Each NHS Trust should have policies in place to ensure that all medications are stored and kept at the correct temperature according to the licensing guidelines. Examples of these are insulin and antibiotic liquid solutions – which must be kept in a locked refrigerator.

Standard 7

Registrants may transport medication to patients including CDs, where patients or their carers/relatives are unable to collect them, provided the registrant is conveying the medication to a patient for whom the medicine has been prescribed (e.g. from a pharmacy to the patient's own home).

(NMC 2008b p. 25)

Although this is permissible it is not considered good practice that it is undertaken routinely. This is more likely to affect nurses working in the community or specialist nurses who perform outreach duties. Medicines must be kept out of sight during transportation and not left in cars or at risk of theft. Where CDs are collected from a pharmacy the nurse will be asked to provide some form of identity which will usually be identification concerning professional practice, for example a PIN card or identity badge from a current employer. The nurse will also be asked to sign a receipt of Controlled Drugs at the pharmacy.

Standard 8

As a registrant, in exercising your professional accountability in the best interests of your patients:

- *You must be certain of the identity of the patient to whom the medicine is to be administered.*
- *You must check that the patient is not allergic to the medicine before administering it.*
- *You must know the therapeutic uses of the medicine to be administered, its normal dosage, side effects, precautions and contraindications.*
- *You must be aware of the patient's plan of care (care plan/pathway).*
- *You must check that the prescription or the label on the medicine dispensed is clearly written and unambiguous.*
- *You must check the expiry date (where it exists) of the medicine to be administered.*
- *You must have considered the dosage, weight where appropriate, method of administration route and timing.*
- *You must administer or withhold in the context of the patient's condition (e.g., digoxin not usually to be given if pulse below 60) and co-existing therapies e.g., physiotherapy.*
- *You must contact the prescriber or another authorised prescriber without delay where contraindications to the prescribed medicine are discovered, where the patient develops a reaction to the medicine, or where assessment*

of the patient indicates that the medicine is no longer suitable (see Standard 25).

- *You must make a clear, accurate and immediate record of all medicine administered, intentionally withheld or refused by the patient, ensuring the signature is clear and legible; it is also your responsibility to ensure that a record is made when delegating the task of administering medicine.*

In addition:

- *Where medication is not given the reason for not doing so must be recorded.*
- *You may administer with a single signature any Prescription Only Medicine (POM), general sales list (GSL) or pharmacy (P) medication.*

In respect of controlled drugs:

- *These should be administered in line with relevant legislation and local standard operating procedures.*
- *It is recommended that for the administration of Controlled Drugs a secondary signature is required within secondary care and similar health care settings.*
- *In a patient's home, where a registrant is administering a Controlled Drug that has already been prescribed and dispensed to that patient, obtaining a secondary signatory should be based on local risk assessment.*
- *Although normally the second signatory should be another registered health care professional (for example doctor, pharmacist, dentist) or student nurse or midwife, in the interest of patient care, where this is not possible a second suitable person who has been assessed as competent may sign. It is good practice that the second signatory witnesses the whole administration process. For guidance go to: www.dh.gov.uk and search for Safer Management of Controlled Drugs: Guidance on Standard Operating Procedures.*
- *In cases of direct patient administration of oral medication e.g. from stock in a substance misuse clinic it must be a registered nurse who administers, signed by a second signatory (assessed as competent), who is then supervised by the registrant as the patient receives and consumes the medication.*
- *You must clearly countersign the signature of the student when supervising a student in the administration of medicines.*

These standards apply to all medicinal products.

(NMC 2008b pp. 26–27)

This standard clearly sets out not only what must be checked when administering medications to patients, but also the level of knowledge about each individual medicine, and patient. Practices such as undertaking a medicine round or administering intravenous medicines on other clinical areas present problems as the nurse may not be aware of care plans for the patients.

Clearly a substantial level of knowledge of both drugs and patients is required to comply with this standard, and medicine administration will take some time. It can be difficult to concentrate on a medicine round when the ward is busy, and numerous demands are placed on the nurse. It is imperative that nurses ensure that medicine rounds are given the necessary time for providing a safe environment. This has been recognised in the NHS Institute of Innovation and Improvement with their 'Productive Ward' initiative which emphasises getting everything ready and ensuring that medicine rounds do not clash with other ward activities. For example, keeping the trolley tidy so that medicines can be found easily will prevent delays. In order to comply with Standard 8 of medicines management it is suggested that nurses develop a structured system of administration that adheres to both Standard 8 and individual Trust policy. The medicine administration records used varies between trusts but many are designed to facilitate checking. A suggested routine is set out in Box 14.3.

Box 14.3 Suggested checking routine
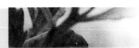

- Check patient's name on the front of the chart and on the inside if double-paged. Confirm the name with the patient.
- Check for allergies.
- Check to see if there are any once-only medicines outstanding.
- Read the chart from left to right by checking the date of the prescribed medicine, which medicine, what time should it be administered, has it been signed by a prescriber? Are there any special instructions e.g. before or after meal? What is the duration of prescription and what time was it last given?
- Does the patient's condition give cause for concern based on your knowledge of the medicines and the individual patient? Ask how the patient is. Many side effects are symptoms rather than signs. Symptoms (nausea, dizziness) are felt by the patient. Signs (high or low BP) can be observed or measured. Check the observation chart. Open and closed questions can be used.
- Then find the medication, check the correct dosage and expiry date. Place medication in a pot and return the box or bottle to the correct place.
- Check the patient's name band against the patient details on the medication record chart to ensure it is the correct patient, remembering also to ask the patient, if they are able, to confirm their identity. Be prepared to answer any questions.
- Administer the medication, check it has been taken and sign the chart.

This may seem a long-winded method of administering medicines, particularly when the ward is busy and the patients are familiar, but this is the time that most medication errors take place (O'Shea 1999).

How much do nurses need to know?

The standards of proficiency for pre-registration are not explicit about how much needs to be known about the medicines that registered nurses manage. The only proficiency is that students should 'Apply relevant principles to ensure the safe administration of therapeutic substances' (NMC 2004, p. 32). However, since this document was written, essential skills clusters (NMC 2007a) have been introduced clarifying and complementing the standards. Of the 42 statements of patient/client expectation, 10 are concerned with medicines management, and these, unlike all the others, also have indicative content. There are 18 skills relating to medicines management to be met prior to registration including that the student:

    35(iv)   *Questions, critically appraises and uses evidence to support an argument in determining when medicines may or may not be an appropriate choice of treatment.*

36(ii)   *applies knowledge of basic pharmacology, how medicines act and*
            interact in the systems of the body, and their therapeutic action
            related to Branch practice.

(NMC 2007a p. 26)

So the NMC through the standards and skills clusters requires a high level of knowledge and its application, but it does not state exactly what is required. The example that the NMC gives about digoxin in Standard 8 illustrates the point. Digoxin acts by slowing heart rate, and contraindications given in the *British National Formulary* (BNF) include heart blocks, which may result in bradycardia. Heart block is also a side effect of digoxin. However, neither the BNF nor the drug information leaflet offers the advice that digoxin should not be given if the pulse is below 60. Nurses must exercise clinical judgement and accountability in viewing the pulse rate in the individual patient and clinical context.

Details about each drug are given in the BNF, and a copy of this should be available in all clinical areas. The BNF is also available online. You are required to register at the site but it is easy, and following this you have free access to the entire site. Patient information leaflets are available online.

Case 14.3

Martha, a second-year student nurse is asked to second check a controlled drug for Mrs Blackmoor, a 77-year-old woman admitted for pain control following a diagnosis of brain and bone metastases. Mrs Blackmoor is usually orientated in time and place and has not displayed any signs of memory loss or cognitive impairment. Morphine sulphate tablets (MST) 30mg is prescribed for 0800. It is now 0830 and Martha is assisting her patients with washing and dressing. But she agrees to be the second checker. She arrives at Mrs Blackmoor's bedside with the other nurse having already checked the prescription and CD record book in line with hospital policy. Mrs Blackmoor is on the commode by the bedside. The Sister in charge, with whom Martha is checking, tells Martha that she will give the MST to Mrs Blackmoor and she can just sign the CD record book and medicines administration chart and return to her patients. Martha knows the patient on the commode is definitely Mrs Blackmoor, and she has been working with the Sister in charge for several shifts and thinks that she is trustworthy.

This scenario will be familiar to many nurses who may be impatient at having to spend so much time waiting when there is so much to do. Mrs Blackmoor may be some time on the commode (especially if the MST has made her constipated), and she may feel uneasy knowing that the nurses are waiting for her. There are a number of options. The tablet could be returned to the cupboard and signed back in, but this would itself be time-consuming. The tablet could be administered to Mrs Blackmoor while she is on the commode, but this seems undignified and unhygienic, though not completely out of the question depending on the circumstances and the relationship with Mrs Blackmoor; perhaps she has asked for this? What of the suggestion proposed by the ward manager, that Martha signs the book and leaves the MST with the Sister?

The *Standards for Medicines Management* (NMC 2008b) states that 'it is good practice that the second signatory witnesses the whole administration process' (p. 27). The DH document *Safer Management of Controlled Drugs: A guide to good practice in secondary care (England)* states that:

Both practitioners should be present during the whole of the administration process. They should both witness:

- *The preparation of the CDs to be administered*
- *The CD being administered to the patient*
- *The destruction of any surplus drug (e.g. part of an ampoule infusion not required).*

(DH 2007a p. 30)

So it is clear that good practice is that Martha should not do as the Sister asks. However, these documents are detailing good practice rather than legal requirements, and these must be interpreted in the light of the circumstances. As a student Martha is acting under the accountability of the ward sister who may decide that the situation on the rest of the ward allows her not to follow good practice in this case. However, it is clear that the Sister's proposal should not be followed unless there are compelling reasons. If Martha was a registered nurse, she would be accountable for her actions, and would have to make the decision herself. If she did as the Sister asked she would be unable to sign the medicines administration record as she did not witness the tablet being taken. This is a good example of a decision where being an accountable professional requires more than just following instructions from the NMC or anyone else. It is also a good reason why Martha should know what is in the NMC standards, as they are not presented in a way which readily allows reference at the time a decision is needed. She should also be aware of other relevant documents like those from the DH. These can be referred to when Martha reflects on the experience later.

Standard 9

As a registrant you are responsible for the initial and continued assessment of patients who are self-administering and have continuing responsibility for recognising and acting upon changes in a patient's condition with regards to safety of the patient and others.

(NMC 2008b p. 29)

Patients are being encouraged wherever possible to take responsibility for their health. This is increasingly so in relation to self-administration of medicines, supported by many patients and patients' groups. See for example the Parkinson's Disease Society (PDS) 'Get it on Time' campaign (PDS 2008). There is much more to self-medication than simply allowing and expecting patients to get on with it unsupported. The nurse retains a duty of care. Patients need to be assessed as to their ability to be able to undertake self-medicating safely. The NMC recommends that patients are assessed at three levels:

Level 1.   *The registrant is responsible for the safe storage of the medicinal products and the supervision of the administration process ensuring the patient understands the medicinal product being administered.*

Level 2.   *The registrant is responsible for the safe storage of the medicinal products. At administration time the patient will ask the registrant to open the cabinet/locker. The patient will then self-administer the medication under the supervision of the registrant.*

Level 3. *The patient accepts full responsibility for the storage and administration of the medicinal products. The registrant checks the patient's suitability and compliance verbally.*
The level should be documented in the patient's notes.

(NMC 2008b pp. 29–30)

When patients are self-medicating the nurse is not liable in the case of an error providing the risk assessment was completed and documented in accordance with local policy. There is further guidance about exclusion criteria in Annex 4.

Concordance with medication is an important aspect of medicines management, but not directly addressed in the standards. It is known (Carter *et al.* 2005) that there are low levels of concordance across a range of long-term conditions. Like the NMC standard above, the study used the term 'compliance', but this has been criticised as it reinforces the image of a power relationship with the patient complying with the health care professional's instructions. The need for a partnership approach to medicines management is emphasised, and, at the time of writing, NICE is consulting about a guideline to improve practice in involving patients and carers in decisions (NICE 2008).

Standard 10

In the case of children, when arrangements have been made for parents/carers or patients to administer their own medicines prior to discharge or rehabilitation, the registrant should ascertain that the medicinal products have been taken as prescribed.

(NMC 2008b p. 31)

It is recommended that this is performed by direct observation but if appropriate this could be done by questioning the patient, parent or carer. When the nurse has not been involved directly in the administration of the medication the medicines administration record should be initialled and the term 'patient self-administration' documented. Nurses must be aware that whilst parents or carers should be encouraged to administer medicines to their children caution should be applied as doses may be omitted in error.

Standard 11

In exceptional circumstances, where medication (NOT including Controlled Drugs) has been previously prescribed and the prescriber is unable to issue a new prescription, but where changes to the dose are considered necessary, the use of information technology (such as fax, text message or email) may be used but must confirm any change to the original prescription.

(NMC 2008b p. 32)

NMC guidance (2008b) suggests that a verbal order is not acceptable on its own. There should be an accompanying fax or e-mail confirming any new direction and it is recommended that students refer to local policy.

Standard 12

As a registrant, you must ensure that there are protocols in place to ensure patient confidentiality and documentation of any text received include: complete text message, telephone number (it was sent from), the time sent, any response given, and the signature and date received by the registrant.

(NMC 2008b p. 34)

With increasing use of mobile phones and advancing technology it is possible to concede that texts may be used in exceptional circumstances to confirm medication directions. If this does happen it is good practice to ensure that a second nurse observes the text and the subsequent documentation, for example the medicines administration record, to confirm the text message. In line with maintaining confidentiality all text messages of this nature should be deleted from the phone as soon as possible.

Standard 13
Where medication has been prescribed within a range of dosages it is acceptable for registrants to titrate dosages according to patient response and symptom control and to administer within the prescribed range.

(NMC 2008b p. 35)

This refers to medication regimes such as sliding scales of insulin where the amount of insulin to be infused depends on the blood glucose levels at the time of administration. The nurse must ensure that she is competent to interpret test results such as blood glucose levels prior to administration of the medicinal product. She will also need to be competent in using the specific pump or other medical equipment.

Standard 14
Registrants must not prepare substances for injection in advance of their immediate use or to administer medication drawn into a syringe or container by another practitioner when not in their presence.

(NMC 2008b p. 36)

The language in this standard is clear and unambiguous. Practices such as drawing up all the IV drugs in advance are not allowed. There are some exceptions, for example, where an infusion is already running, or where medication has been prepared in the pharmacy.

Case 14.4

Dilip is a staff nurse on a surgical ward. Hannah, one of his colleagues, is finishing her morning drug round and is in the process of drawing up IV medication. Suddenly the emergency call button is activated from one of her patients. Hannah asks Dilip to give the medication telling him that it is the last vial on the ward. She tells him that the medication has been checked by another registered nurse but that the vial has been discarded.

The NMC standard here is unambiguous. Despite an understandable wish to assist his colleague and more importantly ensure that the patient receives timely medication, Dilip should not give the medication, as he has no way of checking the medication against the prescription. Local policy may not require two people to check intravenous injections, though Dilip is aware that Standard 20 states that two registrants should check IV medication wherever possible. He wonders whether this would be considered 'an exceptional circumstance where this is not possible'. Dilip considers putting a sterile cap on the syringe and storing it appropriately in line with the drug information leaflet. However, Standard 14 unambiguously states that substances must not be prepared in advance of their *immediate* use. As in all decisions made by accountable professionals, the details are important; there would be a difference between a minute's delay and an hour's delay. Dilip and Hannah are aware of the importance of ensuring that the patient receives the medicine, and there will be a considerable delay if additional stock has to be ordered and delivered. Perhaps Dilip can assist at the emergency so that Hannah can give the injection. Standard 14 makes it clear that Dilip should not give the medicine, and Hannah may be required to account for her decision if she gives it after a delay.

Standard 15
Registrants should never administer any medication that has not been prescribed, or acquired over the internet without a valid prescription.

(NMC 2008b p. 37)

Many medications are available for purchase over the Internet. Increasingly medicines are bought to save patients time or embarrassment or because a request may have been refused by a prescriber. Examples are slimming pills or phosphodiesterase type-5 inhibitors (e.g. viagra) for erectile dysfunction. In the CD version of the standards, the word 'never' in Standard 15 is emboldened in the text, implying even more certainty than the language in other standards. However, the guidance following the standard goes on to give some circumstances when registrants can give medication purchased abroad without a UK product licence.

In a life-threatening situation or where the patient refuses to take anything but the 'unlicensed product' and he or she is unable to administer him/herself the registrant may administer the medication in conjunction with locally agreed policies. In all circumstances a clear, accurate and contemporaneous record of all communication and administration of medication should be maintained.

(NMC 2008b p. 37)

Standard 16
Registrants must assess the patient's suitability and understanding of how to use an appropriate compliance aid safely.

(NMC 2008b p. 38)

There are many compliance aids available to help with administration of medicines. For example, dosette boxes with individual compartments which are filled at the beginning of the week to include breakfast, lunch, dinner and bedtime dosages, and bubble packs which are pre-packed by a pharmacy usually for a month at a time. Spacer devices can assist the delivery of inhaled medicines. These appliances may be useful for older people or people with mild learning difficulties who may have problems remembering whether or not they have taken their medication, though difficulty remembering whether we have taken our medicine applies to all people. Before considering such aids, the nurse should assess the patient's suitability for such items, for example, can they open the compartments of the dosette box, can they read and understand the days of the week and mealtimes? Can they handle the spacer correctly and use a safe technique?

Standard 17

A registrant is responsible for the delegation of any aspects of the administration of medicinal products and they are accountable to ensure that the patient or carer/care assistant is competent to carry out the task.

(NMC 2008b p. 40)

The guidance following this Standard states that this will require education, training and assessment of the patient or carer/care assistant. Records of training received and outcomes should be kept.

Case 14.5

Naomi is a registered nurse working on a medical ward. It is the early shift and she is undertaking the drug round. Mrs Pilot is a 48-year-old lady who has motor neurone disease and is receiving palliative care. Her daughter Jean aged 18 wishes to be involved in her care as much as possible and has been in hospital for the last few days helping with washing, toileting and feeding. Mrs Pilot has some difficulty swallowing her medication and Jean offers to assist her mother.

Mrs Pilot's views about her daughter are very important; she needs to be willing for her daughter to undertake this role in hospital and at home. As the accountable nurse Naomi needs to be sure that Jean is competent to administer the medication. Naomi should arrange to supervise Jean giving the medicine to her mother and this will involve arranging sufficient time to be able to explain how and when to give the medicine. If there are swallowing difficulties, referral to another practitioner may be required. With Mrs Pilot's permission and co-operation, Jean will also need to know what the medicine is for and what to do if there is a problem in giving it. Naomi must ensure that all discussions with Jean are fully documented.

Standard 19

In delegating the administration of medicinal products to unregistered practitioners, it is the registrant who must apply the principles of administration of medicinal products as listed above. They may then delegate an unregistered practitioner to assist the patient in the ingestion or application of the medicinal product.

(NMC 2008b p. 42)

Delegating aspects of medicines management to unregistered practitioners is similar to delegating any other task. *The Code* (NMC 2008a) states that:

- You must establish that anyone you delegate to is able to carry out your instructions.
- You must confirm that the outcome of any delegated task meets required standards.
- You must make sure that everyone you are responsible for is supervised and supported.

The delegating registered nurse remains accountable to ensure that medicines are correctly administered, and will need to decide if the health care assistant is competent to assist the patient in taking the medicines. For some tasks, there may be local policy which details what training and assessment of competence is required, and personal experience of a fellow team member may help the nurse to decide how trustworthy the health care assistant is, whether for example she is likely to forget to give the medicine. It should be remembered that health care assistants are unlikely to know what the medicine is for and may not be able to prioritise. For CDs, the health care assistant must remain under 'direct supervision'. In an exploratory study in inpatient psychiatric wards, Dickens *et al.* (2008) found that care workers administered 17 per cent of medication, just under half of which was administered out of sight of the accountable nurse.

Standard 20
Wherever possible two registrants should check medication to be administered intravenously, one of whom should also be the registrant who administers the IV medication.

(NMC 2008b p. 43)

The NPSA suggests that the incidence of errors in prescribing, preparing and administering injectable medicines is higher than any other form of medicine (NPSA 2007a, Taxis and Barber 2003). The guidance following Standard 20 suggests that in exceptional circumstances if a second registrant is not available to check the medication then a second person who has been deemed competent to undertake this task should be approached. This may be another health care professional, a parent/carer or the patient. The guidance refers to three other publications. The guidance states that 'registrants should be aware of the risks identified in the NPSA fourth report from the Patient Safety Observatory' (NMC 2008b p. 43, NPSA 2007b). The report is discussed in more detail in Part 3 of this chapter. The guidance goes on to emphasise the duty to monitor the patient and their response during the administration of IV therapy, and suggests that the standards for the administration of IV therapy from the Royal College of Nursing (RCN) should be viewed. The link is to the RCN homepage and the document can be found by searching under its correct name, *Standards for Infusion Therapy* (RCN 2005). This document is 80 pages long but is a comprehensive resource.

The guidance also states that 'registrants should also be familiar with the UK injectable medicines guide currently under development at www.ukmi.nhs.uk/'. The need for a guide of this sort was identified in a patient safety alert from the NPSA in 2007 (NPSA 2007c). The proposal for a two-year project to produce the guide was finalised in January 2008 by UKMI and suggested that the guide be produced on a phased basis, but at the time of writing (December 2008) nothing has been published.

Standard 21
A registrant must dispose of medicinal products in accordance with legislation.
(NMC 2008b p. 44)

Disposal of unwanted/unused or out-of-date medicines is a complex issue governed by legislation. Medicines from a patient's own home and from residential homes are considered household waste. Medicines and clinical waste from hospitals and nursing homes are considered industrial waste. Disposal of medicines into sinks/waste water should be avoided. Hospital and local pharmacies can give advice regarding the safe disposal of medicines.

Standard 22

A registrant may administer an unlicensed medicinal product with the patient's informed consent against a patient-specific direction but NOT against a patient group direction.

(NMC 2008b p. 45)

Unlicensed medicine is one that has no marketing authorisation. Unlicensed medication may be seen for patients who have agreed to take part in research trials of new drugs that have not yet received their product licence from the MHRA. If it is suspected that there has been an adverse drug reaction or there is reason to think that the patient should not be receiving this medicine, the investigator of the trial should be contacted as soon as possible. The nurse has a responsibility to understand potential side effects and contraindications of unlicensed medications before administration. For example, if a patient is taking a trial medicine that is purported to be a new anti-platelet medication then they would not be able to give any prescribed licensed anti-platelet such as aspirin in conjunction with the trial medication unless authorised to do so. Details about administering medicines in clinical trials are given in Annexe 5.

Some patients have swallowing difficulties, for example people who have had a stroke or have head and neck cancer. When people are unable to take medicines it can be tempting to 'help' the patients with their medicines by opening capsules onto food products or to dissolve in water or by crushing medicines and trying to put them into nasogastric tubes or percutaneous gastrostomy tubes. Nurses must be aware that the opening of capsules/crushing of medication can alter the form of the medication so that it is then used in an 'unlicensed' form. The term modified release informs us that the drug is manufactured to allow the medicine to be released over a period of time. Abbreviations in drug names can indicate that their mode of action is modified release (M/R LA, CR, XL, SR, f/c s/c). Words such as slow, continuous or retard in the title also indicate modified release. Opening the capsule for the patient will result in the patient receiving the full dose quicker than intended. Enteric coating (EC) allows the drug to pass through the stomach before being released, so crushing an enteric-coated tablet would negate this.

If a drug which is being used outside of its product licence causes harm, manufacturers will not accept liability. It is poor practice to crush a tablet prior to administration unless written authorisation from the independent prescriber has been obtained. It is also worth noting that even when written permission has been given by a prescriber to use the product unlicensed the administering nurse may still remain partially liable should the patient come to any harm (Wright 2002, 2006).

Guidance about crushing and disguising medication follows Standard 16 (aids to support compliance), and the ethical issues of disguising medication is discussed in some detail in Chapter 2.

Standard 23

Registrants must have successfully undertaken training and be competent to practise the administration of complementary and alternative therapies.

(NMC 2008b p. 46)

444 CHAPTER 14 MEDICINES MANAGEMENT

Many members of the public purchase treatments such as plant remedies or undertake therapies such as massage or reiki. These treatments can be taken alone or combined with more traditional medicine. Increasingly, nurses choose to undertake alternative and complementary practices in their career. *The Code* states that 'You must ensure that the use of complementary or alternative therapies is safe and in the best interests of those in your care' (NMC 2008a, p. 7). However, the NMC regulates the practice of nursing and midwifery and is not responsible for overseeing other types of training and education. Therefore nurses must take responsibility in deciding whether they have sufficient qualifications and education to offer such therapies to people in their care. Furthermore, they must ensure that they have sufficient insurance and/or vicarious liability in the therapy they intend to practise within their existing employment.

In relation to administration of alternative remedies, nurses must be aware that it is being administered and its possible effects, for example, St John's wort may interact with orthodox medicines.

Standard 24

As a registrant, if you make an error you must take any action to prevent any potential harm to the patient and report as soon as possible the prescriber, your line manager or employer (according to local policy) and document your actions. Midwives should also inform their named Supervisor of Midwives.

(NMC 2008b p. 47)

According to the NPSA (2007a) 59.3 per cent of the medication incidents reported between January 2005 and June 2006 were related to administration errors. The majority of these incidents were related to the patient being given the wrong dose, strength or frequency, the wrong medicine or the dose was omitted. Drug errors are discussed in more detail in Part 3 of this chapter. *The Code* (NMC 2008a, p. 9) states that 'You must act immediately to put matters right if someone in your care has suffered harm for any reason'.

Standard 25

As a registrant, if a patient experiences an adverse drug reaction to a medication you must take any action to remedy harm caused by the reaction. You must record this in the patient's notes, notify the prescriber (if you did not prescribe the drug) and notify via the Yellow Card Scheme immediately.

(NMC 2008b p. 49)

Any drug has the potential of causing an adverse drug reaction and causing an unintended harmful effect. Nurses should be aware of potential side effects of all drugs they are administering (see Standard 8), and these are stated in the BNF and in information leaflets. This is important as nurses should understand the difference between possible disease progression and potential side effects. Reporting adverse drug reaction is an easy process. Yellow cards can be found in the BNF and reporting can also be undertaken online at http://yellowcard. mhra.gov.uk/. The yellow card is shown in Figure 14.5.

Standard 26

Registrants should ensure that patients prescribed Controlled Drugs are administered these in a timely fashion in line with the standards for administering medication to patients. Registrants should comply with and follow

In Confidence

YellowCard*

MHRA

SUSPECTED ADVERSE DRUG REACTIONS

If you are suspicious that an adverse reaction may be related to a drug or combination of drugs please complete this Yellow Card. For reporting advice please see over. Do not be put off reporting because some details are not known.

PATIENT DETAILS Patient Initials:_____ Sex: M/F Weight if known (kg):_____
Age (at time of reaction):_____ Identification number (Your Practice/Hospital Ref.)*: _____

SUSPECTED DRUG(S)
Give brand name of drug and
batch number if known

	Route	Dosage	Date started	Date stopped	Prescribed for

SUSPECTED REACTION(S)
Please describe the reaction(s) and any treatment given:

Outcome
Recovered ☐
Recovering ☐
Continuing ☐
Other ☐

Date reaction(s) started: _____ Date reaction(s) stopped:_____
Do you consider the reactions to be serious?   Yes/No
If *yes*, please indicate why the reaction is considered to be serious (please tick all that apply):

Patient died due to reaction ☐   Involved or prolonged inpatient hospitalisation ☐
Life threatening ☐   Involved persistent or significant disability or incapacity
Congenital abnormality ☐   Medically significant; please give details:_____

OTHER DRUGS   (including self-medication & herbal remedies)
Did the patient take any other drugs in the last 3 months prior to the reaction?   Yes/No
If yes, please give the following information if known:

Drug (Brand, if known)	Route	Dosage	Date started	Date stopped	Prescribed for

Additional relevant information   e.g. medical history, test results, known allergies, rechallenge (if performed), suspect drug interactions. For congenital abnormalities please state all other drugs taken during pregnancy and the last menstrual period.

REPORTER DETAILS
Name and Professional Address: _____

Post code: _____ Tel No: _____
Speciality: _____
Signature: _____ Date: _____

CLINICIAN (if not the reporter)
Name and Professional Address: _____

Post code: _____
Tel No: _____ Speciality:_____

If you would like information about other adverse reactions associated with the suspected drug, please tick this box ☐

* This is to enable you to identify the patient in any future correspondence concerning this report
Please attach additional pages if necessary

COMMISSION ON HUMAN MEDICINES (CHM)

Figure 14.5 A YellowCard form for suspected adverse drug reactions.

the legal requirements and approved local Standard Operating Procedures for Controlled Drugs that are appropriate for their area of work.
(NMC 2008b p. 50)

The use of controlled drugs (CDs) in England, Wales and Scotland is governed by the Misuse of Drugs Act (1971), and the Misuse of Drugs Regulations 2001. The Act provides the statutory framework for the control and regulation of controlled drugs (DH 2007a), which are addictive and produce dependence

Class	Example	Penalties for ...	
		Possession	**Dealing**
A	Ecstasy, LSD, heroin, cocaine, crack, magic mushrooms, amphetamines (if prepared for injection).	Up to seven years in prison or an unlimited fine or both.	Up to life in prison or an unlimited fine or both.
B	Amphetamines, methylphenidate (ritalin), pholcodine.	Up to five years in prison or an unlimited fine or both.	Up to 14 years in prison or an unlimited fine or both.
C	Cannabis, tranquillisers, some painkillers, gamma hydroxybutyrate (GHB), ketamine.	Up to two years in prison or an unlimited fine or both.	Up to 14 years in prison or an unlimited fine or both.

Figure 14.6 Penalties for unlawful possession of controlled drugs.

(Downie *et al.* 2008). CDs are permitted for use in medicine by the Misuse of Drugs Regulations (MDR). CDs are classified according to the potential harm they can cause if abused (Home Office 2008), and there has been much debate in the media concerning the reclassification of cannabis from class B to class C. Unlawful possession of CDs is a criminal offence and carries stiff penalties, more so on conviction of dealing. Penalties for possession and dealing in CDs are given in Figure 14.6.

New government guidelines relating to CDs were published in 2007 (DH 2007b). These were drawn up following the Shipman Inquiry's Fourth Report (DH 2004b). All NHS Trusts, Foundation Trusts and other independent health care organisations such as nursing homes are accountable for all aspects of monitoring the usage and disposal of CDs. They are required to identify an accountable officer who is responsible. The accountable officer remains responsible for the management of controlled drugs including safe storage, usage, auditing and the investigation of any concerns or untoward incidents involving controlled drugs. The accountable officer should be a senior executive who is not routinely involved in the prescribing, supply, administration or disposal of controlled drugs. This could be a director of nursing, chief pharmacist or medical director.

Although each organisation has a nominated accountable officer, each registered nurse in charge of a ward or department is responsible for the safety and management of the controlled drugs in their clinical area/department. As a registered nurse you can allow access to the CDs by another registered health care practitioner, but the legal responsibility for the CDs remains with you at all times throughout your shift (DH 2007a). Nurses are strongly advised to familiarise themselves with their local policies before undertaking this responsibility, and also should refer to *Safer Management of Controlled Drugs* (DH 2007a).

The guidance which follows Standard 26 is comprehensive, detailing specific arrangements for ordering, transporting and administering CDs. Some Trusts exceed the minimum legal requirements by, for example, extending the arrangements to other medicines. Guidance about administering CDs is contained in Standard 8.

Access to the standards

In some ways the *Standards for Medicines Management* is a frustrating document, posing as many questions as it answers. However, a feature of professional practice is that professionals must be accountable for the decisions that they make, and this precludes a list of actions which must always be followed. Even where wording is apparently unambiguous, cases can be constructed to cast doubt on such certainty. The standards are those against which registrants will be compared in justifying decisions and if for this reason alone, all students should have access to them. Unfortunately paper copies are currently not available, but the document and a summary version can be downloaded from the NMC website, and free CDRoms are also available. As students progress through their programmes, they will be required to take on a greater role in medicines management, and discussions with their mentors must refer to the standards.

Part 3: Exploring medicines management

Non-medical prescribing

Non-medical prescribing is a relatively new area of prescribing. The concept originates from the Cumberledge Report (Department of Health and Social Security 1986) which examined the care given to people in their own homes by district and community nurses. The report found that a lot of time was wasted by nurses in requesting prescriptions from the GP for their patients. The report concluded with recommendations for community nurses to be able to prescribe. In 1989 Dr June Crown was asked to chair an advisory group to investigate the possibility of nurse prescribing (DH 1989). This report made several recommendations suggesting items and situations in which suitably qualified nurses could prescribe. The primary legislation, the Medicinal Products: Prescribing by Nurses Act (1992) allowed nurses to prescribe from a limited formulary for specific conditions. A further Crown Report (DH 1999) recommended that prescribing authority should be made available to other non-medical professionals with appropriate training and expertise.

Government investment (DH 2001) finances education at higher educational institutions to ensure nurses and therapists are able to prescribe safely and effectively. At the present time nurses who have undergone further education and are registered with the NMC as independent and supplementary prescribers can prescribe from the BNF within their sphere of competency.

Supplementary prescribing is a voluntary prescribing partnership between the independent prescriber (doctor or dentist) and a supplementary prescriber, to implement an agreed patient-specific clinical management plan (CMP) with the patient's permission (DH 2006). Examples of clinical management plans are available at http://www.cmponline.info/. **Independent prescribing** allows nurse prescribers to prescribe any licensed medication, including some CDs, for any medical condition that she is competent to treat.

Supplementary prescribing is a voluntary prescribing partnership between the independent prescriber (doctor or dentist) and a supplementary prescriber, to implement an agreed patient-specific clinical management plan (CMP) with the patient's permission

Independent prescribing allows nurses to prescribe any licensed medicine for any medical condition that a nurse prescriber is competent to treat, including some controlled drugs.

Podiatrists, physiotherapists, radiographers and optometrists can qualify as independent and supplementary prescribers although at present they are only permitted to prescribe as supplementary prescribers. Pharmacists can also qualify as independent and supplementary prescribers but are currently not able to prescribe CDs (DH 2006).

In order to be able to undertake a training programme enabling nurses to prescribe, eligibility criteria, set by the NMC must be satisfied (NMC 2006). There are three different qualifications that can lead to nurses being able to prescribe:

- The V100 is a training programme integral to the education programme leading to a Specialist Practitioner Qualification/Specialist Community Public Health Nurse Qualification. To be entitled to undertake this programme:
  i   You must be a registered nurse or midwife
  ii You intend to practise in an area of clinical need for which prescribing from the Community Practitioners Formulary will improve patient/client care and service delivery.

(NMC 2006 p. 7)

This qualification allows the community practitioner nurse prescriber to prescribe from the Nurse Prescribers Formulary for Community Practitioners only (NPF 2007). This contains preparations including nicotine replacement therapy, elastic hosiery and peak flow meters.

- The V150 qualification allows nurses without the Specialist Practitioner Qualification to undertake a prescribing course which once successful allows them to prescribe from the Nurse Prescribers Formulary for Community Practitioners. Examples of nurses who may wish to undertake this qualification are community nurses and staff nurses especially those in Community Hospitals.
- The V200/300 allows nurses to become independent/supplementary prescribers.

In order to be eligible to undertake the education programme leading to qualification as an independent and supplementary prescriber, the following criteria must be satisfied:

i   You must be a registered first level nurse, midwife and/or specialist community public health nurse.
ii You must have at least three years experience as a practising nurse, midwife or specialist community public health nurse and be deemed competent by your employer to undertake the programme. Of these three years, the year immediately preceding application to the programme must have been in the clinical field in which you intend to prescribe, e.g. neonates, mental health. Part-time workers must have practised for a sufficient period to be deemed competent by their employer.
iii You must provide evidence via the Accreditation of Prior and Experiential Learning (APEL) process of your ability to study at the minimum academic level three (degree).

In addition you will need to have written confirmation from:

iv Your employer of their support for you to undertake the preparation programme.

v The programme lead about your selection onto the preparation of prescribers education programme. This should be given to you and your employer.

vi A designated medical practitioner who meets eligibility criteria for medical supervision of nurse prescribers and who has agreed to provide the required term of supervised practice.

(NMC 2006 pp. 7–8)

In 2007 the NMC advised that 'Employers must also have the necessary clinical governance infrastructure in place (including a Criminal Records Bureau [CRB] check) to enable the registrant to prescribe once they are qualified to do so (NMC 2007b p. 2). The CRB check should have been within 3 years of commencing the prescribing programme. Furthermore the NMC requires that the nurse must declare they are in good health or if in ill health it does not affect their ability to practise safely and effectively, that they will comply with *The Code*, have no convictions or cautions from the police, that they have not been found guilty of misconduct or lack of fitness to practise and that they are not currently suspended by any other regulatory or licensing body (NMC 2007b). The educational programme must be approved by the NMC and be of a minimum duration of 26 days plus 12 additional days of supervised learning in practice. There are also standards concerning assessment for the programme, including an examination and a numerical assessment for which the pass mark is 100 per cent.

Legislation is set to change in the near future to allow nurse independent prescribers to prescribe any medication including CDs from the BNF within their sphere of competence. Registered nurses and students working in primary, secondary or tertiary care, will need to be aware of the limitations of the independent prescribers. For instance, a nurse prescriber will not prescribe medication for a patient that the prescriber has not assessed, or that has a condition outside of the prescriber's specialist area. You will also need to be aware of who is a non-medical prescriber so that you are able to recognise their signatures and refer any issues relating to the medication to the prescriber.

Case 14.6

Abdul is a community psychiatric nurse with the early intervention service for adolescents. He has undertaken the independent and supplementary educational training programme and has this qualification recorded on the NMC Register. Among his caseload is William, a 17-year-old with newly diagnosed bipolar disorder. As an independent prescriber Abdul is able to see William regularly in his own home and prescribe valproic acid, a medication licensed for use in manic episodes associated with bipolar disorder. Abdul is able to titrate this medication according to clinical need. By doing this as an independent prescriber, Abdul takes responsibility for clinical assessment and diagnosis of William's presenting condition. He is also accountable for the prescribed clinical management William requires. If Abdul was unable to prescribe then William would need to make frequent visits to the psychiatric hospital to see the medical team. By prescribing independently, Abdul saves William time and also ensures that he gets the right treatment as early as possible.

Research focus 14.1

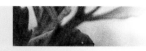

Pilot sites for nurse prescribing were established in 1994 so there has been nearly 15 years experience in the UK. In a review of the literature of the effectiveness of nurse prescribing, Latter and Courtney (2004) reviewed 18 research-based publications on the first phase of nurse prescribing until 2002. At this time nurse prescribing was restricted to the Nurse Prescribers' Formulary. The review highlighted that nurse prescribing has generally been well evaluated, though in a commentary on the review, Barrett (2004) noted that the studies reviewed were predominantly small in scale, resulting in encouraging but unsurprising results. There were no large-scale quantitative studies that included data on cost and clinical effectiveness of nurse prescribing.

Nurse prescribing from the extended range is relatively recent in the UK, and papers in this area are largely limited to studies of setting up services and education (for example Clegg *et al.* 2006). An Australian paper studied the attitudes of patients with schizophrenia towards independent non-medical prescribing of antipsychotic drugs by mental health nurses (McCann and Clark 2008). A non-probability sample of 81 patients with schizophrenia attended an interview where a questionnaire containing 68 closed response questions was completed. Three questions seeking opinions about specially trained mental health nurses prescribing antipsychotic medication were included, and 53 per cent 'agreed or strongly agreed with this form of prescriptive authority' (p. 118): 31 per cent disagreed. The study concluded that prescribing was acceptable to a small majority of patients, and claimed that more attention 'needs to be paid to the pharmacological component of pre-registration' (p. 120) courses, and supporting Barrett's (2004) view, that more research on the efficacy and cost-effectiveness of nurse prescribing is required.

Managing medication errors

The NPSA (2007a) document *Safety in Doses: Improving the use of medicines in the NHS* reports that between January 2005 and June 2006 NHS staff had reported 59,802 medication safety incidents via the National Reporting and Learning System (NRLS). Approximately 80 per cent of these incidents occurred in acute general and community hospitals: 83 per cent of these errors did not result in any harm, 16.6 per cent caused low and moderate harm and 0.2 per cent resulted in severe harm (54 in total) and there were 38 deaths (NPSA 2007a). The NPSA (2007a) found that the wrong dose, strength or frequency of medication accounted for over a quarter of all medication incidents reported to them (28.7 per cent), indicating that perhaps there are problems in numeracy among nurses. This is corroborated by O'Shea (1999) who found that a number of American studies identified poor mathematical skills as the cause of medication errors (Bayne and Bindler 1988, Chenger *et al.* 1988, Worrell and Hodson 1989).

Another common error is giving the wrong medicine, responsible for 11.5 per cent of incidents reported to the NPSA (2007a). This may be attributed to the nurse giving the medication to a patient with a similar name or indeed a similar-sounding medication. It may also be because the nurse was unable to read the writing on the medication administration record. If in doubt as to the prescription you should *never* administer the medication. If handwriting is illegible the prescriber must be contacted and asked to rewrite the prescription clearly.

Errors can also occur because the incorrect drug formulation is prepared, for example antibiotics not correctly diluted with water for injection or administered as a bolus injection instead of via an infusion with sodium chloride

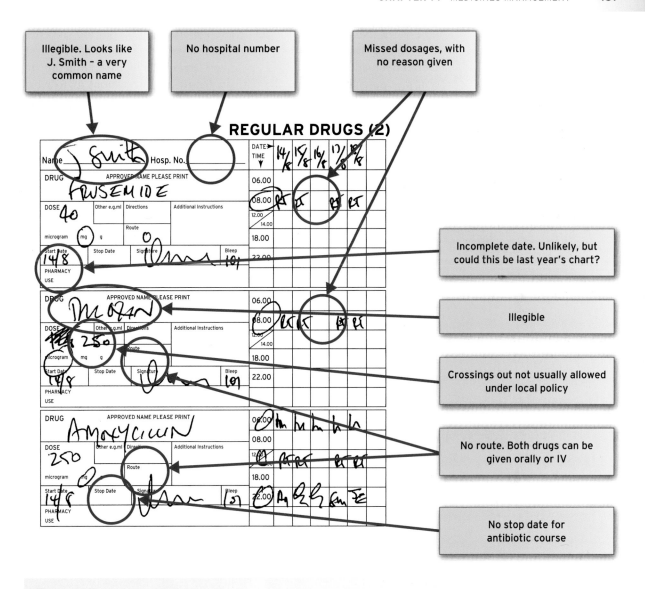

Figure 14.7 Answers to Activity 14.3.

0.9 per cent. A drug may be administered via the wrong route for example, given orally instead of rectally, or may be written intramuscularly but given intravenously by mistake.

Unfortunately nurses and midwives do make medication errors despite the policies, standards and procedures that are in place to minimise their occurrence. The NPSA (2007b) notes that international research suggests a significant level of under-reporting of errors. A Californian study estimated approximately half of medication errors are not reported for fear of disciplinary procedures (Mayo and Duncan 2004), but there is also some confusion about what constitutes a medication error; over half of the nurses in Mayo and Duncan's study admitted to failing to report a drug error because they did not think that it was sufficiently serious to report. Errors can result from genuine mistakes, but failure to report a known error can indicate dishonesty and a breach of *The Code* (NMC 2008a, p. 6) which clearly states that 'you must act without delay if you believe that you, a colleague or anyone else may be putting someone at risk.' If you discover a medication error or indeed realise that you have inadvertently made a medication error you are required to take action to prevent any potential harm to the patient. Below are suggestions as to what you should do in the event of a medication error, but these should be read in conjunction with your local policies.

1. Check that the patient is not in immediate danger, for example, anaphylaxis, respiratory distress. If this occurs start emergency procedures. You must remember to inform the doctors what drug has caused this reaction.
2. A full assessment of the patient must be undertaken, paying particular attention to signs of medication activity. For example if an antihypertensive drug is given in error to a person who is normally hypotensive, blood pressure will need to be closely monitored.
3. If the patient is not in need of immediate clinical assistance you should inform the nurse in charge of the ward without delay of the error that has occurred.
4. The prescriber/doctor should be informed as soon as possible so that they may take any clinical action necessary. The error and subsequent action should be recorded in the patient's notes.
5. A clinical incident form must be completed. It is a requirement that all serious errors and near misses are reported to the NPSA (DH 2004a).
6. The error should be discussed with the patient concerned and/or where appropriate with their next of kin. This is following a recommendation to promote a more open culture within the NHS when things go wrong (DH 2006).
7. Making a drug error can be very upsetting for the nurse, and you may benefit from discussing it with an experienced colleague, or representative. An investigation may be undertaken, and it is to be hoped that the nurse making the error reflects on the experience and learns from it. Evidence of learning may be required by the employer.

Case 14.7

Jenny is a newly qualified staff nurse working night duty on a medical ward. She is undertaking the medication round at 2300 hours. Mrs Patel is a 45-year-old woman who has recently been admitted with a deep vein thrombosis. She has been treated with clexane subcutaneously and has now been commenced on a loading dose of warfarin. When Jenny gets to Mrs Patel she discovers that the warfarin due at 1800 has not been signed for on the medication administration chart. Mrs Patel is sleepy and English is not her first language. Due to Mrs Patel's limited understanding, Jenny is unable to ascertain whether Mrs Patel has taken the warfarin. Jenny knows that the nurse on the previous shift has been working for the last 4 days and is due in again the next morning. She is also aware that this nurse is extremely tired and is probably asleep at home. What should she do?

The NMC (2008b, p. 47) in Standard 24 says you 'must take any action to prevent any potential harm'. Will Mrs Patel be at risk of potential harm if the warfarin is omitted? The answer here is yes, there is potential harm. Jenny must contact the on-call doctor to ask what action should be taken. Jenny should record all of her actions in the patient's notes and complete a clinical incident form as she has discovered a medication omission which constitutes an error. In an attempt to seek more information, Jenny should also consider ringing the staff nurse on duty the previous evening, depending on the exact circumstances.

Although it may seem daunting to admit to a medication error, you are bound by the NMC *Code* and your employer to minimise the risk to the patient and to report the incident. It is acknowledged that managers in the NHS historically blame individuals for errors (DH 2000). However, increasingly the managers are being urged to look at the numerous complex causes of administration errors (DH 2004a) and use education and retraining as opposed to punitive measures.

Conclusion

Administering medicines has been a part of nursing practice for many years. Recently the role of the nurse has extended to management of medicines requiring considerable knowledge and skills. Prescribing medicine is part of practice for more experienced nurses, and research evaluating this important development is awaited. The growing responsibilities of nurses in the area of medicines management, partly as a result of changes in health policy and technology, have been recognised by the NMC with the publication of a comprehensive set of standards. This chapter has reproduced and discussed these standards in some detail, and they must be considered required reading for all students and nurses.

Suggested further reading

Websites

A table of organisations and websites is given in Part 1 of this chapter (Figure 14.2). All of these have valuable resources.

The NMC *Standards for Medicines Management* are required reading. Available at http://www.nmc-uk.org

The collection of patient information sheets for drugs is available at http://www.emc.medicines.org.uk.

The NPSA report *Safety in Doses: Improving the use of medicines in the NHS*, London: NPSA is available at the website http://www.npsa.nhs.uk Free hard copies can also be ordered.

There are some good pharmacology textbooks for nurses available including:

Downie, G., Mackenzie, J., Williams, A. and Hind, C. (2008) *Pharmacology and Medicines Management for Nurses* (4th ed.), Edinburgh: Churchill Livingstone.
Greenstein, B. and Gould, D. (2009) *Trounce's Clinical Pharmacology for Nurses*, (18th ed.), Edinburgh: Churchill Livingstone.

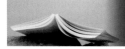

References

Barrett, D. (2004) Commentary on Latter, S. and Courtney, M. (2004) Effectiveness of nurse prescribing: a review of the literature *Journal of Clinical Nursing* **13**, 26–32. *Journal of Clinical Nursing* **13**, 776–778.

Bayne, T. and Bindler, R. (1988) Medication calculation skills of registered nurses. *Journal of Continuing Education in Nursing* **19** (6), 258–262.

Carter, S., Taylor, D. and Levenson, R. (2005) *A Question of Choice – compliance in medicine taking – a preliminary view*. London: Medicines Partnership (http://www.npc.co.uk/med_partnership/assets/research-qoc-compliance.pdf).

Chenger, P., Conklin, D., Hirst, S., Reimer, H. and Watson, L. (1988) Nursing students in Alberta: their mathematical abilities. *AARN* **44** (1), 17–22.

Clegg, A., Meades, R. and Broderick, W. (2006) Reflections on nurse independent prescribing in the hospital setting. *Nursing Standard* **21** (12), 35–38.

DH (Department of Health) (1989) *Report on the Advisory Group on Nurse Prescribing* (Crown Report) London: DH.

DH (1999) *Review of Prescribing, Supply and Administration of Medicines* (Crown Report) London: DH (http://www.dh.gov.uk).

DH (2000) *An Organisation with a Memory*. London: DH (http://www.dh.gov.uk).

DH (2001) Patients to get quicker access to medicines (press release). London: Department of Health, http://www.dh.gov.uk/en/Publicationsandstatistics/Pressreleases/DH_4010748 (last accessed 17 March 2009).

DH (2002) *Supplementary Prescribing*. London: DH (http://www.dh.gov.uk).

DH (2004a) *Building a Safer NHS for Patients: Improving medication safety*. London: DH (http://www.dh.gov.uk).

DH (2004b) *Safer Management of Controlled Drugs: The Government's response to the Fourth Report of the Shipman Inquiry*. London: DH (http://www.dh.gov.uk).

DH (2006) *Medicines Matters. A guide to the mechanisms for the prescribing, supply and administration of medicines*. London: DH (http://www.dh.gov.uk).

DH (2007a) *Safer Management of Controlled Drugs, A guide to good practice in secondary care (England)*. London: DH (http://www.dh.gov.uk).

DH (2007b) *Safer Management of Controlled Drugs: Guidance on standard operating procedures for controlled drugs*. London: DH (http://www.dh.gov.uk).

DH (2008) *Medicines Management: Everybody's business. A guide for service users, carers, and health and social care practitioners*. London: DH (http://www.dh.gov.uk).

Department of Health and Social Security (1986) *Neighbourhood Nursing: A focus for care (Cumberledge Report)*. London: DH.

Dickens, G., Stubbs, J. and Haw, H. (2008) Delegation of medication administration: an exploratory study. *Nursing Standard* **22** (22), 35–40.

Downie, G., Mackenzie, J., Williams, A. and Hind, C. (2008) *Pharmacology and Medicines Management for Nurses* (4th ed.). Edinburgh: Churchill Livingstone.

Healthcare Commission (2007) *The Best Medicine. The management of medicines in acute and specialist trusts*. (http://www.healthcarecommission.org). London: Commission for Healthcare Audit and Inspection.

Home Office (2008) *Class A, B, and C drugs* (http://www.homeoffice.gov.uk/drugs/drugs-law/Class-a-b-c/) last accessed 1 January 2009.

Latter, S. and Courtney, M. (2004) Effectiveness of nurse prescribing: a review of the literature. *Journal of Clinical Nursing* **13**, 26–32.

Mayo, A.M. and Duncan, D. (2004) Nurse perceptions of medication errors: what we need to know for patient safety. *Journal of Nursing Care Quality* **19** (3), 209–217.

McCann, T.V. and Clark, E. (2008) Attitudes of patients towards mental health prescribing of antipsychotic agents. *International Journal of Nursing Practice* **14**, 115–121.

MHRA (Medicines and Healthcare Products Regulatory Agency) (2007) *A Guide to what is a Medicinal Product*. London: MHRA (http://www.mhra.gov.uk).

NICE (National Institute for Health and Clinical Excellence) (2007) (http://www.nice.org.uk/aboutnice/) last accessed 10 January 2009.

NICE (2008) *Medicines Concordance and Adherence: Involving adults and carers in decisions about prescribed medicines. NICE Guidance – draft for consultation.* (http://www.nice.org.uk). London: National Institute for Health and Clinical Excellence.

NMC (Nursing and Midwifery Council) (2004) *Standards of Proficiency for Pre-registration Nursing Education*. London: NMC.

NMC (2006) *Standards of Proficiency for Nurse and Midwife Prescribers*. London: NMC (http://www.nmc-uk.org).

NMC (2007a) *Essential Skills Clusters for Pre-registration Nursing Programmes*. London: NMC (http://www.nmc-uk.org).

NMC (2007b) *Strengthened Requirements on Criminal Records Bureau Checks for Eligibility to Undertake Preparation to Prescribe as a Nurse Independent Prescriber*. London: NMC (http://www.nmc-uk.org).

NMC (2008a) *The Code: Standards of conduct, performance and ethics for nurses and midwives*. London: NMC (http://www.nmc-uk.org).

NMC (2008b) *Standards for Medicines Management*. London: NMC (http://www.nmc-uk.org).

NPC (National Prescribing Centre) (2008) *About us* (http://www.npc.co.uk/about_npc.htm) Last accessed 10 January 2008.

NPF (2007) *Nurse Prescribers' Formulary for Community Practitioners*. London: Bnf (http://www.bnf.org).

NPSA (2007a) *Safety in Doses: Improving the use of medicines in the NHS*, London: NPSA (http://www.npsa.nhs.uk).

NPSA (2007b) *Safety in Doses: Medication safety incidents in the NHS. The Fourth Report from the Patient Safety Observatory*. London: NPSA (http://www.npsa.nhs.uk).

NPSA (2007c) *Patient Safety Alert 20: Promoting safer use of injectable medicines (Alert 3 of 5)*, http://www.npsa.nhs.uk.

O'Shea, E. (1999) Factors contributing to medication errors: a literature review. *Journal of Clinical Nursing* **8** (5), 496–504.

PDS (Parkinson's Disease Society) (2008) *Get it on Time Campaign*. London: Parkinson's Disease Society (http://www.parkinsons.org.uk).

Royal College of Nursing (2005) *Standards for Infusion Therapy*. London: Royal College of Nursing (http://www.rcn.org.uk).

Royal Pharmaceutical Society of Great Britain (2008) *RPS e-PIC References on Prescription-only Medicines Reclassified to Pharmacy-only Medicines*. London: Royal Pharmaceutical Society of Great Britain (http://www.rpsgb.org.uk).

Taxis, K. and Barber, N. (2003) Ethnographic study of incidence and severity of intra-venous medicine errors. *British Medical Journal* **326**, 684–687.

Worrell, P. J. and Hodson, K. E. (1989) Posology: the battle against dosage calculation errors. *Nurse Educator* **14** (2), 27–31.

Wright, D. (2002) Swallowing difficulties protocol: medication administration. *Nursing Standard* **17** (14–15), 43–45.

Wright, D. (2006) Tablet crushing is a widespread practice but it is not safe and may not be legal. *The Pharmaceutical Journal* **269** (7208), 132.

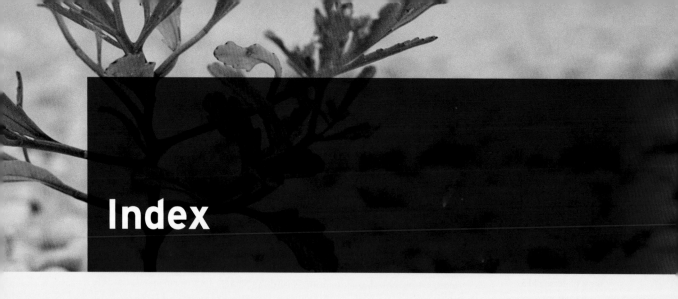

Index

Note: Figures are indicated by *italic page numbers* and definitions by **emboldened numbers**

abortion 5–6
accountability 4–5, 14, 16–17, **357**
  in law 16–17, 93
  line management 352
  professional 17, 352
  students and 20–1
  to employers 17
Acheson Report **305**
act-centred moral theories 53–4, 58
active listening 266–71
activist learning style 338
acute care *see* secondary care; tertiary care
acute care sector, interface with primary care sector 162
adaptation 319
administration of medicines 420, 421
  by health care assistants 441–2
  NMC Standards 433–5
advance decision(s) 46, 81–2
  meaning of term **81**
advance preparation of medicines, NMC standard on 439–40
adverse drug reactions (ADRs) 444
  reporting 444, *445*
aesthetic knowing 396, 404
agency, meaning of term **44**
Agenda for Change 126, 310, 348
agent-centred moral theories 58–61
alternative and complementary therapies 443–4
analytical judgements and decisions 242–5
anxiety, therapeutic relationship affected by 274–5
appearance of patient 206–7
aspirational codes of conduct 12
assessment 198–226
  action preceded by 201–2
  case study 200, 203, 211, 218, 220, 221, 223, 224
  checklist approach 201, 203
  comprehensive 202
  explaining 203–15
  exploring 215–24

harmful consequences of ineffective assessment 202
  importance 201
  nursing process and 204
  outlining 200–3
  skills 202, 204–6
    interviewing 205
    measurement 205
    observations 204–5
  for transfer of patient 220–4
  see also physical assessment
assessment-driven students **324**, 339
attending skills **267**
attention **238**
Audit Commission
  on clinicians' engagement in financial management 378
  on payment by results 133
augmentative and alternative communication (AAC) systems 276
auscultation 218
  respiratory system 219–20
authority **357**
  of managers 349
autonomy
  meaning of term **44**
  of nurses 246
  respect for 44–7, 56

'being accountable' **5**
beneficence **50**
  application in case study 56
blood pressure 210–11
  cuff size **210**
  factors affecting 211, 212
BNF *see* British National Formulary
board meetings 352
body language 257, 259–60
body temperature
  factors affecting 211
  measurement of 208
Bolam Test (for duty of care) 95
Bolitho case (on duty of care) 95

books, as information sources 178
Boud, Keogh and Walker's reflective model 395
bradycardia 209
breath sounds 219–20
British National Formulary (BNF) 436, 444
British Nurses' Association 4
budgets 366

capacity to give consent 77–9, *80*
  assessing 78–9
  factors restricting 77
  research on 82–3
capital expenditure 113–14
  meaning of term **113**
cardiac rehabilitation nurse, public health and 290–2
care ethics 58–60
  compared with ethics of justice 60–1
Care Quality Commission 121, 124, 129, 369
Care Trusts 118
carers, role in interprofessional working 157
caring, meaning of term 59–60
Carper's ways of knowing 404
  in Johns' reflective model 395, 396
CASP package 187
  see also critical appraisal
causal judgements *239*
CDs *see* controlled drugs
change management 189, 364–5
changing practice 189–95
  barriers to change 192–3
    nurse-related barriers 192
    organisation-related barriers 192
    profession-related barriers 193
    research-related barriers 192
  commitment-maximising activities 194–5
  levels of change 190
  ways of implementing change 191
chief executive *351*
children **83**
  consenting for 85–6
  interdisciplinary models 152–3
Children Act (1989) 83, 85
chronic obstructive pulmonary disease (COPD) 219
circular questions 268
civil law 71–2, 94
civil service 105
claim right **44**, 45
clarification, as active listening skill 269
clients, alternative terms **141**
clinical governance 128, 368–9
  components 368–9
  meaning of term 368
clinical guidelines 150, 183–5
  critical appraisal frameworks for 186, 187
  as information sources 180
clinical management plans (CMPs) 447
clinical negligence 94–7
closed questions **268**

closed-mindedness 190
code(s) of conduct 12–13, 23
  NMC Code as 24, 41
code(s) of ethics 23–4
  NMC Code not recognised as 24, 41
  in practice 25–6
cognitive task analysis (CTA) interviews 245–6
collaboration 144–6
  NMC Code on 28
  relationships and communication affecting 157–60
collaborative practice **141**, 146
collaborative working 141, 146
colleagues, as information sources 178–9
Commission for Health Improvement (CHI) 368, 369
commissioning, meaning of term **116**
commissioning organisation, NHS as 116–18
common law 71
communication
  circular transactional model 256–7
  components 257–60
    non-verbal/bodily communication 257, 259–60
    para-verbal/vocal communication 257, 258–9
    verbal communication 257–8
  linear model 255–6
  nursing and 255–7
  patient satisfaction and 255
  in public health 300–1
communication difficulties, therapeutic relationship
    affected by 275–6
communication and interpersonal skills 252–83
  case studies 254, 263, 272
  explaining 257–66
  exploring 266–79
  outlining 254–7
communication mechanisms, interprofessional working
    affected by 149, 159
communication skills
  active listening 266–71
  importance of developing 255
community care
  future development 129
  interprofessional working 154–5, 161
  leadership in 160–1
community of practice 323, 336
competence 328
  assessing when delegating 358–9
  complaints about 20
  Race's model 328–35
competent person **357**
complaints 377
  NMC Code on 30–1
complementary and alternative therapies 443–4
compliance aids 440
compulsory detention, Mental Health Act provisions
    86–7
computer literacy 177
  see also Internet
concordance **292**

confidentiality 43, 88–90
  circumstances when breach is permitted 89–90
  NMC Code/guidelines on 28, 88, 262
congruence between non-verbal and verbal
    communication **265**
connected knowers/knowing 403
consent
  case study 70, 75, 76, 81
  children and 85–6
  documenting 82
  features
    appropriate information 76–7
    capacity to give consent 77–9, *80*
    voluntary agreement 75
  legal aspects 74–86
  meaning of term **75**
  NMC Code on 28–9
  young people and 83–5
consequentialism 54, *59*
  application 55
constructed knowledge 403–4
consultants, new contract for 126
Control of Substances Hazardous to Health (COSHH)
    regulations 296, 300
controlled drugs (CDs) *424*
  administration by health care assistants 442
  classification 446
  legislation on use 445–6
  new government guidelines 446
  NMC Standards 444–6
  standards for administration 434, 436–7, 444–5
  transportation of 433
coordination, in interprofessional collaboration 161, 162
core standards (NHS) 121, *122*
cost-effectiveness 366–7
Council for Health Care Regulatory Excellence (CHRE)
    10, 124
covert administration of medicines
  case study 39, 43, 46, 49, 50, 53, 54, *56*
  NMC advice sheet on *56*
creativity, reflective models and 411–13
credulousness 190
criminal acts 16
criminal law 71–2, 94
Criminal Records Bureau (CRB) 21
  check for nurse prescribers 449
critical appraisal 185–9
critical care, decision-making in 237
critical decision method (CDM) 245–6
critical reflection 391
critiquing frameworks 172–3, 186
  meaning of term **172**
  typical questions 188
Crown Report(s) 447
crushing tablets, advice on 443
cue acquisition and interpretation *243*, 244, 246
Cumberledge Report 447
cyanosis 219

damages, clinical negligence claims 97–8
Darzi review 108, 128–30, 134
Data Protection Act (1998) 91
  withholding information under 91
decision
  meaning of term **230**
  types *235*, 236
decision-making
  aids supporting 234–5, 242
  covert influence of nurses 236–7
  factors affecting quality 234
  in interprofessional working 155
  see also judgement and decision-making
degree-level courses 14
delegation 357–9
  meaning of term **357**
  in medicines management 441–2
  NMC Code on 29, 358, 441
  professional issues 29, 357–8
  steps to effective delegation 357–9
deontology 54
  application(s) 55
Department of Health (DH)
  Chief Nursing Officer (CNO) 105–6
  code of practice for Mental Health Act 87
  on confidentiality 89, 90
  on consent 75, 76, 85, 86
  framework for system reform *127*
  guidance documents 107
  on medicines management 421
  ministers 105
  policy papers 107
  on safer management of controlled drugs 436–7, 446
  strategic objectives 108
  website 33, 105, 106, 135, 180, 196
  World Class Commissioning programme 116, 117
descriptive judgements 239
descriptive model of judgement and decision-making
    233–4
devolution, effects on health policy 130, 311
dialogic teaching 328
digoxin 436
discharge planning 220–4
disengagement from therapeutic relationship 278
dispensing medications 431–2
disposal of medicinal products 442–3
Do Not Attempt Resuscitation (DNAR) orders 45
doctrine of double effect (DDE) 47–8
drug chart 428
  errors *431*, *451*
  see also patient medicines administration chart
duty-based moral theory 54, *59*
duty of care 94–5
  breach in standard 95–6

E. coli outbreak, public health aspects 295–6
economic, meaning of term **366**
education, public health 301

educational assessment **324**
    approaches to 324
educational courses, quality assurance of 14
effective, meaning of term **367**
efficient, meaning of term **366**
electronic databases and indexes, as information sources
    179
email (for administration of medicines) 438
emancipatory reflection 398
emergency treatment, consent for children 86
emotional intelligence **276–7**
empathy 264–5, 277
emphysema 219
empirical knowing 396, 404
employers
    accountability to 17
    duty to 98
empowerment 261, **294**
England
    health policy 117–19
    public health provision 311
England and Wales, basis of law 70–2
enteric-coated medications 443
environment, management of 368–73
environmental health officers 290
epidemiology **287**
episodic memory **243**
error criterion 184
ethical knowing 396, 404
ethical standards 5, 6
ethics 37–67
    debating/discussing 41
    explaining 41–56
    exploring 56–62
    four principles approach 41–55
        application to case study 55, 56
        individual moral judgements 42
        moral theories 53–5
        principles 44–53
        rules 43–4
    meaning of term 40
    morals and 39–40
    outlining 39–41
    see also codes of ethics
Europe, codes of ethics, research study on 26
European Convention on Human Rights (ECHR)
    88, 92
    see also Human Rights Act
euthanasia 47, 49
evaluative judgements 239
evidence
    appraising 180–1
    critical appraisal of 185–9
    error criterion test 184
    hierarchies **173**, *181*, 182–3
    in law 172
    in professional practice 172–5
    searching for 176–80

evidence-based care
    factors affecting choices 175
    NMC Code on 30
evidence-based management 379
evidence-based policy making in health care 131
evidence-based practice 167–97
    case study 169, 176, 186, 189
    changing practice 189–95
    examples 170
    explaining 171–80
    exploring 180–95
    finding evidence 176–80
    importance for nurses 171
    meaning of term **170**
    outlining 169–71
    reason for 170–1
    reviewing practice 176
executive directors *351*
Expected Utility theory of human behaviour 232–3
experimental knowledge 207, 237–8
experiential work-based learning 323–4
expert nurses
    assessment ability 207
    knowledge-based performance 240
Expert Patient Programme 125
extended role of nurses 216
eye contact 259

facial expressions 259
fairness, ways of addressing 51
fax (for administration of medicines) 438
fidelity 43
financial flows, NHS reforms 115–16
financial management and control 366
first-person inquiry see personal reflection
fitness-to-practise complaints 18–19
    standard of proof 19
flexibility, in learning process 341
food poisoning outbreak, public health aspects 295–6
foreseeable risks 97
formal learning **321**
formal learning environment **322**
formative assessment 324
Foundation Trusts see NHS Foundation Trusts
four principles approach (ethics) 41–55
    application 55, 56
Fraser Guidelines (on young people's treatment) 84
Freedom of Information Act (2000) 91
funding for health services 111–14

Gardner's theory of multiple intelligences 412
General Medical Council 9, 124, 143
General Nursing Council 4
general practitioners (GPs), new contract for 126
general sales list (GSL) medicines *424*, *425*
General Social Care Council (GSCC) 143
genuineness 265–6
gestures (body language) 259

Gibbs' reflective model 395, *396*

Gillick competence 83–4

  meaning of term **83**

Gilligan's ethics of care 60, 401

Gold Standard Framework (GSF) 154–5

'good character'

  registered nurses 22–3, 24–5, 32–3, 58

  students 21–2, 31–2

'good health' (of students) 21–2, 24

'good nurse', research on meaning of term 62

government departments, structure 105

government expenditure, health spending as percentage
    112

government priorities and targets 126–8

Green Paper(s) 107

'hard' information/evidence 173, 174

harm resulting from clinical negligence 96–7

hazards **371**

  examples *371*

head-to-toe examination 201, 216–20

health, WHO definition 144

Health for All strategy 305

health care assistants, medicines administered by 441–2

Health Care Commission 120, 121–3

  annual reports 133–4

  complaints procedures 377

  criteria for assessing core standards 369

  see also Care Quality Commission

health care policy 108

health care providers, developing 118–20

health care regulation 120–4

  meaning of term **120**

Health Development Agency 150

health expenditure

  as percentage of GDP, in various countries 113

  in UK 112, 132

health improvement 293, 298

health intelligence **287**

  early example 288

health policy 102–37

  current policy 114–26

  discussion on future policy 134

  explaining 109–31

  exploring 131–4

  information sources 135–6

  meaning of term **104**

  outlining 104–9

  regional differences in UK 130–1

Health Professional Council (HPC) 9, 143

health promotion **288**, 298

  in (adult) nursing practice 290–2

  compared with public health 288

health protection 293, 299

Health and Safety Executive (HSE), on stress at work
    355

Health Service Ombudsman 377

Healthy Cities initiative **305**

hearing, distinguished from listening 266–7

HEARTFELT initiative 151

heuristic thinking 240–2

heuristics **233**, 241–2

hierarchical structures, interprofessional working affected
    by 148, 156, 159–60

hierarchies of evidence 173, *181*, 182–3

High Quality Care for All (White Paper) 108, 129, 348

history

  NHS 109–11

  nursing 3–4

  public health in UK 298

Holm and Stephenson's reflective model (student's
    perspective) 397

homely remedy protocols 429

hospitals, funding of 115–16

Human Fertilisation and Embryology Authority 124

Human Rights Act (1998) (HRA) 92–3

  see also European Convention on Human Rights

hypothesis generation and interpretation *243*, 244

hypothetico-deductive thinking 243–5

  compared with intuitive thinking 245

  meaning of term **243**

hypoxia 219

impartiality, NMC Code on 31

implied consent **82**

improvement/change

  anatomical approach 364, *365*

  model for improvement *375*, 376

  physiological approach *365*, 377

Improvement Leaders' Guides 364, 374–5

indemnity insurance 31, 97

independent prescribing **447**

independent sector treatment centres (ISTCs) 119

individual learning style **337**

individual moral judgements 42

individuals, people as 28

industrial settings, public health in 296–7

infection control 288, 356

inferential judgements *239*

influence **349**

informal learning 318, **322**, 328

informal teaching 318

information and communication technology (ICT),
    effect on health care services 133

information overload 177

information processing **233**

information sharing, NMC Code on 29

information sources 177–80

  books and journals 178

  clinical guidelines 180

  colleagues 178–9

  electronic databases and indexes 179

  Internet 177, 179

  local policies and procedures 178

  policies and reports 180

  professional organisations 179

infusion therapy
  NMC standards 439–40, 442
  RCN standards 442
inspection 217
  respiratory system 219
instrumental understanding of education **339**
insurance
  health care funded by 112
  professional indemnity insurance 31, 97
integrated care pathways 142
  see also interprofessional working
integrity, NMC Code on 30
intensive care, decision-making in 237
Intermediate Care Teams 221, 222
internal listening 271
internal market 110
International Council of Nurses (ICN) 4
International Council of Nursing (ICN), definition of
        judgement 230
Internet
  as information source 177, 179
  medication acquired over 440
interpersonal skills
  interprofessional working affected by 149–50
  see also communication and interpersonal skills
interprofessional working 138–66
  case studies 140, 144, 145, 148, 149, 154, 157, 158
  contrasted with multiprofessional working 146
  contribution of support workers **146**
  evidence base for 150–3
  explaining 142–53
  exploring 153–62
  factors affecting effective collaboration 146–50
    communication mechanisms 149, 159
    hierarchical structures 148, 156, 159–60
    interpersonal skills 149–50
    practitioner's point of view **147**
    professional priorities and boundaries 147, 158, 159
    understanding of others' roles and obligations 147–8
  importance for nurses 142
  meaning of term **141, 146**
  nurses' involvement in leadership and coordination
        160–1
  in nursing practice 154–5
  outlining 140–1
  reason for 140–1
  research on 151, 152, 152–3
  skills and attitudes needed 141
  skills needed by nurses 155–6
interviewing skills 205
intravenous (IV) medication, NMC standards 439–40,
        442
intuition **238**
intuitive judgement and decisions 207, 238–40
  trade-off between speed and error 240
intuitive thinking, compared with hypothetico-deductive
        thinking 245
ipsative assessment 324

Jehovah's Witnesses 79
Johari window 410–11
Johns' reflective model 395–7
  see also Carper's ways of knowing
journals, as information sources 178, 185
judgement
  meaning of term **230**
  types 239
judgement and decision-making 227–51
  analytical stages 243
  case study 229, 232
  examples 231
  explaining 232–8
  exploring 238–46
  factors affecting effectiveness 231
  influence of organisation 236–8
  models 232–5
    descriptive model 233–4
    normative model 232–3
    prescriptive model 234–5
  in nursing practice 235–6
  nursing research on 246
  outlining 229–31
  quality determined in nursing 245–6
justice 50–3
  application in case study 56
  meaning of term **50**
justice ethics 58
  compared with ethics of care 60–1
justified claims 44–5

Kant, Immanuel 54
knowing-in-action 342
knowledge
  nursing practice and 400–5
  see also ways of knowing
Knowledge Audit 246
knowledge base 4
  in public health 299–300
knowledge update, NMC Code on 30
Kohlberg's theory of moral development 60

lasting power of attorney (LPA) 46, **81**
law 68–101
  basis of (in England and Wales) 70–2
  explaining 74–93
  exploring 93–8
  outlining 70–4
leadership
  distinct from management 349–50
  in interprofessional team 160–1
  meaning of term **349**
  see also management and leadership
leadership relationship 356
League of Nations Health Organisation 143–4
learners
  effective 339
  ineffective 339–40

learning
  developing attitudes to 340–2
  meaning of term **318**
  in practice 319
  social aspect of **322**
  as social collaborative process 327
learning community **323**
learning disability nursing, public health and 292–3
learning environment
  building relationships within 326–8
  factors contributing to 335–6
learning styles 337, 338–40
learning and teaching 315–44
  case studies 317, 320, 334, 337
  explaining 320–35
  exploring 335–42
  factors affecting effectiveness 335–6
  interactive approach 327–8
  outlining 317–20
  professional obligations 16, 318
  when they occur 319–20
  see also learners; teachers
learning-to-learn **322**
legal standards 5, 6
liberty 44, 45
liberty right **44**, 45
life expectancy 132
lifestyle changes (health promotion) 291–2
listening, distinguished from hearing 266–7
listening skills 266–71
  in interprofessional working 150
Local Authority Overview and Scrutiny Committees 125
local initiatives for health care services 120
Local Involvement Networks (LINks) 125
local policies and procedures, as information sources 178
long-term memory **243**

McGill Pain Questionnaire 215
management
  costs 378
  distinct from leadership 349–50
  levels 350–1
  meaning of term **349**
management and leadership 345–82
  case study 347, 354, 361, 362, 367, 376
  explaining 353–77
  exploring 378–80
  as help in work 348
  outlining 347–52
  reason for studying 347–8
  see also leadership
manager–clinician tensions 378
managerial relationship 356
manual handling incident (reflective poem) 386–7
material fact **73–4**
measurements 205
media influences 303
medical profession, primacy in health care 4, 143, 158

medical technology 133
medication administration errors 450
  factors affecting 450–1
  management of 444, 451–3
Medications Act exemption 429
medicinal product(s)
  definition 421
  nurse prescribing 447–50
Medicinal Products: Prescribing by Nurses Act (1992) 447
medicine categories *424*
medicines administration record/chart (MAR) **428**
Medicines and Health Care Products Regulatory Agency
        (MHRA) 425
  definition of medical product 421
medicines management 418–55
  case studies 420, 423, 436, 439, 441, 449, 452
  direct and indirect supervision 423, 424
  explaining 426–47
  exploring 447–53
  knowledge needed by nurses 435–6
  local policies 425
  meaning of term **421**
  NMC Standards 421, 422–4, 426, 427, 428–47
  organisations involved 425–6
  outlining 420–6
  students and 422–4
  see also Nursing and Midwifery Council (NMC),
        Standards for Medicines Management
medicines rounds/trolleys 434
meetings 353–4
mental capacity **77**
Mental Capacity Act 2005 (MCA) 45, 78, 79, 83, 88
  code of practice 78, 79, 81
  guides 78
  holding power of nurse 87–8
mental disorder, definition 86
Mental Health Act (1983, 2007) (MHA) 86–8
  compulsory detention provisions 86–7
Mental Health Act Commission 121, 124
mental health nursing, public health and 293–5
mentor **323**
  role of 319, 320–1
meta-analyses **182**
middle managers *351*
Mill, John Stuart 54
Ministry of Justice, Mental Capacity Act guides 78
Minnesota (public health nursing) model 302
misconduct allegations 16
Misuse of Drugs Act (1971) 445
modern public health *see* new public health
modernisation, attitudes of clinicians and managers *379*
modified-release medications 443
Monitor (Independent Regulator for NHS Foundation
        Trusts) 120, 123
moral judgements, individual 42
moral responsibility 15, 16
moral standards 5–6
moral theories 53–5

morals, ethics and 39–40
multiple intelligences 412
multiprofessional working 145
  contrasted with interprofessional working 146

National Health Service (NHS)
  core principles 51
  draft Constitution (guiding principles) 108–9
  first formed 109, 143, 298
  history 109–11
  structure (in England) *115*
National Institute for Health and Clinical Excellence
    (NICE) 123, 425
  clinical guidelines 150, 180, 183
  QALY calculations 52
  website 123, 196
National Occupational Standards for public health
    practice 310
National Patient Safety Agency (NPSA) 123, 369, 425
  on injectable medicines 442
  medication incidents reporting and analysis 425, 442,
    450, 451
  reporting and learning system 369, 450
  risk matrix 373, *374*
National Prescribing Centre (NPC) 425–6
naturalistic research **187**
  critical appraisal frameworks for 187
new public health 298–9, 303–4
NHS *see* National Health Service
NHS Confederation, report on management in NHS
    378
NHS Constitution 108–9, 129
NHS Foundation Trusts **118**, 125
  independent regulator 120–1, 123
NHS Institute for Innovation and Improvement 124,
    128, 364
  Improvement Leaders' Guides 364, 374–5
  priority areas (2008/09) 374
  'Productive Ward' initiative 434
NHS Knowledge and Skills Framework 310, 348
NHS Litigation Authority 124
  standards for risk management 369
NHS Modernisation Agency 128, 364, 374
  see also NHS Institute for Innovation and Improvement
NHS Plan 110, 125, 133, 373–4
NHS Production Pathway 366, *367*
NICE *see* National Institute for Health and Clinical
    Excellence
Nightingale, Florence 4, 288
NMC *see* Nursing and Midwifery Council
non-maleficence 47–8
  application in case study 56
  meaning of term **47**
non-medical prescribing 447–50
non-verbal/bodily communication 257, 259–60
normative, meaning of term **232**
normative model of decision-making 232–3
Northern Ireland, health policy 130

novice(s)
  checklist approach to assessment 201, 203
  knowledge-based performance 240
NPSA *see* National Patient Safety Agency
'nurse', meaning of term 11
nurse–patient relationship *see* therapeutic relationship
Nurse Prescribers Formulary for Community Practitioners
    448, 450
nurse prescribing 447–50
  qualifications 448
  research on 450
nurse's anxiety, therapeutic relationship affected by
    274, 275
Nurses and Midwives Act (1979) 8
Nurses' Registration Act 4
Nursing and Midwifery Council (NMC) 9, 10–21, 124
  accountability to 17
  advice sheets 23, 56
  Code (of professional conduct) 5, 12–14, 16, 17, 21,
    23–4, 27–31, 53, 70, 88, 273, 358
    on medicines management 441, 444, 451–2
  committees 10–11
  competence complaints 20
  composition of council 10
  core function 10, 17
  on covert administration of medicines 56
  essential skills clusters, for pre-registration nursing
    programmes 435–6
  first established 4
  fitness-to-practise complaints 18–19
  on 'good character' 22
  on 'good health' 21–2
  key tasks 11–17
    consideration of allegations of misconduct, etc.
      14–21
    maintenance of professional register 11
    quality assurance of education 14
    setting standards 12–14
  practice committees 10, 18
  Register 11, 302, 311
  services 23
  on specialist community public health nursing 302, 311
  Standards for Medicines Management 421, 426, *427*
    access to standards 447
    on advance preparation of medicines 439–40
    on adverse drug reactions 444, 452
    on complementary and alternative therapies 443–4
    compliance aids 440
    on controlled drugs 444–6
    on delegation 441
    on dispensing 431–2
    on disposal of medicines 442–3
    on IV medication 439–40, 442
    on medication acquired over Internet 440
    on medication administration errors 444
    method of supplying/administration of medicines
      428–30
    on patients' own medicines 432

Nursing and Midwifery Council (NMC) (*continued*)
    on remote (email/fax/text message) prescriptions
      438–9
    on self-administration of medicines 437–8
    standards for administration of medicines 433–5
    on storage of medications 433
    student nurses/midwives 422–4
    on titration of doses 439
    on transcribing medication 430–1
    on transportation of medications 433
    on unlicensed medicines 440, 443
    on unregistered practitioners 441–2
  Standards of Proficiency
    for Nurse and Midwife Prescribers 448
    for Pre-registration Nursing Education 2, 38, 69,
      103, 139, 168, 199, 228, 253, 285, 316, 346,
      384, 419, 435
    for Specialist Community Public Health Nurses 303
  website 33
nursing process **204**
  assessment and 204
nursing profession, development of 3–6

objective data **204**
objectives **357**
  setting 359
observational skills 204–5
observations **208**
  blood pressure 210–11
  pulse rate 209–10
  respirations 210
  temperature 208
occupational health nursing, public health and 296–7
occupational therapists
  professional body representing 9
  viewpoint 223
open questions **267**, 268
opening capsules, advice on 443
open-mindedness 190, 341
operational managers *351*
organisational chart 351–2
organisational culture, patient safety and 371
organisational reflection 388, 393
organisational structures 350–2
Organization for Economic Cooperation and Development
    (OECD), health expenditure data 113
Ottawa Charter **305**
Our Health, Our Care, Our Say (White Paper) 111

pain
  assessment of 212–15
  factors affecting 214–15
  location 214
pain scales
  self-reporting scales 213–14
  subjectivity 214
palliative care services, Gold Standard Framework
    154–5

palpation 217–18
  abdomen 218
  pulse 209, 217
  respiratory system 219
paraphrasing, as active listening skill 269
para-verbal/vocal communication 257, 258–9
parental responsibility 85
participation 144–6
paternalism **46**
patient, alternative terms for **141**
Patient Advice and Liaison Service (PALS) 125
patient assessment *see* assessment
patient choice 118
patient empowerment 261
patient group direction (PGD) **428**, 429
patient medicines administration chart **428**
patient and public involvement 124–5
patient safety, core standards 369–70
patient-specific direction (PSD) **428**
patient's anxiety, therapeutic relationship affected by
    274, 275
patients' charter 110
patients' own medicines 432
patterns of knowing
  Carper's 395, 396, 404
  women's 401–4
payment-by-results system **115**, 117
  Audit Commission report 133
peer assessment 324
people as individuals, NMC Code on 28
Peplau's theory of nursing 255
percussion 218
  respiratory system 219
personal development, improvement through 386
'personal health budgets' 129
personal knowing 396, 404
personal and professional development 383–417
  case study 385, 389
  explaining 389–99
  exploring 399–413
  outlining 385–9
personal reflection 388, 392
personal responsibility for health 52, 306–9
  basis of discriminatory view 307
  limitations of approach 307–9
    genetic aspects 307
    individual's priorities 308
    'reasonableness' view 308
    risk-taking viewpoint 309
    social factors 307–8
    wider considerations 308–9
pharmacy (P) medicines *424*, 425
physical assessment 206–12, 216–20
  head-to-toe approach 201, 216–20
  novice's compared with expert's observations
    207
  see also observations
physiological measurements 208–12

Plan/Do/Study/Act (PDSA) cycles **376**, 377
policy, definition(s) **104**, 106–7
'polyclinics' 129
portfolio 324, 409–10
posture, as non-verbal communication 259–60
power of attorney 46, 81
practical knowledge, distinct from theoretical knowledge 400
practical reflection 398
practice-based commissioning 117, 129
practitioner's point of view, interprofessional working affected by 147
pragmatist learning style 338
pre-registration nursing education 319
    NMC Standards of Proficiency 2, 38, 69, 103, 139, 168, 199, 228, 253, 285, 316, 346, 384, 419
prescription forms 429
prescription-only medicine(s) (POM) *424*, 425
prescriptions, checking 430
prescriptive codes of conduct 12
prescriptive model of decision-making 234–5
presence skills **267**
prima facie rules 43
primary care **109**
    future development 129
    management of 117–18
    public health and 295–6
primary care sector, interface with acute care sector 162
Primary Care Trusts (PCTs) *115*, 124
    funding of 115
    targets and priorities 126–7
primary sources of evidence/information **180**
principles, rules of ethics based on 44–53
principlism 41
    critiques 56–62
        agent-centred ethics 58–61
        'insufficient philosophy' critique 57
        procedural critiques 57–8
prioritisation of tasks 354
privacy 43
Private Finance Initiative (PFI) schemes 114
probabilistic terms **243**
problem-solving
    NMC Standard of Proficiency 228
    see also judgement and decision-making
procedural knowledge 403
process mapping **375**
productive, meaning of term **366**
profession
    characteristics defining 7
    nursing as 7–9
professional accountability 5, 6, 14, 17
professional boundaries 273, 278
    NMC Code on 29, 273
    testing by patient(s) 274
professional indemnity insurance 31, 97

professional issues 1–36
    explaining 7–23
    exploring/critiquing 23–6
    outlining 3–6
professional organisations, as information sources 179
professional priorities and boundaries, interprofessional working affected by 147, 158, 159
professional regulatory bodies 9, 142–3
professional standards 5, 6
professions
    interaction between 142–4, 147–8
    self-regulation of 9
propositional knowledge 400
proximal development zone (in learning) 327
proximity (physical closeness) between communicators 260
public health 284–314
    case studies 286, 288–9
    compared with health promotion 288
    development 304–6
    explaining 288–97
    exploring 298–312
    future of 311–12
    history 298
    hospital-based 293–5
    in industrial setting 296–7
    meaning of term **287**
    media influences 303
    mental health nursing and 293–5
    nursing and 297
    outlining 286–8
    purpose of 309–11
    reasons for importance 288–90
    reducing health inequalities 128
    skills 299–301
    vulnerable groups 292–3
    see also health promotion; new public health
public health nurses, on NMC Register 302
public health nursing
    qualification 302
    as specialism 302
    in UK 302–3
public interest
    confidentiality and 89–90
    freedom of information and 91
pulse rate 209–10
    factors affecting 211

qualitative research **184**
    critical appraisal frameworks for 186
quality, effect of time taken 353–4
quality-adjusted life years (QALY) 51
    example of calculation 52
quality improvements 129
quantitative research **182**
    critical appraisal frameworks for 186
questions, in 'active listening' 267–8

Race's competence model 328–35
  competence/uncompetence line 328–30
  conscious competence quadrant 330, 331
  conscious uncompetence quadrant 330, 331–2
  unconscious competence quadrant 331, 332
  unconscious uncompetence quadrant 331, 333–5
  unconscious/conscious line 330
randomised controlled trials (RCTs) **181**
  critical appraisal frameworks for 186, 187
'reasonableness', meaning in law 72–3
received knowledge 402
record-keeping
  legal aspects 73–4
  NMC Code on 30
reflecting feelings, as active listening skill 270–1
reflection 341–2
  creative ways 412–13
  definition(s) 390
  language used 388
  models 394–8
    Boud, Keogh and Walker's approach 395
    creativity and 411–13
    Gibbs' model 395, 396
    Holm and Stephenson's model 397
    Johns' model 395–7
    Taylor's model 397–8
  organisational 388, 393
  as part of personal and professional development
    386, 405
  personal 388, 392
  relational 388, 392
  terms used to describe 389–90
reflection-in-action 342, **392**, 393
reflection-on-action 342, **392**, 393
reflective diary 406–7
  guidelines on starting 408–9, 410
  poem on writing 408
  research on 407
reflective learning 390
reflective portfolio 409–10
reflective practice
  benefits 398
  effects 387–8
  meaning of term **387**
  public health and 309
  research on 398–9
  typology for 309, *310*
reflective process *407*
reflector learning style 338
refusal of treatment, by children and young people 84–5
regional differences in health policy 130–1
registration of nurses 11
  first introduced 4
regulation
  health care 120–4
  meaning of term **120**
  medicines 425–6
  professions 9, 142–3

regulatory bodies 9
relational reflection 388, 392
remote (email/fax/text message) prescriptions
  438–9
reports, as information sources 180
reputation of profession, NMC Code on 31
research, definitions, in ethics studies 49
resource management 365–7
respect 263–4
respirations 210
  factors affecting 212
respiratory system, examination 219–20
responsibility 15–16
restating, as active listening skill 269
revenue expenditure 113–14
  meaning of term **113**
reviewing practice 176
right(s), meaning of term **44**
risk assessment **372**
  NPSA risk matrix 373, *374*
risk management 371–2
  NMC Code on 29
risks **371**
  examples *371*
role responsibility 15, 20
Royal College of Nursing (RCN) 8
  on delegation and accountability 358
  medicines management guidelines 426
  Standards for infusion therapy 442
  Team Effectiveness Guides 360
  website 135, *426*
rules (in ethics) 43

safety of health care 369–71
saline bath, research on 171
scenario planning 234
schemas **234**
Scotland
  health policy 130
  public health provision 311
Scottish Intercollegiate Guidelines Network (SIGN)
  183–5
  hierarchy of evidence 183
  level of evidence table *185*
seamless care 142
  see also interprofessional working
search engines (Internet) 177, **179**
search strategy **177**
searching for information/evidence 176–80
  effective use of time 177
second-person inquiry *see* relational reflection
secondary care **109**
secondary sources of evidence/information **180**
self-assessment 333
self-awareness 271–2
  of learning process 340–1
self management 353–6
self-regulating professions **9**

self-regulation
  of individuals 277
  of professions 9–10
self-study 392
  see also personal reflection
self-understanding, Johari window used 410–11
separate knowers/knowing 403
serious crime, confidentiality and 90
service improvement 373–7
service redesign 128
service reform(s) 128
  attitudes of clinicians and managers *379*
  meaning of term **114**
service users, alternative terms **141**
'Shaping the future of Health Promotion' project 311
short-term memory **243**
side effects of medicines 435, 436, 444
silence
  as active listening skill 269–70
  as way of knowing 401–2
single assessment process 142
  see also interprofessional working
Skills for Health organisation **306**
  on public health 306, 309–10
skills update, NMC Code on 30
SMART objectives 359
social aspect of learning **322**
social collaborative process, learning as 327
'soft' information/evidence 173, 174
special interest groups (SIGs) 323
specialist community public health nurses 302–3,
  311
staff empowerment 379–80
standard of proof
  in legal cases 72, 172
  in NMC fitness-to-practise hearings 19
Standing Nursing and Midwifery Advisory Committee
  (SNMAC), on public health 298
standing orders (for medicines) 429
statute law 71
stethoscope
  bell side 218
  flat (diaphragm) side 218, 219
'stopping rules' (in decision-making) 241
storage of medications 433
Strategic Health Authorities (SHAs) *115*
strengths/weaknesses/opportunities/threats (SWOT)
  analysis 333
stress **355**
  factors affecting *355*
    management behaviour and 355–6
striking-off order (NMC) 18, 19
students, accountability 20–1
subjective data **204**
subjective information **174**
subjective knowledge 402–3
summative assessment 324
supplementary prescribing **447**

support workers, contribution to interprofessional
  working **146**
surgical morning meetings (interprofessional working) 152
systematic reviews **182**
  critical appraisal frameworks for 186, 187
systems reform(s) 114–26
  developing providers and patient choice 118–20
  financial flows 115–16
  meaning of term **114**
  NHS as commissioning organisation 116–18
  patient and public involvement 124–5
  regulation 120–4
  success 133–4
  workforce development 125–6

tachycardia 209
tacit knowledge 400
taxation, NHS funded by 111, 112
Taylor's reflective model 397–8
teachers
  good 325, 326
  poor 326
teaching
  approaches 322
  meaning of term **318**
team **359**
team development, stages 361–2
Team Effectiveness Guides 360
team leaders *351*
team performance curve 360
  characteristics of identified points *361*
team roles 362
team working 359–63
  factors affecting 362–3
technical reflection 398
tender loving care (TLC) 60
tertiary care **109**
text messages (for administration of medicines) 438–9
theoretical knowledge, distinct from practical
  knowledge 400
theorist learning style 338
therapeutic boundaries **273**
therapeutic relationship 260–6
  barriers to 274–6
  developing and maintaining 261–6
  disengaging from 278–9
  meaning of term **260**, 261
  setting and maintaining personal boundaries in 272–4
third-person inquiry *see* organisational reflection
time management 353–4
time taken for task, quality and 353–4
titration of doses 439
transcribing medications **431**
transfer of patient, assessment for 220–4
transportation of medications 433
trust **262**
  building and maintaining 262
tympanic thermometers 208

UK Medicines Information (UKMI) service 426
underarm lift, case study on 169, 176, 186, 189
unforeseeable risks 97
Unison 8
 website 135
United Kingdom Central Council for Nursing, Midwifery
 and Health Visiting (UKCC) 12
 see also Nursing and Midwifery Council (NMC)
unlicensed medicinal products 440, 443
unrecognised learning needs 333–4
unregistered practitioners, administration of medications by
 441–2
utilitarianism 54
utility, meaning of term **232**

V100 qualification (for nurse prescribers) 448
V150 qualification (for nurse prescribers) 448
V200/300 qualification (for nurse prescribers) 448
value for money 366–7
veracity 43
verbal communication 257–8
vicarious liability **98**
virtue ethics 58, 59
vital signs 208–12
vocal communication 257, 258–9
vocalisations **258**

waiting-time target 127
Wales
 health policy 130
 public health provision 311
walk-in centres 129
Wanless report(s) 112, 132–3
'ways of knowing'
 Carper's 395, 396, 404
 women's 401–4
White Paper(s) 107
women's ways of knowing 401–4
 constructed knowledge 403–4
 procedural knowledge 403
 received knowledge 402
 silence 401–2
 subjective knowledge 402–3
workforce development 125–6, 133
working memory **243**
Working for Patients (White Paper) 110
World Health Organization (WHO) 143, 144, **304**
 public health initiatives 305

YellowCard system (for reporting suspected adverse drug
 reactions) 444, *445*
young people **83**
 consent and 83–5